# Continuous Quality Improvement in Health Care

*Theory, Implementations, and Applications*

## Third Edition

**Curtis P. McLaughlin, DBA**
Professor Emeritus of Business Administration
Kenan-Flagler Business School
Professor Emeritus of Health Policy and Administration
School of Public Health
Senior Research Fellow Emeritus
Cecil B. Sheps Center for Health Services Research
University of North Carolina at Chapel Hill
Chapel Hill, NC

**Arnold D. Kaluzny, PhD**
Professor Emeritus of Health Policy and Administration
School of Public Health
University of North Carolina at Chapel Hill
Chapel Hill, NC

JONES AND BARTLETT PUBLISHERS
*Sudbury, Massachusetts*
BOSTON    TORONTO    LONDON    SINGAPORE

*World Headquarters*

Jones and Bartlett Publishers
40 Tall Pine Drive
Sudbury, MA 01776
978-443-5000
info@jbpub.com
www.jbpub.com

Jones and Bartlett Publishers
Canada
6339 Ormindale Way
Mississauga, Ontario
L5V 1J2
CANADA

Jones and Bartlett
Publishers International
Barb House, Barb Mews
London W6 7PA
UK

Jones and Bartlett's books and products are available through most bookstores and online booksellers. To contact Jones and Bartlett Publishers directly, call 800-832-0034, fax 978-443-8000, or visit our website www.jbpub.com.

Substantial discounts on bulk quantities of Jones and Bartlett's publications are available to corporations, professional associations, and other qualified organizations. For details and specific discount information, contact the special sales department at Jones and Bartlett via the above contact information or send an email to specialsales@jbpub.com.

**Production Credits**
Publisher: Michael Brown
Production Director: Amy Rose
Associate Production Editor: Daniel Stone
Editorial Assistant: Kylah McNeill
Associate Marketing Manager: Marissa Hederson
Composition: Graphic World
Manufacturing Buyer: Therese Connell
Cover Design: Timothy Dziewit
Printing and Binding: Malloy, Inc.
Cover Printing: Malloy, Inc.

**Library of Congress Cataloging-in-Publication Data**
Continuous quality improvement in health care / [edited by] Curtis McLaughlin, Arnold Kaluzny.—3rd ed.
  p. ; cm.
  Includes bibliographical references and index.
  ISBN 0-7637-2712-1 (hardcover)
  1. Medical care—United States—Quality control. 2. Total quality management—United States.
  [DNLM: 1. Delivery of Health Care—organization & administration. 2. Total Quality Management—methods. W 84 AA1 C66 2006] I. McLaughlin, Curtis P. II. Kaluzny, Arnold D.
  RA399.A3C66 2006
  362.1'068'5—dc22

                                                                          2005007393

Printed in the United States of America
09  08  07  06  05                                    10  9  8  7  6  5  4  3  2  1

*To Barbara Nettles-Carlson
and Barbara Kaluzny
for the patience, trust,
and love for which
we are most grateful.*

# TABLE OF CONTENTS

**Chapter 12—Quality Improvement in Primary Care: The Role of Organization, Collaboratives, and Managed Care . . . . . . 297**
*Leif I. Solberg, Thomas E. Kottke, and Milo L. Brekke*

**Chapter 13—CQI in Contract Research Organizations . . . 318**
*William A. Sollecito and Kaye H. Fendt*

**Chapter 14—Continuous Quality Improvement in Public Health Organizations . . . . . . . . . . . . . . . . . . . . . . . . 357**
*Glen P. Mays and Paul K. Halverson*

# CONTRIBUTORS

## EDITORS

**Curtis P. McLaughlin, DBA**
Professor Emeritus of Business
  Administration
Kenan-Flagler Business School,
  University of North Carolina
  at Chapel Hill
Professor Emeritus of Health
  Policy and Administration
School of Public Health
Senior Research Fellow
  Emeritus
Cecil B. Sheps Center for Health
  Services Research
University of North Carolina at
  Chapel Hill
Chapel Hill, NC

**Arnold D. Kaluzny, PhD**
Professor Emeritus of Health Policy
  and Administration
School of Public Health
Senior Research Fellow
  Emeritus
Cecil B. Sheps Center for Health
  Services Research
University of North Carolina
  at Chapel Hill
Chapel Hill, NC

## CONTRIBUTORS

**Paul Batalden, MD**
Professor, Department of
  Pediatrics, Community
  and Family Medicine
Director, Health Care
  Improvement Leadership
  Development, Center for
  Evaluative Clinical Sciences
Dartmouth Medical School
Hanover, NH

**Paul Barach, MD, MPH**
Associate Professor
Department of Anesthesiology
Medical Director of Quality
  and Safety
Jackson Memorial Hospital,
  and Director, Miami Center
  for Patient Safety
University of Miami
Miami, FL

**Shulamit L. Bernard, PhD, RN**
Director, Program on Health Care
    Quality and Outcomes
RTI International
Research Triangle Park, NC

**Richard M.J. Bohmer,
    MBChB, MPH**
Assistant Professor
Harvard Business School
Boston, MA

**Milo L. Brekke, PhD (deceased)**
Brekke Associates, Inc.
Minneapolis, MN

**William R. Carpenter,
    MHA, PhD**
Post-Doctoral Fellow
UNC Lineberger Comprehensive
    Cancer Center
University of North Carolina
    at Chapel Hill
Chapel Hill, NC

**Richard B. Colletti, MD**
Vice-Chair and Professor of
    Pediatrics
Associate Physician-in-Chief,
    Vermont Children's Hospital
University of Vermont College
    of Medicine
Burlington, VT

**Susan I. DesHarnais, PhD**
Assistant Director, Health Services
    Evaluation and Policy Research
    Section
Buehler Center on Aging
Feinberg School of Medicine
Northwestern University
Chicago, IL

**Amy C. Edmondson, PhD**
Professor
Harvard Business School
Cambridge, MA

**Laura R. Feldman, BA**
Research Associate
Harvard Business School
Cambridge, MA

**Kaye H. Fendt, MSPH**
Department of Pediatrics
School of Medicine
University of North Carolina
    at Chapel Hill
Chapel Hill, NC

**Bruce Fried, PhD**
Associate Professor
    and Director, Residential
    Master's Program
Department of Health Policy
    and Administration
School of Public Health
University of North Carolina
    at Chapel Hill
Chapel Hill, NC

**Paul K. Halverson, MHSA,
    DrPH**
Professor and Chair
Department of Health Policy
    and Management
College of Public Health
University of Arkansas for
    Medical Sciences
Little Rock, AR

**Brent James, MD, MStat**
Director
IHC Institute for Health Care
    Delivery Research
Salt Lake City, UT

**Susan Paul Johnson, MBA, PhD**
Visiting Associate Professor
Economics Department
Agnes Scott College
Decatur, GA

**Linda C. Jordan, RN, MSN**
Administrator, Risk Management
   and Compliance Office
Brody School of Medicine
East Carolina University
Greenville, NC

**William Q. Judge, PhD**
Professor of Strategic
   Management
College of Business
University of Tennessee at
   Knoxville
Knoxville, TN

**Diane L. Kelly, DrPH, MBA, RN**
Assistant Administrator
   for Quality
St. Mark's Hospital, Salt Lake
   City, UT
Adjunct Assistant Professor
College of Nursing,
   University of Utah
Adjunct Assistant Professor
School of Public Health
University of North Carolina
   at Chapel Hill
Salt Lake City, UT

**David C. Kibbe, MD, MBA**
Director, Center for Health
   Information Technology
American Academy of Family
   Physicians
Washington, DC

**Thomas E. Kottke, MD,
   MPH, FACC**
Regions Heart Center and
HealthPartners Research
   Foundation
Minneapolis, MN

**Peter A. Margolis, MD, PhD**
Professor of Pediatrics and
   Epidemiology
Department of Pediatrics
School of Medicine
University of North Carolina
   at Chapel Hill
Chapel Hill, NC

**Glen P. Mays, MPH, PhD**
Associate Professor and Director
   of Research
Department of Health Policy
   and Management
College of Public Health
University of Arkansas
   for Medical Sciences
Little Rock, AR

**Beth Melcher, PhD**
North Carolina Service
   to Science Project
Durham, NC

**Paul V. Miles, MD, FAAP**
Vice-President, Quality
   Improvement
American Board of Pediatrics
Chapel Hill, NC

**Julie J. Mohr, MSPH, PhD**
Assistant Professor
Department of Medicine
University of Chicago
Chicago, IL

**Robert Perelman, MD**
Deputy Executive Director
Director, Department of Education
American Academy of Pediatrics
Elk Grove Village, IL

**Christina Rausch, MSW**
Project Director
NC Service to Science Project
Durham, NC

**Lucy A. Savitz, PhD, MBA**
Senior Health Services Researcher
Program on Health Care Quality
  and Outcomes
RTI International
Research Triangle Park, NC

**Kit N. Simpson, DrPH, MPH**
Professor of Health Adminis-
  tration, Pharmacy and Biometry
  Medical University of South
Carolina
Charleston, SC

**Donna J. Slovensky, PhD**
Professor
Department of Health Service
  Administration
School of Health Related
  Professions
University of Alabama
  at Birmingham
Birmingham, AL

**Leif I. Solberg, MD**
HealthPartners Research
  Foundation
Minneapolis, MN

**William A. Sollecito, DrPH**
Director, Public Health Leadership
  Program
Department of Health Policy and
  Administration
School of Public Health
University of North Carolina at
  Chapel Hill
Chapel Hill, NC

**Vaughn M. Upshaw, EdD, MPH**
Lecturer, Public Administration
  and Government
School of Government
University of North Carolina
  at Chapel Hill
Chapel Hill, NC

**Joseph G. Van Matre, PhD**
Professor, School of Business
Senior Scientist, Center for
  Outcomes and Effectiveness
  Research and Education,
  University of Alabama
  at Birmingham
Birmingham, AL

# PREFACE

Quality management has come of age in health care. This book presents an interdisciplinary perspective on quality management in health care, taking into account the disciplines of operations management, organizational behavior, and health services research. Graduate students in health services management, and in the health professions, are the primary audience. This book will also be of interest to those in undergraduate and extended degree programs, and executive education, as well as continuing educational activities involving medicine, nursing, and allied health.

Our approach to quality management is integrative. Special attention has been given to the underlying tools and approaches fundamental to Total Quality Management/Continuous Quality Improvement (TQM/CQI). The challenges of implementation and institutionalization are addressed using examples from a variety of health care organizations, including primary care clinics, hospital laboratories, public health departments, and academic health centers. TQM/CQI is a "body-contact sport," and understanding its concepts and its application requires studying its implementation in a real setting. The book concludes with eight case studies that track the development of CQI in a variety of settings and show how these organizations have adapted TQM/CQI concepts to their particular needs and strategies. Each case describes in detail the implementation in that context and is accompanied by study questions that highlight the important discussion points and link the case back to specific chapters in the text.

Figure 1 represents the basic structure of the book. Chapter 1 outlines the underlying philosophy of TQM/CQI with its structural elements, its health-care associated elements, and the context within which these

**Figure 1**

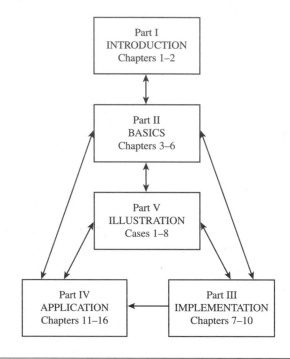

elements must presently function. It also develops the interaction between CQI at the institutional level, the professional level, and the national policy level. Chapter 2 summarizes in a balanced way the theoretical and empirical evidence that CQI can work and can improve the safety, cost, and quality of health care.

The remaining chapters are divided into four parts: Part II, Basics (Chapters 3–6); Part III, Implementation (Chapters 7–10); Part IV, Application (Chapters 11–16); and Part V, Illustration (Cases 1–8). As presented in Figure 1, the book's structure reflects a continuous process in that the basics lead to implementation, and implementation leads to application. Application of TQM/CQI provides an opportunity for further refinement and understanding of the basics through studying illustrative cases and conducting research.

Part II, Basics, deals with the tools and approaches fundamental to TQM/CQI. Chapter 3 presents this within an outcomes model. The chapter outlines the existing quality movement within health care and the specific measurement issues that health care improvement programs must address. Chapter 4 presents the fundamentals of measurement and statistical analysis applied in CQI efforts. Various techniques are presented here and in the cases in Part V with specific examples taken from the health care setting. Chapter 5 discusses issues of meeting customer satisfaction requirements together with methods and instrumentation required for assessing satisfaction. Again, specific illustrations are presented in the cases. Chapter 6 focuses on the role of teams within the context of CQI implemented locally and through collaboratives.

Part III, Implementation, presents the challenges associated with the implementation and institutionalization of CQI within the health care setting. The five chapters in this part address the challenges that a manager is likely to face in implementing CQI in the professional environment, including managing a number of transitions during the implementation process, making sure that there is a high level of physician involvement, assuring patient safety, and providing an appropriate information infrastructure. Chapter 7 discusses the challenge of CQI in a clinical environment and shows how effective CQI requires that managers and physicians are involved in a "learning organization." Chapter 8 considers the systems currently required to address the issues of patient safety that have received much attention recently, while Chapter 9 presents some of the psychological constructs behind the identification and avoidance of adverse events. Chapter 10 outlines the management information system requirements of CQI and suggests how to develop such a resource at the institutional and community levels.

Part IV, Application, deals with the specific application of CQI to a variety of health care settings. Chapter 11 suggests that for CQI to truly have an impact requires that it be incorporated into professional development efforts, including graduate education and recommends inclusion of training that uses the clinical microsystems approach to quality improvement. Further discussions involving the application of CQI include primary care and managed care settings (Chapter 12), contract organizations (Chapter 13), public health departments (Chapter 14), and academic medical centers (Chapter 15). Part IV concludes in Chapter 16 with a look at how health care quality improvement, which started out as a strictly professional concern, moved on to encompass institutional learning and knowledge management, and more recently has become the focus of much national policy debate and investment. However, the chapter concludes out that ultimately, all three levels must be involved, and that clinician involvement remains a necessary condition of quality health care.

Part V, Illustration, presents a series of eight cases of CQI activity in real settings. All are intended for the purposes of classroom discussion of the philosophy and techniques of CQI as applied in a real context. These case studies both illustrate the applications of the methods and provide a basis for discussing ways of applying the concepts discussed in earlier chapters. Intermountain Health Care (Case 1) shows many of the same issues with special emphasis on changing physician behaviors and the impact of technology and the external environment on respected CQI efforts. Quality in Pediatric Subspecialty Care (Case 2) is a contemporary effort by the medical profession to incorporate the improvement of treatments and processes into the credentialing process for specialists, a radical departure from past roles and responsibilities.

Community-Based Quality Improvement Efforts in Kingsport, Tennessee (Case 3) follows one community's efforts to apply these techniques throughout the community even when environmental turbulence in the town, its primary employer, and its provider community is extensive. This new case subsumes some of the material presented in the Holston Valley Hospital and Medical Center case in the 2nd Edition of this book. This initial trio of cases illustrates many of the key issues at the three levels: institutional, professional, and societal. The next two cases reinforce the study of institutional approaches, while the remaining three cases focus on the interests of private and governmental purchasers of care. West Florida Regional Medical Center (Case 4) outlines parts of the CQI activity followed early on in the CQI movement by a Hospital Corporation of America hospital in response to serious price competition in its community. Rex HealthCare and Service Line Teams (Case 5) illustrates the organizational structure that this institution has been developing to implement productivity improvement include both CQI and establishing service line teams. Dr. Johnson, Market Medical Director (Case 6) describes the role of a medical director in managing both quality and cost in a very large HMO within an overall quality management structure. It also considers some issues of quality improvement from a payer point-of-view.

NC Science to Service (Case 7) reports on a recent federally-funded planning project designed to disseminate and implement evidence-based treatment practices in a state's community mental health system which is in a period of major transition. Transforming Health Care: The President's Health Information Technology Plan (Case 8) illustrates the expanding influence of national policy initiatives that represent a political response to growing public concerns about patient safety and health care quality and the tendency of policy makers to focus on information technology as the primary means to those objectives.

*Curtis P. McLaughlin*
*Arnold D. Kaluzny*

# FOREWORD

Arthur Schopenhauer noted that "Every truth passes through three stages before it is recognized. In the first it is ridiculed, in the second it is opposed, and in the third it is regarded as self-evident. On May 1, 1994, *Continuous Quality Improvement in Health Care* first appeared before a health care world where clinical quality improvement was, at best, skeptically questioned. Ideas that today are widely accepted could then still provoke impassioned debate. This volume brought together ideas, principles, and people to help create a new vision of health care delivery.

At its heart, quality improvement argues that all health delivery activities—structure, data systems, planning, accountability, etc.—should build up from value-adding work. Value-adding work occurs through defined (and, hopefully, designed) work processes. On that foundation, improvement is prediction about transformation. It starts with a vision of what could be. Iterative experimentation, informed by quantitative and qualitative measurement and integrated learning, builds a better reality over time. It is a race without a finish line. No process is ever perfect; so it is always possible to conceive and test changes that could make it better.

You hold in your hands an example of continuous improvement principles applied to the explication of the principles themselves. In its Third Edition, *Continuous Quality Improvement in Health Care* adds new insights and findings. When it first appeared it was well before its time. In truth, rereading it with the benefit of ten years of hindsight I am delighted that it essentially got the entire structure right. McLaughlin and Kaluzny not only laid out the core principles of process management and improvement, but they correctly anticipated much of the fine detail—the elegant subtleties—that later years would validate. It remains clear, concise, and well organized—a treat to read and a key reference. Francis Bacon observed that "Some books are to be tasted, others to be swallowed, and some few to be chewed and digested." Any serious student of quality improvement owes it to themselves to make this volume a main course in their intellectual diet.

Ackoff wrote about "power over" versus "power to." "Power over" is the exercise of authority, to punish or reward. "Power to" is the force of ideas to inspire, coordinate, and transform. As a workforce increases in education, the success of organizations shifts from "power over" to "power to," from management to leadership. While there is little question that quality improvement lies at the heart of a major shift in how people think about and execute health care delivery, it is a massive transformation that could well span a full generation. The ideas in this book could not be more timely. It presents a road map and a "how to" guide for the leadership of a health care transformation that is the core work of this generation of caring professionals.

*Brent James*
*IHC Institute for Health Care Delivery Research*

# ACKNOWLEDGMENTS

Throughout the development of the third edition, we have again had the privilege and good fortune to work with many individuals whose considerable talent, dedication, and good humor made it possible for the chapters to be delivered on target and on time. Our faculty and student colleagues at the University of North Carolina at Chapel Hill reaffirmed our long-standing conviction that it is a privilege to work at a university where interdisciplinary efforts are encouraged and faculty members from various departments actually communicate with one another. Specifically, Tim Carey, the director of the Cecil G. Sheps Center for Health Services Research; Jayashankar Swaminatham, chair of the Operations, Technology and Innovation Management Area, Kenan-Flagler Business School; Peggy Leatt, chairperson of the Department of Health Policy and Administration, School of Public Health; and Bill Sollecito of the school's Public Health Leadership Program, were instrumental in maintaining an environment that continued to support our collaborative efforts. This spirit of interdisciplinary cooperation allowed us to bring together a group of clinicians, health services and management researchers and health administrators, all of whom brought a unique set of skills and perspectives to the book.

In addition to working with our contributing authors, who some would say "thrive on abuse," we have had extraordinary support from many other individuals—here in Chapel Hill and elsewhere. The case writing effort was initially supported in part by a grant from the American College of Healthcare Executives, the Whelan Fund of the UNC-CH Kenan-Flager Business School, and the Physician Executive MBA Program at the University of Tennessee, Knoxville. Special thanks must go to Chantal Donaghy, Paul Frellick, Damian Gallina, Adrienne Terrell, and Willie

Williamson at the UNC-CH Public Health Leadership Program and Bessie Neville at the UNC-CH Sheps Center for their assistance in the preparation of the manuscript. Thanks are also due to Marjorie Satinsky, who assisted in the preparation of the Rex Healthcare case by helping to gather illustrative materials. At Jones and Bartlett we thank Mike Brown, who offered us the opportunity to produce this third edition, and Kylah Goodfellow McNeill, Elizabeth J. Mills, and Dan Stone, who provided able editorial support during the production process.

*Curtis P. McLaughlin*
*Arnold D. Kaluzny*
*Chapel Hill, North Carolina*

# PART I

# Introduction

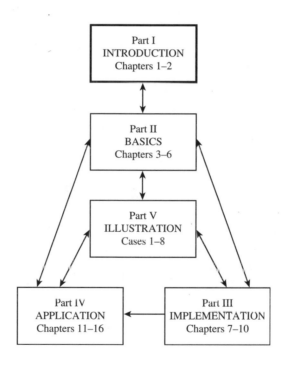

# CHAPTER 1

# Defining Quality Improvement

*Curtis P. McLaughlin and Arnold D. Kaluzny*

Continuous quality improvement in health care comes in a variety of shapes, colors, and sizes and is referred to by many names. Don't be confused—whether it is called total quality management (TQM), continuous quality improvement (CQI), or some other term. TQM/CQI is a structured organizational process for involving personnel in planning and executing a continuous flow of improvements to provide quality health care that meets or exceeds expectations. In this book the terms CQI and TQM are used interchangeably. TQM more often refers to industry-based programs and CQI typically refers to programs designed for clinical settings. The latter term will be used most frequently to encompass quality improvement efforts and philosophies.

While quality improvement has various names, it usually involves a common set of characteristics, including

- a link to key elements of the organization's strategic plan,
- a quality council made up of the institution's top leadership,
- training programs for personnel,
- mechanisms for selecting improvement opportunities,
- formation of process improvement teams,
- staff support for process analysis and redesign, and
- personnel policies that motivate and support staff participation in process improvement.

In the course of that process analysis, rigorous techniques of the scientific method, including

- assessing the state of the art in theory and
- methods and statistical process control

are typically applied. The purpose of this chapter is to present the distinguishing characteristics and elements of performance improvement of all types, and describe their underlying philosophies.

## INSTITUTIONAL IMPROVEMENT

Quality improvement under the labels of TQM and CQI is both an approach and a set of activities applied at various times to one or more of the four broad types of performance improvement initiatives undertaken within a given institution:

1. localized improvement efforts
2. organizational learning
3. process reengineering
4. evidence-based medicine and management

Localized improvement occurs when an ad hoc team is developed to look at a specific process problem or opportunity. Organizational learning occurs when this process is documented and results in the development of policies and procedures, which are then implemented. Examples include the development of protocols, procedures, clinical pathways, etc. Process reengineering occurs when a major investment blends internal and external resources to make changes, often including the development of information systems, that radically impact key organizational processes. Evidence-based medicine and management involves the selection of best clinical and management practices; these are determined by examination of the professional literature and consideration of internal experience. The lines of demarcation between these four are not clear because performance improvement can occur across a continuum of project size, impact, clinical content, external consultant involvement, and departure from existing norms.

## SOCIETAL LEARNING

In recent years, the emphasis on quality has increased at the societal level. The US Institute of Medicine (IOM) has issued a number of reports critical of the quality of care and the variability of both quality and cost across the country (2000, 2001). This concern has increased with mounting evidence of the societal cost of poor quality care in both lives and dollars (Brennan, Leape *et al.* 2004). It is not limited to the United States and the United Kingdom; similar evidence and quality concerns have been reported from Canada, Australia, and New Zealand (Baker *et al.* 2004; Kable, Gibbard, and Spigelman 2002; Davis *et al.* 2002). This newer emphasis has played out in studies, commissions, and reports as well as the efforts of regulatory organizations to institutionalize quality through their standards and certification processes. As you will see throughout this book, concern for quality and cost as a matter of public policy carries risk: having everyone in charge of quality may end up with no one in charge, especially in a culture where so much, including health care, is presumed to be market-driven.

## PROFESSIONAL RESPONSIBILITY

Health care as a whole is often likened to a cottage industry with overtones of a medieval craft guild, including its monopoly of access to and implementation of technical knowledge, which reached its zenith in the mid-twentieth century, but has been under pressure ever since (Starr 1982; McLaughlin and Kaluzny 2002; Schlesinger 2002; Rastegar 2004). This was reinforced by the concept of professionalism, in which service providers are assumed to have exclusive access to knowledge and competence and, therefore, take full responsibility for self-regulation and for quality. However, much of the public policy debate has centered on the weaknesses of the professional system in improving quality of care. Critics point to dominance of the need for professional autonomy; protectionist guild practices, such as secrecy, restricted entry, and scapegoating; lack of capital accumulation for modernization; and economic self-interest as major problems. As we will see, all of these issues impinge on the search for improved quality. However, we cannot ignore the role of professional development as a potential engine of quality improvement, despite the popular emphasis on institutional improvement and societal learning. This too will be addressed in subsequent chapters.

## RATIONALE AND DISTINGUISHING CHARACTERISTICS

As health care organizations and professions develop their own performance improvement approaches, their managements must lead them through a decision process in which activities are initiated, adapted, and then institutionalized. Organizations embark on CQI for a variety of reasons, including accreditation requirements, cost control, competition for customers, and pressure from employers and payers. Linder (1991), for example, suggests that there are three basic CQI strategies: conformance to requirements, competitive advantage, and true process improvement. Some institutions genuinely desire to maximize their quality of care as defined in both technical and customer preference terms. Others wish simply to increase their share of the local health care market. Still others wish to do whatever is necessary to maintain their accreditation status with bodies such as the Joint Commission on Accreditation of Healthcare Organizations (JCAHO), National Committee on Quality Assurance (NCQA), and others, after which they will return to business as usual. As you might imagine, this book is written for the first group—those who truly wish to excel in the competitive health care market by giving their customers the quality care that they deserve.

Although CQI comes in a variety of forms and is initiated for a variety of reasons, it does have distinguishing characteristics and functions. These characteristics and functions are often defined as the essence of good management. They include: (1) understanding and adapting to the external environment; (2) empowering clinicians and managers to analyze and improve processes; (3) adopting a norm that customer preferences are important determinants of quality and that the term "customer" includes both patients and providers in the process; (4) developing a multidisciplinary approach that goes beyond conventional departmental and professional lines; (5) adopting a planned, articulated philosophy of ongoing change and adaptation; (6) setting up mechanisms to ensure implementation of best practices through planned organizational learning; and (7) providing the motivation for a rational, data-based, cooperative approach to process analysis and change.

What is perhaps most radical vis-à-vis past health care improvement efforts is a willingness to examine existing health care processes and rework these processes collaboratively using "state-of-the-art" scientific and administrative knowledge and relevant data-gathering and analysis methodologies. Many health care processes have developed and expanded in a complex, political, and authoritarian environment, acquiring the patina of science. The application of data-based management and scientific principles to the clinical and administrative processes that produce patient care is what CQI is all about. Even with all the public concern about medical error and patient safety, improvement cannot occur without both institutional will and professional leadership (Millenson 2003).

CQI is simultaneously two things: a management philosophy and a management method. It is distinguished by the recognition that customer requirements are the key to customer quality and that ultimately customer requirements will change over time because of changes in education, economics, technology, and culture. Such changes, in turn, require continuous improvements in the administrative and clinical methods that affect the quality of patient care. This dynamic between changing expectations and continuous efforts to meet these expectations is captured in the Japanese word, *kaizen*, translated as continuous improvement (Imai 1986). Change is a fundamental of the health care environment, and the organization's systems must have both the will and the way to master such change effectively.

The use of the term "customer" presents a special challenge to many health professionals. For many it is a term that runs contrary to the professional model of health services and the idea that "the doctor knows best." Some health professionals would prefer terms that connote the more dependent roles of "client" or "patient." In CQI terms, "customer" is a generic term referring to the end user of a group's output or product. The customer can be external or internal to the system—a patient, a payer, a colleague, or someone from another department. User satisfaction then becomes one ultimate test of process and product quality. Consequently, new efforts and new resources must be devoted to ascertaining what the customer wants through the use of consumer surveys, focus groups, interviews, and various other ways of gathering information on customer preferences, expectations, and perceived experiences. If one encounters resistance and challenges to the use of such words as "customer," perhaps the best strategy is to demur, since the real issue is the concept and not the labels.

CQI is further distinguished by its emphasis on avoiding personal blame. The focus is on managerial and professional processes associated with a specific outcome. The initial assumption is that the process needs to be changed and that the persons already involved in that process are needed to help identify how to approach a given problem or opportunity.

Therefore, CQI moves beyond the ideas of participative management and decentralized organizations. It is, however, participative in that it encourages the involvement of all personnel associated with a particular work process to provide relevant information and become part of the solution.

CQI is also decentralized in that it places responsibility for ownership of each process in the hands of its implementers, those most directly involved with it. Yet this level of participation and decentralization does not absolve management of its fundamental responsibility; in fact, it places additional burdens on management. Where the problem is with the system (the usual case), management is responsible for change. CQI calls for significant amounts of management thought, oversight, flexibility, and responsibility.

CQI inherently increases the dignity of the employees involved because it not only recognizes the important role belonging to each member of the process improvement team, but also involves them as partners and even leaders in the redesign of the process. In some cases, professionals can also serve as consultants to other teams and to management itself. Not surprisingly, organizations using CQI often experience improvements in morale. When the level of quality is being measured, workers can rightly take pride in the quality of the work they are producing.

Another distinguishing feature of CQI is the rigorous belief in fact-based decision making, captured by the saying, "In God we trust. All others send data." Facts do include perceptions, and decisions cannot all be delayed to await the results of scientifically correct, double-blind studies. However, everyone involved in CQI activities is expected to study the multiple causes of events and to explore a wide array of system-wide solutions. It is surprising and rewarding to see a team move away from the table-pounding, "I'm right and you're stupid" position (with which so many meetings in health care start), by gathering data, both hard and soft, to see what is actually happening and why. Multiple causation is assumed and the search for answers starts with trying to identify the full set of factors contributing to less than optimal system performance.

Later in this book, we will also refer to some of the built-in stresses that accompany CQI implementation. These include the tension between the professionals' need for autonomy and control and the objectives of organizational learning and conformance to best practices. Organizations can also oversimplify their environment, as sometimes happens with clinical pathways. Seriously ill patients do not fit the simple diagnoses often assumed when developing such pathways. There may also be a related tendency to try to over-control processes. Health care is not like manufacturing and it is necessary to understand that patients (anatomy, physiology, psyche, family setting), providers, and diagnostic categories are inherently highly variable and that variance reduction can only go so far. One has to develop systems that properly handle the inherent variability (called common cause variability) after unnecessary variability (called special cause variability) has been removed (McLaughlin 1996).

## ELEMENTS OF CQI

Together with these distinguishing characteristics, CQI is usually composed of a number of elements including

- philosophical elements, which for the most part mirror the distinguishing characteristics cited above;
- structural elements, which are usually associated with both industrial and professional quality improvement programs; and
- health-care-specific elements, which add the specialized knowledge of health care to the generic CQI approach.

The philosophical elements are those aspects of CQI that, at a minimum, have to be present in order to constitute a CQI effort. The structural elements also are usually associated with CQI, but are not defining and might occasionally be omitted for one reason or another. The health-care-specific elements are those not often included in lists of elements of CQI initiatives, but are particularly relevant to the health care setting.

### Philosophical Elements

The philosophical elements that are representative of continuous quality improvement include:

1. Strategic Focus—Emphasis on having a mission, values, and objectives that performance improvement processes are designed, prioritized, and implemented to support.
2. Customer Focus—Emphasis on both customer (patient, provider, payer) satisfaction and health outcomes as performance measures.
3. Systems View—Emphasis on analysis of the whole system providing a service or influencing an outcome.

4. Data-driven (evidence-based) Analysis—Emphasis on gathering and use of objective data on system operation and system performance.
5. Implementer Involvement—Emphasis on involving the owners of all components of the system in seeking a common understanding of its delivery process.
6. Multiple Causation—Emphasis on identifying the multiple root causes of a set of system phenomena.
7. Solution Identification—Emphasis on seeking a set of solutions that enhance overall system performance through simultaneous improvements in a number of normally independent functions.
8. Process Optimization—Emphasis on optimizing a delivery process to meet customer needs regardless of existing precedents and on implementing the system changes regardless of existing territories and fiefdoms. To quote Dr. Deming: "Management's job is to optimize the system."
9. Continuing Improvement—Emphasis on continuing the systems analysis even when a satisfactory solution to the presenting problem is obtained.
10. Organizational Learning—Emphasis on organizational learning so that the capacity of the organization to generate process improvement and foster personal growth is enhanced.

### Structural Elements

Beyond the philosophical elements cited above, a number of useful structural elements can be used to structure, organize, and support the continuous improvement process. Almost all CQI initiatives make intensive use of these structural elements, which reflect the operational aspects of CQI and include:

1. Process Improvement Teams—Emphasis on forming and empowering teams of employees to deal with existing problems and opportunities (see Chapter 6).
2. Seven Tools—Use of one or more of the seven quality tools so frequently cited in the industrial and the health quality literature: flow charts, cause-and-effect diagrams, histograms, Pareto charts, run charts, control charts, and correlational analyses (see Chapter 4).

3. Parallel Organization—Development of a separate management structure to set priorities for and monitor CQI strategy and implementation, usually referred to as a quality council (see Chapter 2).
4. Top Management Commitment—Top management leadership to make the process effective and foster its integration into the institutional fabric of the organization (see Chapter 2).
5. Statistical Analysis—Use of statistics, including statistical process control, to identify and reduce unnecessary variation in processes and practices (see Chapter 4).
6. Customer Satisfaction Measures—Introduction of market research instruments to monitor customer satisfaction at various levels (see Chapter 5).
7. Benchmarking—Use of benchmarking to identify best practices in related and unrelated settings to emulate as processes or use as performance targets (see Chapter 4).
8. Redesign of Processes from Scratch—Making sure that the end product conforms to customer requirements by using techniques of quality function deployment and/or process reengineering (see Chapter 4).

**Health-Care-Specific Elements**

The use of CQI in health care is often described as a major management innovation, but it also resonates with past and ongoing efforts within the health services research community. The health care quality movement has its own history, with its own leadership and values that must be understood and respected. Thus in health care there are a number of additional approaches and techniques that health managers and professionals have successfully added to the philosophical and structural elements associated with CQI, including:

1. Epidemiological and clinical studies, coupled with insurance payment and medical records data, often referred to as the basis of evidence-based medicine
2. Involvement of the medical staff governance process, including quality assurance, tissue committees, pharmacy and therapeutics committees, and peer review

3. Use of risk-adjusted outcome measures
4. Use of cost-effectiveness analysis
5. Use of quality assurance data and techniques and risk management data.

## THE PAST AND FUTURE OF HEALTH CARE QUALITY MANAGEMENT

Quality has been and continues to be a central issue in health care organizations and among health care providers. The classic works of Avedis Donabedian, Robert Brook, and Leonard Rosenfeld, to name a few, have made major contributions to the definition, measurement, and understanding of health care quality. However, the corporatization of health care in the United States (Starr 1982) and health care change have redefined and will continue to redefine how we manage quality. Given the increasing proportion of the gross national product allocated to health services and the redefinition of health care as an "economic good," health care organizations are influenced to a growing extent by organizations in the industrial sector. As part of this process, health care organizations have become more and more isomorphic with the organizations that finance most of the services that they provide. This conformity is reflected by the increasing tendency to refer to hospitals as "corporations"; by the development of "product lines" rather than service areas; by the replacement of planning by marketing; by the use of titles such as President, Chief Executive Officer, or Chief Operating Officer rather than Administrator; and, in the area of quality, by a nomenclature and perspective known as total quality management (TQM).

The long-held perception of health care as a cottage industry persisted into the 1960s and 1970s. In this view, health care was seen as a craft or art delivered by individual professionals who had learned by apprenticeship and who worked independently in a decentralized system. These practitioners tailored their craft to each individual situation using processes that were neither recorded nor explicitly engineered, and they were personally accountable for the performance and financial outcomes of the care they provided.

The 1980s and 1990s witnessed a distinct change, which is often described as the "industrialization of health care" (Kongstvedt 1997). This change affected almost all aspects of health care delivery, influencing ways that risks are allocated, how care is organized, and how professionals are motivated and incentivized. Figure 1–1 outlines this industrialization process utilizing the dynamic stability model of Boynton, Victor, and Pine (1993). One route, marked A, follows the traditional route of industrialization as illustrated by the bundling of cataract operations into a few high-volume, specialized centers. However, most health care activities have followed the B route, bypassing mass production due to the high variability in patient needs and using techniques of CQI and process re-engineering.

The Victor and Boynton (1998) model for the organization suggests an appropriate path for organizational development and improvement. As presented in Figure 1–2, health care processes and product lines have begun to move from the craft stage to positions in all of the other three stages of that model. Each of the four stages requires its own approach to quality.

1. Craft requires that the individual improve with experience and use the tacit knowledge produced to develop a better individual reputation

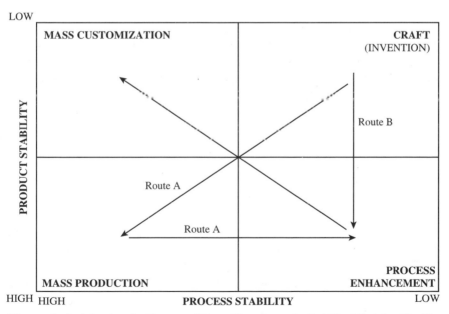

**Figure 1–1** Adapting the Boynton-Victor-Pine dynamic Stability Model to Health Care.
Figure appeared in *OR/MS Today*, Vol. 25, No. 1. Reprinted with permission.

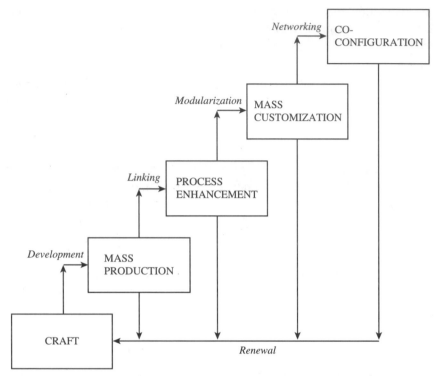

**Figure 1–2** The Right Path Transformations Are Sequenced Along the Way. From *Invented Here: Maximizing Your Organization's Internal Growth and Profitability* by B. Victor and A.C. Boynton, Harvard Business School Press, 1998. Reprinted by permission.

---

and group reputation. Craft activities can be leveraged to a limited extent by a community of cooperating and teaching craftspersons.

2. Mass production requires the discipline that produces conformance quality in high volume at low cost. Critics sometimes refer to this approach using the terms such as "industrialization" or the "deskilling" of the profession and occasionally mention Henry Ford's assembly lines as a negative model.

3. Process enhancement requires that processes be analyzed and modified to develop a best practice approach using worker feedback and process-owning teams within the organization.

4. Mass customization requires that the organization takes that best practice, modularizes and supports it independently, and then uses

those modules to build efficient, low-cost processes that are responsive to individual customer wants and needs.

Because health care is a complex, multiproduct environment, various types of care can be found at each of the four stages, depending on the state of the technology and the strategy of the delivery unit. The correct place to be along that pathway depends on the current state of the technology. The revolution in health care organization is driven not only by economics, but also by the type of knowledge work that is being done. As described in Victor and Boynton (1998):

> Managers take the wrong path when they fail to account for the fact that (1) learning is always taking place, and (2) what learning is taking place depends on the kind of work one is doing. The learning system we describe along the right path requires that managers leverage the learning from previous forms of work.... If managers attempt to transform without understanding the learning taking place..., then transformation efforts will be at best slightly off the mark and at worst futile. In addition, if managers misunderstand what type of work (craft, mass production, process enhancement, or mass customization) is taking place in a given process or activity when transformation starts, then they may use the wrong transformation steps (development, linking, modularization, or renewal). (p. 129)

These authors, however, were referring to a single commercial firm with a relatively limited line of goods and services. In health care, a single organization such as a hospital might contain examples of multiple stages due to the variety of its products. The various DRG systems offer almost 500 categories by which to describe health care products. These rather loose product designations have been the basis of managed care and disease management because they allowed us for the first time to collect and compare outcomes and costs across organizations and processes for many purposes, including process enhancement.

However, these definitions are not very precise. Even where clinical pathways are institutionalized, one hears complaints that the definitions apply to patients with only one diagnosis, whereas most very sick patients, especially the elderly, have multiple diagnoses. Therefore, the prevailing quality and performance enhancement systems have to be prepared with much greater levels of variability—in patient problem constellations, anatomy, physiology, and preferences, as well as in provider potentials and preferences (McLaughlin 1996). Furthermore, increased availability of genetic information will further fractionate many disease categories, making the definitions of disease even more complex.

Figure 1–3 suggests how this has and will occur in health care. As scientific information about a health care process accumulates, it shifts from the craft stage to the process enhancement stage. After the process is codified and developed further, it may shift into the mass production mode if the approach is sufficiently cut and dried, the volume is high, and the patients will accept this impersonal mode of delivery. If there is still too much art or lack of science to justify codification, the enhanced process can be returned to the craft mode or moved into the mass customization and co-configuration pathway.

The craft mode contains multiple delivery alternatives. If, for example, one were to decide to commission an artist to make a custom work of art, one has two ways to specify how it is to be controlled. The first is to say, "You are the artist, do your thing and I will pay whatever it costs." This is fee-for-service indemnity. The other is to say, "You can decide what to do, but here is all that I can afford to pay." This is capitation. In both cases, the grand design and the execution are still in the hands of the artist. However, that does not preclude the artist from learning by doing or from vendors of materials and equipment or from observing and collaborating with colleagues. However, one does not commit to a one best way to do things, because one is not able either to articulate or agree on what is the best way.

The mass customization pathway is the way that is best suited to the production of satisfied health care customers at low or reasonable relative costs. The organization develops a series of modular approaches to prevention and treatment, highly articulated and well supported by information technology, so that they can be deployed efficiently in a variety of places and configurations to respond to customer needs. Clinical pathways represent one example of modularization. They represent best practice as known to the organization and they are applied by a configuror (the health care professional) to meet the needs of the individual patient. This requires an integrated information system that will give the configuror, usually a generalist, access to specialized information; to full information about the patient's background, medical history, and status; and to synchronize the implementation of the modules of service being delivered. In a sense, mass customization represents a process that simulates craft, but is highly science-based, coordinated, integrated with other process flows,

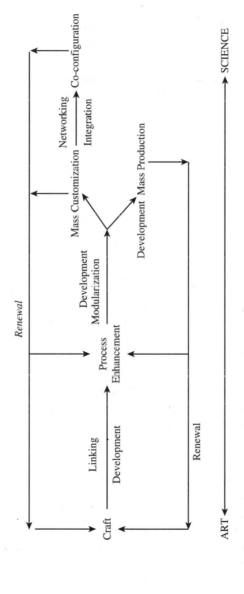

**Figure 1-3** Revised Boynton and Victor Model for Health Care

and efficient. How does this differ from the well-run modern hospital or clinic? As described by Victor and Boynton (1998):

> the tightly linked process steps developed under process enhancement are now exploded, not into isolated parts, but into a dynamic web of interconnected modular units. Rather than the sequential assembly lines ... work is now organized as a complex, reconfigurable product and service system.
>
> Modularization breaks up the work into units that are interchangeable on demand from the customer. And everything has to happen fast... Modularization transforms work by creating a dynamic, robust network of units.
>
> Within some of these units ... there may still be active craft, mass production, or process enhancement work taking place, but all the possible interfaces among modules must be carefully designed so that they can rapidly, efficiently, and seamlessly regroup to meet customer needs. (pp. 12–13)

Where does science come in? Victor and Boynton refer to architectural knowledge, a much deeper process understanding than that needed for earlier stages of their model. Also at a practical level it takes hard science to legitimize the conformance by providers required to make such a system work.

The remaining and most futuristic stage of this model is what they call "co-configuration"—a system in which the customer is linked into the network and customer intelligence is accessed as readily as the providers'. In a futuristic sense, one should also be able to include the patient in the decision-making network to a high degree.

## The History of Continuous Quality Improvement (The Performance Enhancement Stage)

The explosion of medical and technical knowledge in the last 60 years has moved much of medicine away from art and toward science. However, this movement has occurred at a very uneven pace. Even within a single disease entity, the scientific bases for prevention, diagnosis, treatment, and aftercare may be at quite different levels. Therefore, some activities in the organization are still very much an art form and still suited to the craft approach. Others have become so routinized and are done in such high volumes that the centers of excellence and focused factories that are the health care equivalent of mass production seem appropriate. However, the recent past, the present, and still much of the future of health care focus on performance enhancement. This has emphasized the adaptation of TQM approaches from industry, especially the work of Deming, Juran, and others. Here the tacit craft knowledge in use is examined, codified, compared to best practices elsewhere, reworked, tested (often using a variant of the PDCA cycle outlined below), implemented, and institutionalized. Such efforts produce individual and group learning and, if properly implemented, become organizational learning.

Because this TQM/CQI process takes a great deal of time to implement and relies on information available only to the participants, information drawn from benchmarking, and the skills inherent in the organization, some organizations have adopted the business process reengineering approach. This approach calls for much bigger investments, especially in outside information technology talent, to provide a better process faster, but at a much greater financial and organizational cost. These processes use teams of inside and outside individuals to produce totally new processes on relatively tight timetables. Both the TQM/CQI processes and the reengineering processes can produce tightly articulated processes and procedures such as: clinical protocols, clinical pathways, and clinical guidelines.

The processes under consideration can be administrative and/or clinical. The approaches to clinical process enhancement have many names, including the currently popular clinical quality improvement, evidence-based medicine, outcomes management, and disease management. Each of these terms also represents a reliance on clinical epidemiology and joint organizational and professional learning.

Approaches to organizational forms for delivery and strategies of implementation vary widely. HMOs and other managed care organizations are very much involved in process enhancement, especially where decision-making is based on continuous review of best practice and of one's own billing, costing, and patient record files. However, they are often guilty of a one-size-fits-all control system that tries to use the same approach to all levels of art and science. Figure 1–4 illustrates that control mechanisms need to vary at the very least with the degree of art versus science involved.

| Delivery Mode Continuum / Disease Knowledge Status Continuum | Individual Choice of Methods (Craft) | Organizational Learning (Mass Customization) |
|---|---|---|
| | ←——— Continuous Quality Improvement ———→ | |
| Art | • Professional autonomy needed<br>• Fits well with either fee-for-service (PPO) or capitation<br>• High cost/high quality<br>• Apprenticeship effective | • Conflict over autonomy and efficiency<br>• Conflict over costs<br>• Highly variable quality<br>• Peer review effective |
| Science | • High Costs<br>• Highly variable quality<br>• Conflict over autonomy versus efficiency<br>• Continuing medical education effective | • Best practice protocols<br>• Managed care fits well<br>• Low cost/high quality<br>• Procedural inservice training effective |

**Figure 1–4** Relationship between Delivery Mode and Degree of disease Knowledge
Figure appeared in *OR/MS Today*, Vol. 25, No. 1. Reprinted with permission.

## EMERGENCE OF TQM

The fundamentals of TQM are based on the scientific management movement developed in the early 20th century. Emphasis was given to "management based on facts," but with management assumed to be the master of the facts. It was believed to be the responsibility of management to specify one correct method of work for all workers and to see that personnel executed that method to ensure quality. Gradually that perspective has been influenced by the human relations perspective and by the recognition of the importance and ability of the people in the organization. Building on those perspectives, Figure 1–5 presents the major US contributors to the emergence of TQM.

### Walter Shewhart

Most histories of TQM credit statistics pioneer Walter Shewhart, at Bell Laboratories, with the first published efforts in this area. His best known contributions are the control chart and the Plan, Do, Check, Act (PDCA) cycle illustrated in Figure 1–6. Although the PDCA cycle is often attributed to Deming, he attributes it to Shewhart (Deming 1986).

Shewhart was aware of and promoted the idea that price alone was no indication of value. He wrote that price, without an understanding of quality, was meaningless. Shewart taught that decisions based on price alone were almost certain, in the long run, to be more expensive than necessary and to lead to undesirable results. He also was aware that there were inherent difficulties in defining quality, although he felt that reasonable people could develop operational definitions, that is, standards.

Furthermore, it was Shewhart's idea that statistical control (also called statistical process control) of stable or "in control" processes is the foundation of all empirical CQI activities. If a process exhibited variation, then the cause of that variation had to be discovered and removed. Determining variation and analyzing its causes in order to remove them is one primary function of TQM.

### W. Edwards Deming

W. Edwards Deming is the best known of the proponents of TQM. In 1950 he was invited by representatives of Japanese industry to suggest

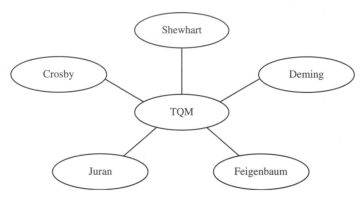

**Figure 1–5** Major U.S. contributors to TQM

how they might best rebuild their war-ravaged economy. Although he had been advocating his statistical approach to quality for some time, the Japanese were the first to implement his ideas widely.

Over the intervening years, Deming has made enormous contributions to the development of TQM, but he is perhaps best known for the 14-point program of recommendations that he devised for management to improve quality (see Table 1–1). But his focus has always been on processes (rather than organizational structures), on the ever-continuous cycle of improvement, and on the rigorous statistical analysis of objective data.

Arraying data in various ways to facilitate its analysis, Deming sought to identify two types of sources of improvement in processes. The first was elimination of "special" causes of process variation: unnecessary variation associated with specific material(s), machine(s), or individual(s). The second was elimination of "common" causes of variation: those associated with aspects of the system itself such as design, training, materials, machines, or working conditions. Special causes of problems can be addressed by those working directly with the process, whereas common causes of problems are the responsibility of management to correct.

Deming believed that management has the final responsibility for quality. Employees work in the system; management deals with the system itself. He also felt that most quality problems are management controlled rather than worker controlled. This was the basis for his requirement that TQM be based on a top-down, organization-wide commitment.

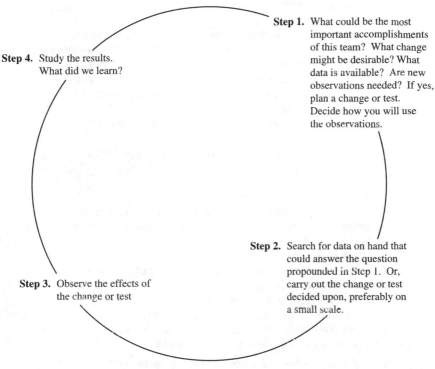

**Step 1.** What could be the most important accomplishments of this team? What change might be desirable? What data is available? Are new observations needed? If yes, plan a change or test. Decide how you will use the observations.

**Step 4.** Study the results. What did we learn?

**Step 3.** Observe the effects of the change or test

**Step 2.** Search for data on hand that could answer the question propounded in Step 1. Or, carry out the change or test decided upon, preferably on a small scale.

**Figure 1–6** Shewhart's PCDA Cycle

## Armand F. Feigenbaum

Building on Deming's statistical approach, Armand F. Feigenbaum and Joseph M. Juran provided theoretical constructs for TQM. Feigenbaum coined the phrase "total quality control," which he defined as an effective system for integrating the functions of quality development (conception, planning, design, and set-up), quality maintenance (production, distribution, and service), and quality improvement (training, data analysis, and user feedback). These functions cut across all activities in the organization (including marketing, production, and finance) and involve all system phases (inputs, transformation, outputs, and outcomes). Both suppliers and customers are drawn into the total quality concept. The goal of quality, according to Feigenbaum, is to meet satisfactorily whatever customers believe to be their requirements for the service or product.

**Table 1-1**  Deming's 14-Point Program

1. Create and publish to all employees a statement of the aims and purposes of the company or other organization. The management must demonstrate constantly their commitment to this statement.
2. Learn the new philosophy, top management and everybody.
3. Understand the purpose of inspection, for improvement of processes and reduction of cost.
4. End the practice of awarding business on the basis of price tag alone.
5. Improve constantly and forever the system of production and service.
6. Institute training.
7. Teach and institute leadership.
8. Drive out fear. Create trust. Create a climate for innovation.
9. Optimize toward the aims and purposes of the company the efforts of teams, groups, staff areas.
10. Eliminate exhortations for the work force.
11a. Eliminate numerical quotas for production. Instead, learn and institute methods for improvement.
11b. Eliminate Management by Objective.
12. Remove barriers that rob people of pride of workmanship.
13. Encourage education and self-improvement for everyone.
14. Take action to accomplish the transformation.

*Source:* Reprinted from *The New Economics for Industry, Government, Education* by W. Edwards Deming by permission of MIT and W. Edwards Deming. Published by MIT, Center for Advanced Engineering Study, Cambridge, MA 02139. Copyright © 1993 by W. Edwards Demig.

(Note that factors outside the organization—cultural, attitudinal, and technological changes—can make customers dissatisfied with a once satisfactory outcome, thereby continuously motivating new quality improvement cycles.)

## Joseph M. Juran

Joseph M. Juran, like Deming, was involved with the Japanese in the 1950s. He argued that the quality improvement process is a never-ending spiral of progress, or "fitness for use," as defined by customers. He further argued that management must focus on two levels within the organization. The first level is the mission (always fitness for use), which is determined by design requirements and by the degree of conformance to the specifications of that design's availability, reliability, and maintainability. The second level is the mission of the individual departments and units within the organization to do their work according to the specifications that have been designed to achieve fitness for use: that is, to go about their work in a way that maximizes the organization's overall attainment of fitness for use. (This may mean that some units must suboptimize their performance in order for the organization as a whole to optimize its performance. This is often a difficult concept for professional personnel to accept.) Juran emphasized the interdependency of all units in achieving the ultimate outcome.

Juran's writings paralleled Deming's concepts of classifying process variations, separating them into "sporadic" and "chronic." Sporadic problems occur when production falls below acceptable standards; chronic problems are inherent in the work setting and require intervention by management. Improvements in chronic problems he called "breakthroughs."

Furthermore, Juran insisted that quality goals be specific. Vague statements like "We are dedicated to improving quality" or "Quality is Job One" are unacceptable. Instead, he insisted on a specific goal such as "We will reduce the number of medical records uncompleted after two weeks to 1% of total discharges by January 1 of next year."

Juran's followers in health care also emphasized Juran's Quality Trilogy of basic quality processes: (1) quality planning, (2) quality control, and (3) quality improvement. These must be supported by an "infrastructure" of measurement systems, buyer-user-supplier relationships, education and training, and information management. These quality processes must rest on a "foundation" of customer focus, management involvement, and strategic planning that links all quality efforts back to the firm's key business goals.

## Philip B. Crosby

Philip B. Crosby, working in the 1980s, developed a different theoretical perspective on quality improvement based on changing the corporate culture and attitudes. He departed from his predecessors' focus on statistical process control techniques and emphasized the concept of "zero defects." He emphasized organization and management theories rather than the application of statistical tools.

Crosby asked two questions: What is quality? What standards and systems are needed to achieve quality? He answered with four "absolutes of quality." The first absolute is "conformance to requirements," often referred to as "Do it right the first time." The second is "Defect prevention is the only acceptable approach." The third is that "zero defects" is the only performance standard. The fourth is that the "cost of nonconformance" is the only appropriate measure of quality. His approach, like Deming's, was to implement a 14-step process, but a process that stresses changes in the organization's culture and attitudes. Crosby's 14 steps are listed in Table 1–2.

Crosby believed that the quality program should go forward on two fronts. Management needs to master a set of skills, including his 14 steps, and to develop the necessary implementation and support systems. At the same time, individuals will need training in a variety of tools, including process and systems modeling, statistical techniques, experimental design, problem solving, and error prevention.

---

**Table 1–2**  Crosby's Fourteen Steps

1. Management commitment
2. Quality improvement team
3. Quality measurement
4. Cost of quality evaluation
5. Quality awareness
6. Corrective action
7. Establish an ad hoc committee for the zero defects program
8. Supervisor training
9. Zero defects day
10. Goal setting
11. Error cause removal
12. Recognition of success
13. Quality councils
14. Do it over again

Source: P.B. Crosby, *Quality is Free: The Art of Making Quality Certain.* 1979, Mentor Books. Reproduced with permission of The McGraw-Hill Companies.

Crosby's writings emphasize developing an estimate of the "cost of nonconformance," also called the "cost of quality." Developing this estimate involves identifying and assigning values to all of the unnecessary costs associated with waste and wasted effort when work is not done correctly the first time. This includes the costs of identifying errors, correcting them, and making up for the customer dissatisfaction that results. Estimates of the cost of quality range from 20% to 40% of the total costs of the industry, a range also widely accepted by hospital administrators and other health care experts.

Crosby's concept of the cost of quality is a good one to use when the top management has not yet accepted the philosophical arguments of CQI. They often can be impressed by arguments that show the specific cost items that poor quality generates, especially when the presenter also shows how these faults can be addressed using standard quality improvement techniques.

## The Japanese

All the individuals mentioned to this point have been Americans (although their ideas were largely ignored in the United States until about 1980). However, the Japanese have made numerous original contributions to CQI thinking, tools, and techniques, especially since the 1960s. The most famous of Japanese experts are Genichi Taguchi and Kaoru Ishikawa. Taguchi emphasized using statistical techniques developed for the design of experiments to quickly identify problematic variations in a service or product; he also advocated a focus on what he called "robust" (forgiving) design. He also emphasized evaluating quality from both an end-user and a process approach. Ishikawa and other Japanese quality engineers refined the application of the foundations of CQI and added:

1. total participation by all members of an organization (quality must be company-wide)
2. the next step of a process is its "customer" just as the preceding step is its "supplier"
3. communicating with both customer and supplier is necessary (promoting feedback and creating channels of communication throughout the system)
4. a participative team emphasis, starting with "quality circles"

5. an emphasis on education and training
6. quality audits; e.g., the Deming Prize
7. rigorous use of statistics
8. "just in time" processes.

New approaches, refinements of older concepts, and different combinations of ideas are occurring almost daily. As more and more organizations adopt CQI, we are seeing increasing innovation and experimentation with CQI thinking and its applications. This is especially true of the health care area, where virtually every organization has had to work hard to develop its own adaptation of CQI to clinical process.

## APPLICATION TO HEALTH CARE ORGANIZATIONS

Around the mid-1980s, CQI was applied in several health care settings. Most notable was the early work done by three physicians following the principles outlined by Deming: Paul Batalden at Hospital Corporation of America (HCA), Donald Berwick at Harvard Community Health Center, and Brent James at Intermountain Health System.

One of Deming's major premises (1993) was that management needs to undergo a transformation. In order to respond successfully to the current challenges to our organizations and their environments, the way to accomplish that transformation, which must be deliberately learned and incorporated into management, is by pursuing what he calls "Profound Knowledge." The key elements of his system of profound knowledge are: (1) appreciation for a system; (2) knowledge about variation; (3) theory of knowledge; and (4) psychology.

A Deming approach, as adopted by the Hospital Corporation of America, is illustrated in Figure 1–7. It was referred to by HCA as FOCUS-PDCA and provided the firm's health care workers with a common language and an orderly sequence for implementing the cycle of continuous improvement.

The Deming process is especially useful in health care because professionals already have knowledge of the subject matter as well as a set of values and disciplines that fit the Deming philosophy. What training in Deming methods adds is knowledge of how to build a new theory using insights about systems, variation, and psychology, and it focuses

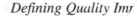
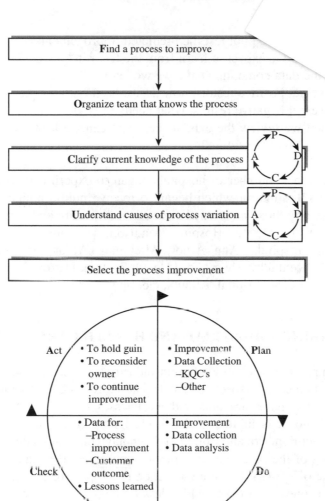

**Figure 1–7** The FOCUS-PDCA® Cycle

on the answers given to the following basic questions (Batalden and Stoltz 1993):

1. What are we trying to accomplish?
2. How will we know when that change is an improvement?
3. What changes can we predict will make an improvement?

4. How shall we pilot test the predicted improvements?
5. What do we expect to learn from the test run?
6. As the data come in, what have we learned?
7. If we get positive results, how do we hold onto the gains?
8. If we get negative results, what needs to be done next?
9. When we review the experience, what can we learn about doing a better job in the future?

In addition, a number of hospitals began to experiment with applications of CQI, some of which began to receive public notice in the late 1980s. Among those mentioned early in the literature and at professional meetings were Meriter Hospital, Madison, Wisconsin; University of Michigan Hospitals, Ann Arbor, Michigan; Alliant Health System, Louisville, Kentucky; Henry Ford Health System, Detroit, Michigan; and West Paces Ferry Hospital, Atlanta, Georgia.

## COMPARING INDUSTRIAL AND HEALTH CARE QUALITY

A comparison of quality from an industrial perspective versus quality from a health care perspective reveals that the two are surprisingly similar and that both have strengths and weaknesses (Donabedian 1993). The industrial model is limited in that it (1) ignores the complexities of the patient-practitioner relationship; (2) downplays the knowledge, skills, and motivation of the practitioner; (3) treats quality as free, ignoring quality-cost trade-offs; (4) gives more attention to supportive activities and less to clinical ones; and (5) provides less emphasis on influencing professional performance via "education, retraining, supervision, encouragement and censure" (Donabedian 1993, pp. 1–4). On the other hand, Donabedian suggested that the professional health care model can learn the following from the industrial model:

1. new appreciation of the fundamental soundness of health care quality traditions
2. the need for even greater attention to consumer requirements, values, and expectations
3. the need for greater attention to the design of systems and processes as a means of quality assurance

4. the need to extend the self-monitoring, self-governing tradition of physicians to others in the organization
5. the need for a greater role by management in assuring the quality of clinical care
6. the need to develop appropriate applications of statistical control methods to health care monitoring
7. the need for greater education and training in quality monitoring and assurance for all concerned. (1993, pp. 1–4)

In reality, there is a continuum of TQM/CQI activities, with manufacturing at one end of the continuum and professional services at the other (Hart 1993). The TQM approach should be modified in accordance with its position along this continuum. Manufacturing processes have linear flows, repetitive cycle steps, standardized inputs, high analyzability, and low worker discretion. Professional services, on the other hand, involve nonstandardized and variable inputs, nonrepetitive operations, unpredictable demand peaks, and high worker discretion. Many organizations, including health care organizations, have processes at different points along that continuum that should be analyzed accordingly. The hospital, for example, has laboratory and support operations that are like a factory and diagnostic and treatment activities that are professional services. The objective of factory-like operations is to drive out variability to conform to requirements and to produce near-zero defects. At the other end, the objectives of diagnosis and treatment are to do whatever it takes to produce customer health and satisfaction and maintain the loyalty of customers and employees.

## The 1990s and Into the 21st Century: A Breakout Period

This historical narrative has a conspicuous feature: relatively little reference to broadly-based activities within the medical professions. While many key figures, e.g., Donabedian, Berwick, Batalden, Leape, and James, have been physicians, the profession as a whole has not been easily galvanized to action (Millenson 2003). The most significant professional recommendations for action were provided in two Institute of Medicine reports (2000, 2001)—*To Err Is Human and Crossing the Quality*

*Chasm*—which have been widely publicized. These works have been the focal point for quality efforts by a host of actors, including professionals, institutions, consumers, employers, insurers, vendors, government programs and regulators, advocacy groups, accrediting bodies, and media organizations. In the first two editions of this book, the editors felt it necessary to justify their concern about quality. In this edition, we recognize a new need—to catalogue the sometimes bewildering array of actors and active interest groups currently undertaking quality initiatives. Figure 1–8 provides an overall schematic of the actors in the complex tug-of-war currently surrounding health care quality and involving consumers, employers, third-party payers, and the professionals and institutions actually providing the care. Figures 1–9 through 1–13 present the mechanisms and processes involved in supporting the interactions outlined in Figure 1–8.

As Figure 1–9 indicates, institutions must measure and report on consumer satisfaction surveys and monitor the demand for services. They must handle complaints effectively because their volume of services depends to a very large degree on their reputation and on the word-of-mouth (WOM) recommendations that their clients give. The consumers feed this information back to the institutions through surveys and complaints. At the same time, institutions must work hard to enhance their reputations and service volumes through advertising, outreach efforts, and satisfactory service levels.

Institutions must also attempt to influence the quality of professional services through the multiple methods outlined in Figure 1–10. Furthermore, the professionals must respond with their own requests for participation in governance and for state-of-the-art equipment and support systems.

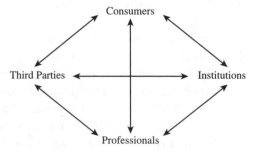

**Figure 1–8** Interactions Among Health Care Quality Actors

As presented in Figure 1–11, the third parties (employers, labor unions, insurers, and government agencies) also monitor many of the same satisfaction indicators that the institutions monitor. HMOs also become aware as people "vote with their feet" by not renewing memberships or requesting transfers from one provider to another. Third parties are increasingly attempting to influence consumer behavior, especially where chronic diseases are involved; they act indirectly through consumer advertising, the media, and personalized Web portals, and directly through case managers. Another method of influence is the report cards distributed by government agencies and employer associations to encourage consumers to seek out higher quality providers and hospitals. Another source of advertising

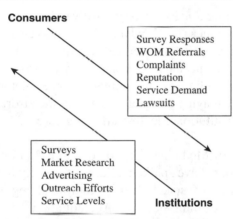

**Figure 1–9** Consumer–Institution Quality Interactions

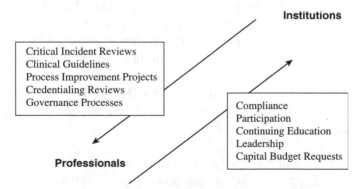

**Figure 1–10** Institution–Professional Quality Interactions

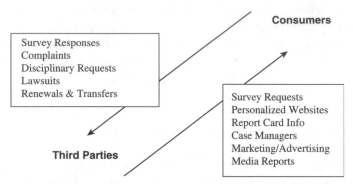

**Figure 1–11** Consumer–Third Party Quality Interactions

which can have either a negative or a positive effect on health care quality is direct-to-consumer (DTC) advertising from vendors of pharmaceuticals, medical devices, and medical equipment. Furthermore, third parties also work to influence one another's efforts through lobbying, advertising, pricing, alliances, and numerous other methods.

Third parties are playing an extensive role in the effort to improve both professional and institutional factors affecting care.

> The Institute of Medicine's reports on patient safety and quality improvement have sparked a flurry of activity in health policy by a range of stakeholders. Traditional regulators such as the Joint Commission on Accreditation of Healthcare Organizations (JCAHO) and Medicare Peer Review Organizations have developed new patient safety requirements. The federal Quality Interagency Coordination Task Force is attempting to synthesize a comprehensive federal approach to medical safety improvement. The nonprofit National Quality Forum is doing much the same, working with insurers, states, and the federal government. Finally, the Agency for Healthcare Research and Quality (AHRQ) is formulating expert evaluations of cost-effective safety practices (Mello *et al.* 2003, p. 46).

Figures 1–12 and 1–13 only just scratch the surface here. Employers through the Leapfrog Group are demanding specific changes in information systems, full-time hospital-based physicians (hospitalists) to provide

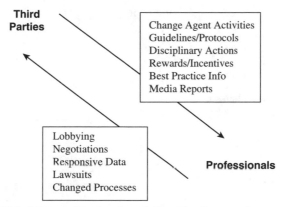

**Figure 1–12**  Third Party–Professional Quality Interactions

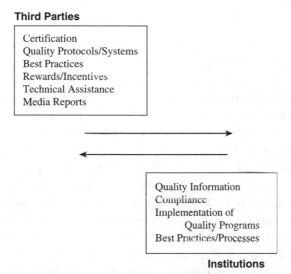

**Figure 1–13**  Third Party–Institution Quality Interactions

twenty-four hour—seven day coverage, and referral of high risk procedures to centers with high volumes and good results. The industrial model has been adapted to health care in the Baldrige National Quality Award standards for health care promulgated in 1998, leading to the first health award in 2002.

One of the big debates in the quality arena is whether or not to tie incentive payments to quality performance (known as pay for performance) and,

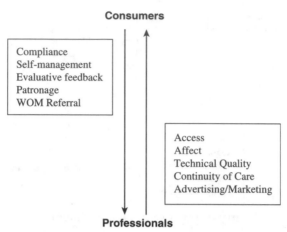

**Figure 1–14** Consumer–Professional Quality Interactions

if done, how best to structure the payments (Mehrotra *et al.* 2003; Leatherman *et al.* 2003; Fernandopulle *et al.* 2003; Eagle *et al.* 2003). There seems to be a consensus that paying for quality makes sense, but that health care quality measurement systems are not yet up to the task of making incentive systems effective or equitable.

We must not forget the primary relationship in health care—the provider–patient relationship. Here in Figure 1–14 we have returned to the four attributes of the Donabedian model as well as the influence of professionals' marketing efforts. (The Donabedian categories could have been incorporated into the consumer–patient relationship diagram as well.) At the same time, patients provide feedback as well as work for the professionals. Hopefully, they comply with the provider's advice, including prescription guidelines; they offer the history of their own attempts at disease self-management (Wagner *et al.* 2001), including their responses to their personal searches for information and to the deluge of health care advertising and marketing that pervades television and other media.

## PROBLEMS, CHALLENGES, AND QUALITY ISSUES IN HEALTH CARE

As is the case with any new approach to the management of organizations, difficulties and conflicts with prior concepts need to be anticipated.

Difficulties and conflicts are likely to center around a number of issues, including the definition of quality, who will define it, how much it will cost, and how it is to be achieved.

## Defining Quality

Although there are many definitions of quality, there are essentially three levels of quality commonly discussed today. These levels are cumulative, with the difficulty in achieving quality increasing at each level.

1. Conformance quality—conforming to specifications; having a product or service that meets predetermined standards.
2. Requirements quality—meeting total customer requirements; having perceived attributes of a service or product that meets or exceeds customer requirements.
3. Quality of kind—quality so extraordinary that it delights the customer; having perceived attributes of a product or service that significantly exceeds customer expectations, thereby delighting the customer with its value (Dumas *et al.* 1987).

CQI is not the same as quality assurance (QA), which focuses on conformance quality, although at times the concepts overlap. The confusion that surrounds the use of the terms CQI and QA stems in large part from the difference in quality as conceptualized in the work of early leaders in the health care quality movement and the somewhat simplistic popularization of TQM by health care groups and organizations. If one reviews carefully the initial quality writings in health care, such as those of Donabedian, there is surprisingly little difference between their conceptualization of quality and what TQM leaders in industry have written.

Patient safety is an important quality of care issue. However, it is only one aspect of quality and should not be confused with the overall quality effort. Safety issues occur in several categories—accidents while receiving care, medical errors, and iatrogenic disease (the side effects and adverse consequences inherent in accepted treatments). All are legitimate concerns of health care quality efforts.

Quality has been an issue in health care for many decades. Quality is inherent in the professional standards, guidelines, and codes of the myriad professions involved in health care, the many associations that represent these professionals, and the health care organizations themselves. A concern for quality is also evident in the many statutes enacted over the years at the local, state, and national levels to "protect" the quality of health care provided to the public. This results in several significant problems. First, conflict can develop between the standards of one group and the standards of another group. Second, there can be conflict between the professionals and the health care organization in which they are working. Third, all these standards can be viewed as "floors" or lowest acceptable limits for quality: as thresholds where quality becomes acceptable but where there is no recognition that some quality levels are better than others. Finally, these standards tend to be static and therefore counter to the "continuous improvement" philosophy of CQI.

## Who Defines It?

Akin to the potential differences among the standards set by professional groups is the tendency of health care professionals, particularly physicians, to think of themselves as operating individually, authoritatively, and situationally. In reality, professionals are contributing members of a group, each of whose members is empowered to correct the actions of others for the good of the customer. Similar difficulties will be encountered between management and those involved in any participative process.

## Will It Help with Malpractice Suits?

There are legal as well as organizational issues involved in CQI. It is not clear whether CQI efforts will be viewed positively or negatively in tort cases such as malpractice suits. Most states have laws that shield quality assurance studies done on behalf of the institution's board of trustees from discovery proceedings related to malpractice cases. Some laws are being amended to cover, under the same principles of law, CQI program data as well. The legal status of practice guidelines and their use is less clear. According to Holzer (1990),

> Although it is possible that such policies and guidelines could be admitted into evidence to show that a provider breached a legal duty or standard of care owed a patient, it is uncertain whether

these risk control standards could ultimately pass the evidentiary
rules of relevancy or materiality in a given law suit. (p. 78)

Borbas *et al.* (1990) cite a case heard in Minnesota that employed the
argument that solid data are more effective for defending physicians'
practices than are expert witnesses.

Although many observers express concern about the use of CQI data
in discovery proceedings associated with malpractice suits, Holzer
(1990, p. 78) suggests that it is more likely that "the consensus-based
process of creating clinical standards and guidelines specifically for
controlling professional liability losses is itself a powerful and emerging standard for health care risk management programs." This would be
especially important should the initial data suggest that the quality of
care is generally enhanced by the use of health care protocols per se.
Already some are concerned about how and when third-party efforts
like the Leapfrog standards and clinical guidelines might become relevant in tort law, displacing local "reasonable and customary" care standards (Mello *et al.* 2003).

## How Much Does It Cost and For Whom?

Another challenge is how to determine the economic impact of quality
improvement on health care organizations. Meaningful cost-benefit and
cost-effectiveness studies are often difficult to do. Yet, as previously indicated, there are costs associated with implementing quality improvement.
Boards, employer groups, and government entities will want to know
what the payoff is for CQI. The costs of quality have typically fallen into
four categories, two of which are somewhat easy to determine—the cost
of prevention (training, team activities, communication, etc.) and the
cost of appraisal (testing and inspection)—and two of which are difficult
to determine—the cost of internal failure (waste, rework, downtime, dis-
ruption, etc.) and the cost of external failure (patients go elsewhere, litigation, ill will, etc.).

With third parties involved in the quality decision, it is likely that there
will be winners and losers. Leatherman *et al.* (2003) show that what
serves public and patient interests does not always serve the economic
interests of the provider or the employer. How does a society or an individual make decisions in such situations?

**How Do We Achieve Quality?**

A number of other issues emerge when CQI is superimposed on a traditional organizational approach; some of these issues are beginning to be
investigated by researchers. For example, what can be done to improve
the acceptance of TQM/CQI by first line supervisors, the group that
seems to have the hardest time adjusting to the changes that CQI calls for?
Many of these "how to" issues will be addressed in subsequent sections
of this book.

# CHAPTER 2

# Does TQM/CQI Work in Health Care?

*Curtis P. McLaughlin and Kit N. Simpson*

Despite widespread use of total quality management/continuous quality improvement (TQM/CQI) methods, its effectiveness in health care remains a legitimate concern. Health care delivery systems are large, decentralized, and complex, yet at their core they involve a fundamental personal relationship between providers and patients. Moreover, if this were not a sufficient challenge, rapid and uncertain changes in the structure and processes of providing and paying for care make measuring the effect of any single management intervention over time very difficult, if not impossible. This chapter reviews the evidence to date concerning the effectiveness of TQM/CQI in health care at a system level. Although evidence continues to accumulate from both controlled trials (Solberg 1993; Goldberg *et al.* 1998; Mehta *et al.* 2000) and survey data (Shortell *et al.* 1998) on the implementation process and perceived impact, much of the evidence remains anecdotal (Arndt and Bigelow 1995; Bigelow and Arndt 1995). Leatherman *et al.* (2003), for example, argue that the "business case" for quality improvement is yet to be proven, even while evidence mounts for the overall societal and economic benefits.

A *business case* for a health care improvement intervention exists if the entity that invests in the intervention realizes a financial return on its investment in a reasonable time frame, using a reasonable rate of discounting. This may be realized as "bankable dollars" (profit), a reduction in losses for a given program or population, or avoided costs. In addition, a *business case* may exist if the investing entity believes that a positive indirect impact on organization function and sustainability will accrue within a reasonable time frame. (p. 18)

The economic case includes the returns to all the actors, not just the individual investing business unit. The social case, as they define it, is one of measuring benefits, but not requiring positive returns on the investment. Right now that is the overriding consideration as health care wrestles with the well documented effects of medical variation, medical errors, and use of outmoded clinical methods (McGlynn *et al.* 2003). As Leatherman *et al.* (2003) imply, the business case for quality improvement suffers from the same negative factors as the business case for other preventive health care measures; namely, all or part of the benefits accruing to other business units or patients, and delayed impacts that get discounted heavily in the reckoning. The regulatory arguments for quality improvement efforts have generally been justified on the basis of social and economic benefits such as lives saved and overall cost reductions, but are not necessarily profitable to the investor. These authors also present a whole array of public policy measures that would overcome the barriers to a positive business case and encourage wider and more assertive implementation of quality improvement methods. These barriers are discussed in Chapter 3.

## EARLY LESSONS FROM THE NATIONAL DEMONSTRATION PROJECT

The National Demonstration Project in Quality Improvement in Health Care, reported on by Berwick, Godfrey, and Roessner in *Curing Health Care* (1990), was the initial effort to launch quality improvement within health services. Although it did not give evidence on the costs and benefits of CQI, this eight-month demonstration project clearly showed that the quality improvement techniques that have succeeded in industry could be applied to the health care setting. The Project provided ten key lessons to guide subsequent efforts, namely:

1. Quality improvement tools can work in health care.
2. Cross-functional teams are valuable in improving health care processes.

3. Data useful for quality improvement abound in health care.
4. Quality improvement methods are fun to use.
5. Costs of poor quality are high, and savings are within reach.
6. Involving doctors is difficult.
7. Training needs arise early.
8. Nonclinical processes draw early attention.
9. Health care organizations may need a broader definition of quality.
10. In health care, as in industry, the fate of quality improvement is first of all in the hands of leaders. (Berwick *et al.* 1990, pp. 145–157)

In the book's afterword, Garvin (1990) suggests that a number of unanswered questions continue to pose problems. These problems include the indirect relationship between inputs and outputs (especially outcomes) in health care, the lack of clear quality standards, and the professionally separate organizational structures of the health care institutions. He also suggests some differences between the quality assurance model and the industrial quality model: (1) variation may be viewed differently; (2) prevention is better than successful inspection; (3) the system, not the individual, is the unit of analysis; (4) the focus is on the customer; and (5) the definition of quality extends beyond the technical dimensions.

## EARLY EMPIRICAL EVIDENCE

The health care literature indicates a number of specific benefits associated with quality improvement and related measures such as customer satisfaction. These benefits include profitability, employee satisfaction, reduced costs, improved patient survival, and better continuity of care. Some of the early evidence relating to each of these criteria is presented below.

### Profitability

There appears to be a clear relationship between profitability and customer satisfaction in hospitals. Harkey and Vraciu (1992), for example, reported on this relationship among the 82 HealthTrust hospitals. They suggest a quality-profitability model that is shown in Figure 2–1. This model shows profitability affected by increased market share and better prices on the market gains side and reduced costs due to productivity improvements and re-duced lengths of stay. They reviewed the literature, which had reached varied conclusions on cost-quality relationships. Then they compared the gross mar-gins of the HealthTrust hospitals with the results that were achieved on the company's standardized customer quality surveys in prior years. These sur-veys were sent to active medical staff, discharged patients, employees, and community members. Each hospital surveyed all of its active medical staff an-nually by mail, with a 60% to 65% response rate; 350 discharged patients every six months by mail, with a 60% to 65% response rate; most employees annually, with an 86% response rate; and up to 300 randomly selected resi-dents in the hospital's market area annually by telephone survey. Financial performance was defined as the net operating income of the hospital, exclud-ing interest, depreciation, ESOP expenses, and corporate management fees. The researchers took the results of all these surveys and looked at the rela-tionship between questionnaire values and financial performance.

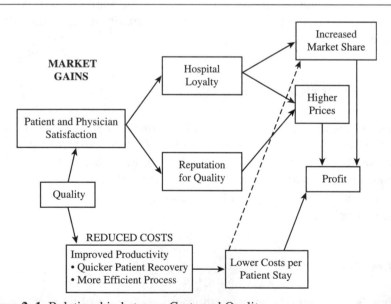

**Figure 2–1** Relationship between Costs and Quality
J. Harkey and R. Vraciu, "Quality of Health Care and Financial Performance: Is There a Link?" *Health Care Management Review*, Vol 17, No. 4, p. 56. Reprinted by permission of Lippincott Williams & Wilkins.

Factor analysis was used to determine whether a quality factor could be developed from the many quality questions. Two quality factors were developed from ten questions. The first seven questions, based on employee, patient, and physician responses, made a very strong factor, accounting for 39.4% of the variance. The second quality factor was made up of three community responses about the hospital's image and explained 11.1% of the variance. The questions used for these two factors are shown in Table 2–1. Other factors developed to control for other attributes of the hospitals were wealth of the community and bed size. Given a reliable factor for quality based on the first seven questions above, the researchers then used regression analysis to estimate the relationship between a quality factor score and net operating margin. The reported regression model uses this quality factor and two other variables, Percent Medicare and Percent Managed Care, to explain 29% of the variance in net operating income. The quality factor was positively associated with net operating income and significant at the 0.02 significance level in this model. The other two dependent variables were negatively associated and significant at the 0.01 significance level. The authors concluded that the perceptions of quality held by employees, patients, and physicians were in strong agreement and that the perception of quality, when controlled for payer mix and managed care, added to profitability.

Nelson *et al.* (1992) have also reported that patients, employees, and physicians have correlated quality perceptions. They determined that quality ratings by 15,095 patients at 51 Hospital Corporation of America (HCA) hospitals explained 10% to 29% of the variation in net operating revenue and return on assets. At that point in time both HCA and HealthTrust used similar questionnaires to measure customer satisfaction.

The finding of a link between perceived quality and profitability is in justifying CQI. Other research can find other intermediate relationships, but it is this meta-relationship that will be of great interest to boards of trustees and to senior management.

## Employee Satisfaction

Rush-Presbyterian-St. Luke's Medical Center in Chicago surveyed 5,174 employees (out of a possible 7,400) in 1990, two years into an extensive TQM program; about half of those surveyed also participated in the program. After adjusting for demographic differences in the participating and nonparticipating groups, the hospital found a statistically significant improvement in intrinsic job satisfaction, in the general opinion

**Table 2–1**  Questions and Responses

| Respondent | Question | Response Used | Mean Value (%) |
|---|---|---|---|
| Employee | "Are you proud of the overall quality of care provided by your hospital?" | Yes (of 5) | 34.9 |
| Employee | "Is good service to physicians a high priority for this hospital?" | Yes (of 5) | 59.4 |
| Employee | "Do you feel the community views the quality of medicine provided by your medical staff as being generally high?" | Yes (of 5) | 24.9 |
| Physician | "My patients typically give positive reports about their experiences at this hospital." | Strongly or somewhat agree (of 5) | 78.8 |
| Physician | "The nursing care delivered to my patients is typically good (competent and caring)." | Strongly or somewhat agree (of 5) | 79.0 |
| Patient | "How well did our nursing staff do their job (skill, competence, helpfulness, and friendliness)?" | Excellent or very good (of 5) | 74.6 |
| Patient | "How would you rate the hospital's overall care?" | Excellent or very good (of 5) | 74.2 |
| Community | "HealthTrust has the best physicians." (Yes or No or Don't Know) | Yes | 14.1 |
| Community | "HealthTrust has the best care." (Yes or No or Don't Know) | Yes | 18.6 |
| Community | "HealthTrust has the most modern technology (Yes or No or Don't Know) | Yes | 12.5 |

of the hospital as a place to be a patient and to work, and in a number of positive attitudes toward TQM. Because of the large sample, however, statistical significance was relatively easy to achieve. Particularly large changes in scale values (1-5) were achieved in the areas of higher organizational standards, worker and management involvement, and especially TQM awareness (the objective of the program) (Counte *et al.* 1992).

## Cost Effects

The University of Michigan Medical Center in Ann Arbor, Michigan, monitored its savings and costs from 19 teams between July 1987 and June 1991. Seventeen of the 19 teams showed a positive net cost saving. The implementation costs were estimated at $2.5 million, of which $1.3 million represented programmatic costs. The combined two-year savings and additional revenues attributed to these teams were $17.7 million. Teams focusing on the turnaround of the center's operating rooms led to added revenues of about $13 million. These were direct costs and did not include the time of the team members while in training or carrying out the team efforts. The value of the time spent in training was valued at $1.5 million. Including the training costs, the return was 4.5 times the investment. One might still ask about the cost of employee time in team activities, but the reported return would be highly favorable, even if that cost were included (Gaucher and Coffey 1993).

Other efforts have also recorded cost savings. Baptist Medical Center in Columbia, South Carolina, found that the suppliers of contrast media solution for radiology were packaging the solution in volumes greater than each patient needed to drink. The team asked the vendor to repackage the material in smaller volumes, reducing costs from wasted product by about $200,000 per year. Yet the bigger part of the saving may be in hundreds of day-to-day small changes. The West Florida Regional Medical Center case in this book shows a reduction in inpatient antibiotic costs of more than $200,000 per year. Additionally, Bluth *et al.* (1982) report that one team reduced outpatient "Stat" lab delays by 76%, reduced patient waiting time 62%, and achieved a one-time saving of $225,000 as well as annual recurring savings of $40,000.

Improvements may not come quickly in the beginning, but may occur in spurts as the approach is internalized and then reoriented. Consultant Thomas H. Breedlove, Senior Vice President of Crosby Associates, argues against a time estimate for full implementation of TQM because he sees it as an always evolving process. However, he does argue that with full consultant experience, the hospital should be getting a three-to-one payback within six months (Burrus 1993a). Northwest Hospital in Seattle, Washington, found this out when its director decided that CQI was a philosophy and not just a procedure. The director began to develop some 40-45 teams around product lines, representing what he calls "The Molecular Structure," and emphasizing statistical process control. In the first few months of the change, the hospital saved about $3 million and the average length of stay dropped by one day. A number of middle management positions were eliminated, as well as a contract management company, at a savings of $750,000 annually (Burrus 1993b).

While the overall evaluations of TQM/CQI programs have had severe limitations, they are more available and better documented than alternative quality improvement approaches (Ovretriet and Gustafson 2002). Their review of the available studies lead to the following findings:

1. Investigators have not effectively or consistently measured the level of implementation in the intervention in terms of depth, breadth, maturity, or length of time.
2. Observations have seldom been validated or corroborated adequately.
3. Data emphasize short-term effects rather than longer term impacts and clinical outcomes.
4. There has been little longitudinal data on CQI programs in health.
5. Cost information is lacking; available information focuses on specific change effects rather than overall programmatic costs and benefits.
6. Studies of interventions fail to test alternatives for implementation or to explain factors behind program effectiveness.
7. There is limited comparability among studies due to lack of standard program definitions and variability in variable specifications and capture methods.
8. Studies have not been aimed at measuring effectiveness nor at developing predictive theories or models for effectiveness.

They go on to observe that no one is going to do a triple blind randomized controlled trial of CQI interventions, but that quasi-experimental and other social science methods represent possible improvements in these evaluations.

## Other Specific Effects

Reduced costs are not the only outcome of CQI efforts. At the University of Utah, for example, the development of a protocol to control life support equipment by using computer systems has increased the survival rate of patients with acute (adult) respiratory distress syndrome (ARDS) from 12% to 42%. A double-blind study was conducted to compare survival rates obtained by two types of equipment. To the researchers' surprise, improvement occurred with both sets of equipment, indicating that it resulted from the rationalized system rather than equipment choices (Morris 1992).

Other effects include increased capacity utilization and improved continuity of care. For example, the Joint Commission on Accreditation of Healthcare Organizations' book, *Striving Toward Improvement* (1992), described the CQI efforts of six hospitals. These hospitals reported improved operating room utilization, a 78% reduction in food waste on a pediatric service, increased utilization of transportation orderlies, and reduced admission and discharge waiting times. The cases in this book and its earlier editions showed increased utilization of capacity, lower supply costs, increased physician continuity, reduced laboratory costs, reduced hospitalization for low back pain, more satisfaction among obstetric patients, and reduced inpatient antibiotic costs. Kibbe *et al.* (1993) showed how CQI techniques were able to improve continuity of care in an academic medical practice.

## Costs of Quality

Crosby (1979) talks about the "cost of quality," meaning the cost of poor quality. Knowledgeable administrators do not hesitate to say that the cost of nonconformance and waste in health care is in the same range—20% to 40% of total costs—that has been seen in American industry. As much as 25% of the cost of care goes into billing, collections, and handling of claims, and the Florida Health Care Cost Containment Commission has warned the public that some 90% of hospital bills contain errors. There are also the costs of clinical errors and of waste as individual employees and groups of employees act to protect themselves from unpleasant situations due to variation in the system. One can legitimately include in that set of unnecessary costs related to both malpractice insurance and defensive medicine. With the costs of health care estimated at about 14% of GNP, the size of these unnecessary costs is staggering.

Why, then, do people so often question the investment costs of a CQI program? First, the data cited above indicate potential savings, thus raising the issue of the probabilities of achieving them and continuing to achieve them over the appropriate time periods. Consultants report that the likelihood that hospital CEOs will maintain a CQI effort is probably about 50-50. Moreover, there appears to be a moment of truth about 18 months into the process when the CEO suddenly realizes that the process does not involve simply changing the corporate culture, but also involves a fundamental change in the way managers, including the CEO, make decisions. Some CEOs never reach that level of understanding; some do and still cannot make the transition.

Another factor limiting the payoff is the fact that only a limited number of quality improvement teams or task forces can be underway at a time, even if everyone has been trained in the basics of CQI. Because only a smaller subset may be actually practicing CQI at one time, the effective increased capacity for change emphasized above is limited. Probably five to twelve teams, depending on the size of the institution, may be active at a given time. The limit on the number of teams is related to the capacity of the facilitators to fully train and support the teams as well as the number of processes that can be in flux at one time without leading to confusion. Thus, although the investment in developing the program and doing the awareness training for large numbers of staff occurs early, the returns come later, mostly in the third year and beyond.

Although the savings on the cost side are relatively easy to quantify, the effects of increased competitiveness are harder to document. An increased occupancy rate quickly improves the bottom line, but one usually cannot tell why a patient chose one hospital over another, and one rarely hears about the patient who didn't come because a neighbor said that the hospital was unfriendly or poorly run. That is why the relationship between customer satisfaction and financial performance is important. The competitive effect cannot be justified based on specific events as can the waste avoidance and cost savings effects. Furthermore, any analysis of competition effects can be confounded by the offsetting marketing efforts of competitors. Hospital A may enhance its image in the community by way of continuous improvement, but the effort may be countered by a heavy advertising campaign by Hospital B or special equipment purchases to attract physicians at

Hospital C. Right now we are virtually in the dark about the relative effectiveness of these three strategies or combinations thereof, so it is nearly impossible to compare the impact of a dollar spent on CQI against the impact of a dollar spent on other market-oriented activities.

There is little longitudinal information about how effective such an effort will be after five or ten years. Prior approaches such as quality circles often started with good results, but these results declined over time as motivation waned. Certainly, it is possible in the early years to "pick the low-hanging fruit," to clear up the obvious quality problems, and to show some immediate improvements. However, that is not likely to be the overall rate of return over several years of activity. One may experience diminishing returns, or one may find a learning effect in which teams and management with experience develop sufficient confidence to tackle some major areas with high potential for payoffs, such as admissions and discharge. We predict that the program will produce savings immediately, then have a decline in savings or contribution to earnings, and then, as clinicians become more involved and management more assertive in looking for high-potential areas, begin to experience some increasing returns. The Quality-Profitability Model in Figure 2–2 shows how these costs and benefits might interact.

Quality efforts can affect a health care process directly and lead to outcome improvements and reduced costs. They should also lead to improved physician and patient satisfaction with the institution, leading to more admissions, more patients, more patient days, and an increased share of the market. Improved quality might also lessen the pressure for reduced prices to compete against other institutions. All of these together could contribute to the observed profitability by both lowering units costs and increasing volume and revenues.

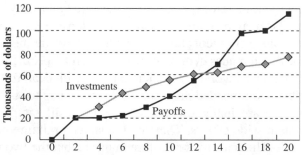

**Figure 2–2** Comparison of Investment and Payoffs of CQI over Time

The costs of a CQI program are not trivial. The organization may pay $20,000 to $200,000 for program development, training materials, trainers, and workshops for senior managers, board members, and key clinicians. Then there is the cost of the facilitators and the time lost by employees attending training sessions and engaging in team tasks. In addition to these costs, there are opportunity costs for the resources that went into the program that might have been used for something else. These efforts are not cheap and are not to be undertaken lightly. Much of the opposition to the Joint Commission requirement for a continuous improvement process has been couched in terms of the costs involved and how they might exceed the returns.

Successful reports of individual interventions have continued. However, retrospective studies with a focus on multiple organizations have been less conclusive. Either they have found little in the way of long-term measurable effects or they have encountered serious measurement difficulties (Bigelow and Arndt 1995; Shortell *et al.* 1998; Blumenthal and Kilo 1998; Ovretreit and Gustafson 2002). However, these studies have strengthened our knowledge base about effective program implementation.

## CQI and Changing Clinical Processes

As CQI has moved from administrative to clinical process change, questions have been raised about its effectiveness in working with medical staff. Goldberg *et al.* (1998) report on a clinical trail of academic detailing (AD) and CQI in improving chronic disease guideline compliance and clinical outcomes. CQI was not a stand-alone alternative in this study, but an add-on to academic detailing. Their rationale was, "We chose this design because we believed most organizations would find it feasible to implement AD. It was important, therefore, to examine the value added by what was hypothesized to be a more complex and labor-intensive CQI program." (p. 133) Their results were inconclusive, for which they cite the confounding factors of local differences in organizational cultures, specific personnel, and disease conditions involved. A later chapter will deal further with changing physician-commanded processes and the barriers to such change.

Here again there are many success stories in the literature, but few which show system-wide effects. They tend to show a mixture of various types of outcomes. The reasons for this are multiple, but the two most important are (1) nomenclature and (2) confounding variables.

*Nomenclature*

Where does CQI leave off and clinical pathways, care management, disease management, actions teams, and reengineering begin? All of these can and have been implemented in a manner consistent with the way that we have defined CQI, while others have gone at them with a command-and-control orientation. There are many, many change programs adopted by consultants and health care organizations that may or may not fit the CQI mold. However, the reporting in the literature usually focuses on one term and sticks with it. With this proliferation of efforts, it is increasingly hard to assess the system-wide effects of any one intervention.

*Confounding Variables*

The health care system does not stand still for the implementation of CQI. At one major health center with a long-standing commitment to CQI, the organization also decided to downsize and knock out one whole layer of middle management. Unfortunately, this layoff included many of those responsible for implementing CQI teams. Was it the layoff or the CQI approach that was at fault for the temporary faltering of the CQI effort? Who can tell? One can go to extremes and claim all of the benefits of clinical pathways for CQI or claim none, whereas the truth lies somewhere in between. Westert and Lagoe (1995) reported on the relatively straightforward variable of length-of-stay for total hip replacement in Syracuse, Onondaga County, NY and Enschede, in the Twente region of The Netherlands. In both cases, quality interventions reduced the length-of-stay, but there was also evidence of a secular downward trend prior to the intervention under the pressure of the reimbursement system in both countries. Coddington *et al.* (1996) looked at a number of large integrated systems and concluded that there were specific team efforts that led to savings in the millions and that it worked to link clinical pathway implementation to multidisciplinary teams and CQI-based processes, but also observed a number of issues to be dealt with, namely:

- Legal reservations have to be overcome
- Supporting information systems must be in place
- Lack of financial incentives to improve clinical performance can slow down the processes

- Clinical guidelines are hard to implement unless physicians are organized
- CQI teams may become too encumbered with processes to achieve results
- Some has to be ready and able to blast through turf battles
- Processes will lose momentum unless the CEO pushes continuously, and is a strong proponent of CQI. (p. 84)

Similarly, Weingart (1998) reports that efforts at Beth Israel Deaconess in Boston to involve house officers in CQI were fruitful, but required strong faculty leadership to achieve results because of resident rotations, long hours, urgent demands, and lack of training in CQI methods. The measurement of system outcomes, therefore, has been difficult and not as enlightening as hoped. However, the economics of quality are rapidly changing. The penalties associated with poor quality, especially those associated with patient safety, have raised the issue to the level of organizational survival rather than return on investment. A single, major adverse event can threaten a hospital's payments for service under government programs, often over half the hospital's revenues.

## ADVANTAGES OF CQI APPLICATION IN HEALTH CARE

Health care personnel are likely to focus on the differences between their service sector and other parts of the economy and society. Although these differences are substantial (Shortell and Kaluzny 2006) and the current focus on medical errors has clearly drawn attention to the importance of improving quality (IOM 2001), it is incumbent on advocates of CQI to explain why and how quality improvement works in health care. Intelligent and articulate professionals need answers to the question, "What is behind the assumption of 'value added' from a health care organization participating in CQI?"

A number of factors contribute to the sustained interest and enthusiasm for CQI for health care, despite the limited empirical evidence regarding impact and cost. The first argument for CQI is its direct impact on quality, usually a net gain to the customer and to the organization. The second is that systems can often be designed or redesigned to give lower costs at the same time and with the same techniques used for quality improvement. The third argument relates to the set of benefits associated with a plan that empowers employees in health care through participation in decision making.

Although some benefits of participatory programs are well understood, the managerial benefits in health care generally come from five sources, several of which are particularly relevant to CQI, including

1. increasing the intrinsic motivation of the workforce;
2. capturing the intellectual capital already developed by the workforce;
3. reducing the managerial overhead necessary to induce managerial change;
4. vastly increasing the capacity of the professionally dominated organization to do process analysis; and
5. creating lateral linkages across highly specialized organizational units to increase effectiveness and reduce the process irresponsibility inherent in most health care settings.

These five benefits are discussed below, with particular emphasis on the provision of health services.

## Intrinsic Motivation

The vast majority of health care workers support the concept of quality care and would like to see improvements and participate in a meaningful quality improvement process. Allowing personnel to work on their own processes, permitting them to "do the right thing," and then rewarding them for that behavior is almost sure to increase intrinsic motivation in employees, if done properly. It is a classic case of job enrichment for health care workers.

## Capturing the Intellectual Capital of the Workforce

Industrial managers are increasingly recognizing that front line workers know their work processes better than the management does. Therefore, management encourages workers to apply that knowledge and insight to the firm's processes. This is especially true in health care, where the professionals employed by or practicing in the institution control the technological core of the organization. Management that does not capitalize on this available pool of professional and specialized knowledge within the organization is naive at best.

### Reducing Managerial Overhead

Some companies have been able to remove layers of management as work groups have taken responsibility over their own processes. The redesign work done by the workforce can also lead to less investment in industrial engineers, quality control specialists, and other overhead staff services. Health care organizations are actually already limited in the number of staff positions, mostly because the professionals rather than the corporate staff have clinical process knowledge. Indeed, one might view the new investments in CQI as a catching-up process for the lack of process-oriented staff that are involved in process enhancement in most other industries. This is but another example of how the incentives in health care are misaligned. Since physicians are not employees in most community hospitals, they are not at risk when processes are suboptimal, unless the situation is so bad that it prompts a lawsuit.

### Increasing Capacity

In health care, the management of the institution often lacks in-depth knowledge of the technological core (medicine, nursing, laboratory chemistry, etc.) of most activities. Therefore management representatives, such as industrial engineers, if they are on the staff, are usually restricted to areas where they have full knowledge and legitimacy, namely administrative activities. By imparting many of those skills to professional staff in their respective departments, units, and centers, CQI can vastly increase the effective capacity of the organization to examine its processes and introduce change. This expansion comes both in personnel hours available and in the areas of operation. For example, a management engineer can participate in and facilitate the process, but would not normally presume to study these processes in the normal hospital setting. Figure 2–3 shows this capacity effect in parallel with the quality program effect. This figure shows how quality efforts and process improvement efforts are mutually reinforcing and how the added capacity induced by involving professionals in

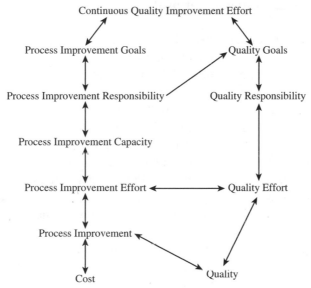

**Figure 2–3** Multiple Effects of CQI in Health Care

process improvement also contributes to the support of the quality effort and ultimately can improve both cost and quality in parallel.

## Lateral Linkages

Health care organizations are characterized by their many medical specialties, each organized into its own professional fiefdom. Galbraith (1973), for example, suggests that specialization is but one response to an information overload in the organization. By specializing, each unit can tend to learn more and more about less and less. One way to offset the effects of this specialization is to provide lateral linkages—coordinators, integrating mechanisms—to get the information moving across the organization as well as up and down the chain of command (Galbraith 1973; Lawrence and Lorsch 1967). So far, that has proved very difficult in health care institutions. CQI, however, through its use of interdisciplinary task forces and its focus on a broader definition of process and system as it affects customers rather than professional groups, presents one way to establish linkages. The technology of CQI focuses as much on coordination of the change process as on its motivation.

**Quality and Organizational Survival**

Once health care organizations have successfully addressed the gross inefficiencies and cost containment, the competitive challenge will shift from one of price to one of value, the combination of cost and quality. In that context we can expect both the visibility and cost of quality problems to rise. More and more report cards will be issued for and by stakeholder organizations. These will be more readily available because of the Internet and they will be used more frequently by the public and their proxies to make decisions and choices about sources of care. Oshel *et al.* (1997) reported over 6,000 users of the National Practitioner data bank disclosure information who, when surveyed, reported very high rates of use of the adverse action reports. A majority of the users reported that this information affected the decisions made. More and more organizations are requiring and publicizing patient satisfaction measures and various oversight and accrediting bodies are insisting on the use of benchmarking systems, including outcome measures.

Increasingly, the surviving health care organizations will be asked to justify their existence on the basis of providing good care at reasonable cost. They will be asked to submit information according to standardized data sets. Current examples include the ORYX systems required by JCAHO and the HEDIS measures developed by NCQA; alternatively, an organization's claims data may be reviewed using a standard set of criteria such as the 22 measures used by the CMS Medicare Quality Improvement Organization. These may involve a combination of organization specific criteria and required outcome measures. For JCAHO's ORYX analysis, the organization is required to meet its own criteria and to report its performance on the required outcome measures. It is likely that over time the self-selected criteria will be replaced by more and more standardized reporting requirements. These requirements have expanded over time and institutions have begun to complain about their complexity and cost to collect and implement.

**More Open Marketplace**

As consumers receive more information about outcome quality, they are increasingly likely to migrate to those centers that show the best results. Even if continuous quality improvement were rigorously applied everywhere, Gawande (2004) notes that there would likely continue to be a bell-shaped curve of outcome performances. One's location on this performance curve is increasingly likely to influence the amount of business and income available to any given institution.

## THE BIG BANG—THE QUALITY CHASM

Quality under the rubric of patient safety suddenly came to dominate the scene following the two significant Institute of Medicine reports *To Err Is Human* (2000) and *Crossing the Quality Chasm* (2001). Virtually all those concerns about cost and benefits and professional autonomy seemed swamped by the documentation of unacceptably high rates of medical error. The recognition that this needless human suffering, loss of life, and wasted resources were related to unnecessary variability in treatment and the lack of implementation of known best practices galvanized professional groups, regulators, and payers into action. Suddenly, quality improvement was acknowledged to be a professional responsibility, a quality-of-care issue rather than a managerial tactic. Current investment and involvement levels are high as evidence has mounted that the variability in clinical processes and the lack of conformance to evidence-based best practices has cost the public dearly. Many of the actors identified in Chapter 1 are demanding accountability for patient safety and for achieving acceptable levels of clinical performance and outcomes achievement. Adverse events are now undergoing extreme scrutiny and a broad range of quality indicators are being reported, followed and compared by payers and regulators. For a while anyway, financial questions have seemed to dissipate as the social costs have taken precedence. Local and regional variability in health care has long been known to exist, but the translation of that variability into missed opportunities for improved outcomes has been slow in coming. With that veil of secrecy about medical errors lifted, the demands for action and professional responsiveness have become extensive. This sea change goes well beyond concerns about malpractice insurance, to issues of clinical governance, professional training, certification, and continuity of care.

This Big Bang has extended beyond the United States. For example, England's National Health Service has launched a mandated quality improvement effort linked to minimum standards of care (quality assurance) called "clinical governance," including the politically powerful general practitioner groups. An early study of this effort showed needed change in terms of a "corporate" approach to quality improvement and sharing of information about performance metrics, complaints, clinical audits, best practices, and benchmarks. This mandated requirement in England's single payer environment, runs the risk of confusing whether it is a quality assurance effort or a continuous improvement process (Campbell *et al.* 2002). Berwick (2004) suggests that CQI can work in developing countries based on experiences in Peru and Russia, provided the promoters "keep targets and measurement processes simple" and "make full use of teams."

## CONVERGENCE

Measurements systems are the key to quality improvement and there is a convergence of the requirements of a number of significant health care regulatory organizations. Led by the American Hospital Association, the Federation of American Hospitals, and the Association of American Medical Colleges, it has become possible to use one set of JCAHO core reporting requirements under ORYX and use the same data to meet the reporting requirements of the Centers for Medicare and Medicaid Services (CMS) and be consistent with the requirements of the National Quality Forum as well. Given the size of the investments required by the new-found concerns about medical errors and accountability for them, it is not surprising that the reporting requirements have become onerous and that those who must do the reporting have pushed for convergence to save resources and achieve comparability. Evaluators also have felt the need for comparability in measures to support meaningful cross-institutional comparisons.

## THIRD PARTY MEASUREMENT SYSTEMS

The Joint Commission (JCAHO) requires that health care organizations it accredits select a number of measures for evaluating their performance. Because some institutions felt that the JCAHO had been heavy-handed in requiring the use of CQI in order to maintain accreditation, in January 1997 JCAHO's Board of Commissioners approved a plan and timetable for integrating outcome measures into the accreditation process for hospitals and long term care organizations.

By mid-2002, JCAHO announced the four core measurement areas that hospitals were required to report on by January 2004: acute myocardial infarctions, heart failure, community-acquired pneumonias, and pregnancy and related conditions. By mid-2004, about 200 contractor organizations were accredited with JCAHO to support hospitals with systems to collect and report these and other non-core performance measurements. JCAHO on-site surveyors are expected to evaluate the organization's use of its performance measure data for quality improvement.

Next on the JCAHO agenda for hospitals are measure sets for surgical infection preventions, ICU care, pain management, and children's asthma care. JCAHO is also working to develop Outcome and Assessment Information Set (OASIS)-derived measure sets for home health agencies, and Minimum Data Set (MDS)-derived measure sets for long-term care facilities. CMS and JCAHO have aligned their requirements to a single set of data reporting requirements concerning acute myocardial infarction, heart failure, and pneumonia.

## Health Plan Employer Data and Information Set-HEDIS

The National Committee for Quality Assurance (NCQA) has been involved in the development of a standardized set of measures called the Health Plan Employer Data and Information Set (HEDIS) for use by the group purchasers of health care coverage. NCQA is a nonprofit organization founded by the managed care industry to develop such an information set in close cooperation with HCFA for Medicare and Medicaid beneficiaries and with the Managed Health Care Association (MHCA), an organization of over 80 FORTUNE 500 companies. The HEDIS system is under continuous refinement. The 2005 HEDIS Summary of Measures and Product Line *(www.ncqa.org)* listed 27 available effectiveness of care measures, 8 access-availability measures, and 27 other measures associated with consumer satisfaction, service utilization, health plan stability, board certification of providers, and other plan characteristics. Each payer can specify a set of measures corresponding to their employees' needs and their plan coverages. For example, in April 2003 the Federal

Employees Health Benefits Program had available on the Internet www.opm.gov/insur/health the following performance measures for some 129 provider plans:

Antidepressant Medication Management
Beta Blocker Treatment
Breast Cancer Screening
Cervical Cancer Screening
Cholesterol Management after Acute Cardiovascular Events
Childhood Immunization Status
Comprehensive Diabetes Care
Follow-Up after Hospitalization for Mental Illness
Prenatal and Postpartum Care

NCQA also sells a data set called *Quality Compass* that employers can use to compare plans. It has an agreement with HCIA, Inc. to market this information product.

> *Quality Compass* not only saves us an inordinate amount of time collecting data, it provides vital information our employees can use to make better plan selection decisions. Having comparable data allows us to make apples-to-apples comparison between health plans, identify strengths and weaknesses and establish realistic performance expectations. (Jon Marie Hautz, Director, Managed Care Plans, Federated Department Stores quoted on NCQA website).

**The Quality Initiative—HQI**

The Quality Initiative was launched nationally by HHS to provide published consumer information coupled with quality improvement support through the Medicare Quality Improvement Organizations (QIOs). It has initiated a Nursing Home Quality Initiative (NHQI), a Home Health Quality Initiative (HHQI) and the Hospital Quality Initiative (HQI) as well as the Doctor's Office Quality (DOQ) project. JCAHO has worked jointly with CMS and the QIOs to develop a public reporting system that meets HHS goals of a set of robust, prioritized and standard quality measures to be used by all private and public purchasers, oversight and accrediting bodies, and payers and providers of hospital care. CMS has also worked with the National Quality Forum (NQF) to develop a consensus-derived set of hospital quality measures appropriate for public reports and with the Agency for Healthcare Research and Quality (AHRQ) to develop the standardized hospital consumer survey instruments (Hospital CAHPS). Related efforts include the Hospital Quality Alliance effort by several hospital and academic medical center associations to develop a voluntary set of reporting standards and the National Quality Measures Clearinghouse, sponsored by AHRQ, a publicly available data base of over 500 evidence-based quality measures and measure sets.

## Contingent Medicare Payments to Hospitals

The Medicare Prescription Drug, Improvement and Modernization Act of 2003 included indexed payments to hospitals based on the cost of a market basket of regularly purchased items in the year 2005 and beyond. However, 4% of the increases was made contingent in the legislation upon the hospitals providing CMS with performance data on 10 quality measures.

## Baldrige National Quality Award for Health Care Organizations

An interesting development has been the emergence of a health care version of the Malcolm Baldrige National Quality Award for health care organizations (Hertz *et al.* 1994). A pilot evaluation was conducted in 1995 with 46 health care organizations as well as with a group of 19 educational institutions. At that time the health care organizations did not score as well on the criteria as the educational institutions nor a comparison group of applying industrial firms (Mayer and Collier 1998).

Because the Baldrige awards are a private–public partnership, it required several years after the pilot to raise the private and public monies to implement the award process. The 1998 criteria for the award process which were available for self-assessments prior to the startup of the award process. A number of years passed before any health care organizations proved ready to receive the award. One organization received the award in 2002 and two received it in 2003. The criteria for the 2003 award competition are included as an appendix to this book. These criteria are very similar to those of the current private sector manufacturing and service company awards except that Organizational Performance Results replaces the Business Results category and Focus on Patients Other Customers, Markets replaces the Customer and Market Focus category. They are included here so that the reader can evaluate whether or not they are the most appropriate criteria for judging a quality system in health care organizations. It is clear that further refinement will be necessary, and the reader is urged to consult with the National Institute of Standards and Technology for updates of the criteria.

Only a few health care organizations could win the award in a single year, making it a government-sponsored claim to being the best in the country. The Baldrige Award criteria are also used for health and education awards in many states and the activation of the national award will certainly push that number higher.

## CONCLUSION

This chapter has summarized some of the theoretical arguments for and empirical evidence about CQI in the health care environment. There is no certainty that a continuous improvement program at a given institution will enhance quality for the patient and the providers and reduce costs for all concerned. However, it is clear that such a program is essential to survival in the current regulatory and competitive market. Later chapters will also identify the need to have such programs and measures in place to respond to the demands of the increasingly hostile health care market.

If CQI is managed properly, it can and will provide such benefits. The challenge is to design, implement, and lead a CQI effort that is successful for a given institution. Each business unit is likely to follow the specific methods of quality improvement that fit its existing culture and comfort levels (Kiassi *et al.* 2004), but that may or may not be the best way to go about implementing efforts. The basics of the successful CQI activity and its implementation are the topic of the remaining sections of this book.

# PART II

# Basics

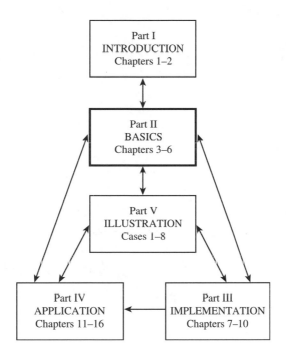

# CHAPTER 3

# The Outcome Model of Quality

*Susan I. DesHarnais and Curtis P. McLaughlin*

A critical question facing most health care continuous quality improvement (CQI) efforts is "Who should evaluate clinical performance, and how?" Controversy often arises over issues of quantity of work performance and its quality. Issues of quantity are relatively easy to address objectively. Issues of quality, however, are much more difficult, both politically and in terms of measurement.

The objectives of this chapter are

- To present a conceptual framework for measuring the quality of health care, and to provide a definition of quality of care that focuses on outcomes of care;
- To present a brief historical overview of outcomes measurement in the US;
- To look at data requirements and risk-adjustment techniques for comparing health outcomes across providers and/or over time;
- To provide an understanding of several possible professional-institutional responses for addressing outcomes measurement issues in health care; and
- To present conclusions.

## A CONCEPTUAL FRAMEWORK AND DEFINITIONS OF QUALITY

Quality may be defined in many ways and from many perspectives. Donabedian (1980, 1982, 1986) observed that definitions of quality ordinarily reflect the values and goals of the current medical care system, as well as those of the larger society of which it is part. He has distinguished three aspects of care that one might choose to measure:

- Structure: Resources available to provide adequate health care
- Process: The extent to which professionals perform according to accepted standards
- Outcomes: Changes in the patient's condition following treatment

In addition, he broadened the definition of quality to include not just technical management, but also management of interpersonal relationships, access, and continuity of care.

The conceptual framework shown in Figure 3–1 allows us to appreciate the complexity of defining and measuring the quality of health care, and provides guidance in what aspects of care we might wish to measure. Dr. Donabedian provided a general framework for thinking about quality of care for those working in the field of quality improvement.

In 1988, the US Office of Technology Assessment (OTA) defined quality of care as "the degree to which the process of care increases the probability of outcomes desired by the patient, and reduces the probability of undesired outcomes, given the state of medical knowledge." (1988)

|  | Structure | Process | Outcome |
|---|---|---|---|
| Accessibility |  |  |  |
| Technical Management |  |  |  |
| Management of Interpersonal Relationships |  |  |  |
| Continuity |  |  |  |

**Figure 3–1** Donabedian's Matrix for the Classification of Quality Measures, Used with permission from *Explorations in Quality Assessment and Monitoring Volume: The Definition of Quality and Approaches to its Assessment Volume 1*, by Avedis Donabedian. (Chicago: Health Administration Press, 1980) pp. 95-99.

This is a useful definition because it makes an explicit connection between the processes of treatment that are used and the resulting outcomes. It demands that evidence-based medicine is the standard of care. Also, the patient's perspective is emphasized. Thus, one is forced to focus on evidence of effectiveness of various treatments from the patient's point of view. Note that it also follows from this OTA definition that neither structure, process, nor outcome measures are meaningful or useful if there is no effective treatment known for a given condition. Thus, one can use quality measures only for those conditions where the technology is reasonably effective.

More recently, the Institute of Medicine discussed quality in the following manner:

> All health care organizations, professional groups, and private and public purchasers should pursue six major aims; specifically, health care should be safe, effective, patient-centered, timely, efficient, and equitable (Committee on Quality of Health Care in America 2003).

This broadens the earlier definitions of quality to recognize that high quality health care must not only focus on the process of care (timeliness); patient outcomes (safety and effectiveness); and the patient's perspective (patient-centered), but must also focus on some of the broader requirements of the social and economic system within which health care is provided (efficiency and equity). While recognizing this broader perspective, this chapter will concentrate on the measurement of health outcomes, a difficult enough task in itself.

Why might one choose to measure or monitor health outcomes when it is so much simpler to monitor structure? In many cases, one can simply do an "inventory" of structural measures by using a checklist. The Joint Commission on Accreditation of Healthcare Organizations (JCAHO) took this approach in its early days because there was some agreement that certain structural elements were needed as minimal standards to ensure an environment in which good care was possible. However, adequate inputs alone do not ensure good outcomes. All that the structural measures can do is indicate whether a facility has the capacity to provide good care.

Then why not focus on process measures, which take into account professional performance? It is often easier to measure provider performance than it is to measure patient outcomes. Processes are generally documented in patient records, as well as in billing or claims data sets, since the procedures that are done usually determine the payment that the professional receives.

There are, however, several problems with process measures. In order to develop useful process measures, there must be agreement or consensus about what the professional should do under defined circumstances. While it is sometimes possible to get agreement among professionals and to develop treatment guidelines, often it is not possible to develop a consensus on explicit process criteria. Moreover, it is virtually impossible to itemize the exceptions to treatment guidelines, i.e., under what circumstances one should not follow the guidelines, due to certain combinations of co-morbidities, advanced age of the patient, patient preferences, or other valid reasons.

Another difficulty of using process measures is that the provider may do the "right thing in the right way," but the patient may be dissatisfied, noncompliant, or may respond poorly to the treatment. Thus, the process, though followed correctly, may not always produce the desired outcome.

## Outcome Measures

Outcome measures are what we would really like to use, since the whole point of treating the patient is, according to the earlier OTA definition, to increase the probability of outcomes desired by the patient and reduce the probability of undesired outcomes, given the state of medical knowledge. Outcome measures are, in effect, the "gold standard" for measuring the quality of care. We would like to monitor the outcomes of care to determine treatment effectiveness, i.e., to measure the effect the treatment has had on the patient's condition. However, it is much more difficult to gather specific outcome data on patients than it is to measure structure or process. Ideally, one would like to start with data on patient health status before and after treatment for a large national sample of hospitals. Instead, what is in our available databases is information on what treatments were used, and, to some extent, information on the adverse consequences of treatments. Data on outcomes are often missing.

There are many reasons that this is so. In most cases there is a time delay until one can assess the effect of a treatment on a patient, since one must wait until the patient has recovered from the treatment itself. It is expensive to try to follow up on patients once they have completed treatment and recovery, and it is difficult to systematically measure the health status of each type of patient after treatment. Moreover, health status following treatment is often not a direct result of the care provided. Outcomes are not determined solely by professional performance. Other patient-related factors (such as the severity of the patient's condition at the time of treatment, comorbidities, patient compliance, patient age, patient financial resources, etc.) also enter into the equation. Unless one can adequately account for these factors, one cannot validly compare the performance of different providers. Outcomes attained by a provider treating more risky patients cannot really be compared with outcomes attained by a provider treating less risky patients unless one can adjust for the impact of the risks when comparing the providers.

To construct valid measures of patient outcomes in hospitals, two separate but related problems must be solved: how to take into account differences across hospitals in the types of patient treated (disease categories), and how to take into account differences across hospitals in the severity and complexity of illnesses in the patients treated within each disease category. These issues will be discussed in more detail below.

## THE HISTORY AND POLITICS IN THE UNITED STATES OF DOING QUALITY ASSESSMENT USING OUTCOME DATA

Consider why the use of outcome measures was not a priority in the United States until recently. This requires a look at the history and politics of measuring and regulating health care in the United States. Although there is much current interest in using measures of patient outcomes (clinical responses to treatment) to evaluate the quality of clinical care, this focus is not new. In the 1860s Florence Nightingale developed and used a systematic approach to collecting and analyzing information on differences in mortality rates across hospitals. She evaluated the effects of introducing improvements in cleanliness and nutrition on the death rates of the sick and wounded soldiers treated during the Crimean War. Fifty years later, Dr. E. A. Codman reported on his study of the end results of care in the United States.

This famous study emphasized the same issues that are being discussed today when examining the quality of care, including the necessity of taking into consideration the severity or stage of the disease; the issue of co-morbidity (two or more illnesses present at one time); the health and illness behavior of the patient; and economic barriers to receiving care. (Graham 1990, pp. 6–7)

American society did not, however, move in a straight path toward using outcome measures to evaluate the quality of care. Outcome measures were not used to measure quality because there were historical-political problems, as well as technical problems.

Since the beginning of the twentieth century in the United States, society has delegated the establishment of quality standards to the medical profession. As Starr (1982) points out,

> Doctors and other professionals have a distinctive basis of legitimacy that lends strength to their authority. They claim authority, not as individuals, but as members of a community that has objectively validated their competence. The professional offers judgments and advice, not as a personal act based on privately revealed or idiosyncratic criteria, but as a representative of a community of shared standards. The basis of those standards in the modern professions is presumed to be rational inquiry and empirical evidence. (p. 12)

Caper (1988) summarized the effect on the medical profession of this delegation of authority:

> Being the perceived custodian of its own standards has distinct advantages for professions such as medicine. First, it has permitted medical professionals to attain, and retain, a very high level of autonomy, both for themselves as a group and for their individual members. Second, it has allowed them largely to determine working conditions and terms of payment. Third, it has helped turn medical decision-making into a 'black box,' which is relatively immune to outside examination. (p. 51)

Given this approach, the responsibility for quality monitoring and improvement was put in the hands of the medical profession. In 1913, the American College of Surgeons (ACS) was formed to develop minimal essential standards of care for hospitals as a first step toward the provision of quality care in American hospitals. The work of this group led in 1918 to the implementation of the Hospital Standardization Program, which developed into an accreditation process that set minimum standards for medical staff credentialing, privileging, and monitoring functions, and for adequate medical records and equipment. At that time, virtually no hospital could meet even those minimal standards, although by 1951 some 3,000 hospitals were accredited by the Hospital Standardization Program. In 1951, the Hospital Standardization Program became the Joint

Commission on Accreditation of Hospitals (Joint Commission). The Joint Commission, created as a private, not-for-profit, voluntary agency, assumed responsibility for the accreditation process, initially using the ACS standards. The Joint Commission standards were later expanded to cover administrative issues. The Joint Commission program gained political acceptance, and accreditation was required for licensure, as well as for Blue Cross participation in many states, and eventually for participation in the federal Medicare and Medicaid programs.

Because the Joint Commission on Accreditation of Hospitals and its successor, the Joint Commission on Accreditation of Healthcare Organizations, assumed a central role in the accreditation of hospitals, many hospitals structured and focused their quality assurance activities primarily toward compliance with the Joint Commission quality assurance survey-guidelines. Quality assurance was defined as a function carried out by clinicians within the hospital. The Joint Commission approach to quality assurance largely reflected the values of society.

The Joint Commission emphasized establishing a proper hospital environment; i.e., the *capacity* for providing high-quality care, rather than determining whether high-quality care was actually being provided. Over many years that focus began to shift from structure measures to some consideration of process. By the 1980s, hospital quality assurance personnel were asked to identify problems, set goals, focus on errors and problems in the process of care, and demonstrate that they had met their own goals. The standards, however, did not indicate how potential problems were to be identified or addressed. There was no requirement that the identification of problems would be based on an examination of data on outcomes. As a result, many hospitals and other facilities focused on issues that could be readily resolved, or on problems that did not reflect the major clinical activities of a department or service (McAninch 1988).

Much important research took place in the mid-1900s studying quality and developing criteria, standards, and protocols, as chronicled by Donabedian (1982). In addition, a substantial body of research documented major variations in medical care practice (Wennberg and Gittelsohn 1973; Paul-Shaheen *et al.* 1987), unnecessary surgery (Leape 1987), and preventable complications (Adams *et al.* 1973; Brook et al. 1975; Roos *et al.* 1985). These studies, along with others, demonstrated the need to monitor and improve medical care practice. There has been strong resistance, however, by many members of the profession when it comes to measuring quality, particularly when the evaluations are performed by nonphysicians, even if the evaluators are using explicit protocols developed by physicians.

By the 1970s and 1980s, conditions had changed. As rapid advances took place in medical technology, as the cost of medical care rose in an unprecedented manner, and as evidence began to accumulate about severe quality problems, the government and the public took a growing interest in measuring the quality of care. A variety of factors created a demand for and availability of data on the outcomes and costs of care.

## Information Technology Changes

In the second half of the twentieth century it became much easier to benchmark and monitor the outcomes of hospital care using computers and large databases. Also, researchers began to develop more sophisticated techniques for modeling risk factors affecting the outcomes of care. The increased availability of data on the use, cost, and outcomes of medical services also enabled consumers, insurance companies, and regulatory agencies to independently analyze trends in the use and costs of health care services, and to draw their own conclusions. Employers, unions, consumers, and insurance companies began to demand access to such data. This change in data availability was significant, making it possible for both professionals and others to compare the performance of various providers.

In addition, public releases of outcomes data began to occur. In the mid-1980s, the Health Care Financing Administration (HCFA) (presently known as the Centers for Medicare and Medicaid Services [CMS]) began releasing information on hospital mortality rates to the public. Because the methods HCFA used to derive these rates had major flaws, the negative findings were invalid in many cases. Hospitals needed to defend themselves against such data releases. In some communities, hospitals received publicity as having high mortality rates when, in fact, their mortality rates were better than what would have been expected, given the severity and complexity of the cases they treated.

By the late 1980s, several states began to gather mortality data for various types of cardiac surgery. In 1989, the New York State Department of Health and its Cardiac Advisory Committee began an effort to reduce mortality from coronary artery bypass grafting (CABG) by collecting clinical data on all patients undergoing that procedure. In 1990, the department made public the data on mortality rates, both crude and risk-adjusted. Surgeon-specific data on mortality were released after a lawsuit by a newspaper. Subsequently, other data releases were made, some of which were likely misleading and superficial (Chassin *et al.* 1996). Understandably, many surgeons and hospitals had unfavorable reactions to these releases. There were concerns with the accuracy of the data, as well as the methods of risk adjustment. Many of these problems have been worked out in subsequent years, as risk adjustment methods have been improved, and public releases of mortality data have become more common.

Pennsylvania has had a similar program of reporting hospital performance. In 1986, the Pennsylvania Health Care Cost Containment Council was established by the General Assembly and the Governor to help improve the quality and restrain the costs of health care. This council developed a series of "Hospital Performance Reports," covering 28 different conditions that are reasons for hospitalization. Reports are divided into regions, and are hospital-specific. These reports have been made available on the Internet for several years.

Other states have moved to public reporting on the Internet. Connecticut, for example, offered measures for ten indicators for three medical conditions in its initial Internet report (Department of Public Health 2004), namely:

| Medical Condition | Performance Measure |
|---|---|
| Heart Attack | Giving an aspirin within 24 hrs. of arrival, if appropriate |
| | Giving a beta blocker within 24 hrs. of arrival, if appropriate |
| | Giving an ACE inhibitor, if function of heart is impaired |
| | Giving a Rx for aspirin on discharge, if appropriate |
| | Giving a Rx for a beta-blocker on discharge, if appropriate |
| Heart Failure | Performing a diagnostic test for heart function impairment, if not done previously |
| | Giving an ACE inhibitor, if function of heart is impaired |
| | Giving an antibiotic within 4 hours of arrival |
| Pneumonia | Performing oxygen assessment test |
| | Screening patient to see if pneumococcal vaccine had been received and administering vaccine, if appropriate |

This data was compared with national median rates from the National Voluntary Hospital Reporting Initiative. Connecticut hospitals appeared to be slightly below the national measures on the use of ACE1 inhibitors and timely antibiotic administration and above on the other seven measures.

In addition, various other sites on the Internet have had an influence on public awareness of outcome measures, including mortality rates. One example is HealthGrades.com, which has been publishing hospital ratings since 1999 as well as quality information on a variety of other health care providers. There are also a variety of other Web sites that have focused a great deal of attention on the quality of health care.

By the end of the 1990s and the early 2000s, another type of information about health care quality was put before the public. Several important reports were issued by the Institute of Medicine (IOM), which brought serious quality problems into the public eye. These included the Committee on the Quality of Health Care in America IOM report, *To Err is Human: Building a Safer Health System* (2000), which focused on patient safety issues, and the 2001 report, *Crossing the Quality Chasm: A New Health System for the 21st Century,* which focused on how the health care delivery system can be designed to improve the quality of care. In addition, the IOM Committee on Understanding and Eliminating Racial and Ethnic Disparities in Health Care published *Unequal Treatment: Confronting Racial and Ethnic Disparities in Health Care* in 2003. This report focused on the clinical encounter that minority patients experience and the processes of care that have resulted in poor care for minority patients. Since these reports have been made public, a variety of other books, research reports, and broadcasts have focused on these quality problems.

Interest in evaluating the quality of care had clearly moved from the professional domain to the public domain. Many physicians felt that the medical profession was under attack from the outside as government and consumers sought to measure and evaluate quality. In particular, governmental, consumer, and industry groups were attempting to measure the value received for their money, to evaluate the relative effectiveness of various treatments, and to compare the quality of care provided by different hospitals and physicians. This interest led to, or paralleled, the development of more sophisticated, complex, and useful models of medical decision making, including computerized decision-making systems, complex treatment protocols for various diseases, and risk-adjusted measures of hospital performance (DesHarnais *et al.* 1997).

As a result, there was an increase in the demand for information about the quality of care, and particularly about the outcomes of care. This interest was manifested in many different ways.

*Consumers Take a More Active Role*

Consumers began to take a much more active role in their own health care. The women's movement in the 1960s and 1970s emerged as a force that was critical of many medical practices. Consumers began to independently analyze trends in the use and costs of health care services. Various consumer interest groups have come forth to question the effectiveness of various practices. Individual consumers, if they have had to share costs, get second opinions, select providers from panels in HMOs, and make decisions concerning treatment options, have become interested in obtaining accurate and useful data on costs in relationship to the outcomes of care.

*Hospitals Become Interested in Outcomes*

Hospitals became much more interested in measuring patient outcomes as a defense against mortality data released by the Health Care Financing Administration (HCFA) as well as state and other agencies. Hospitals also need information on physician performance for appointment and reappointment decisions. Hospitals often lacked the ability to compare physician performance in terms of outcomes produced or resources utilized. As cost-containment pressures increased alongside of concerns for quality, many hospitals wanted objective information on physician performance as part of decision making on privileges.

Hospitals also want information on both quality and costs for planning and marketing. Many facilities are developing integrated management information systems that provide data on both inputs and outcomes. These information systems can integrate medical records, risk management, quality management, and financial management systems.

*Professional Societies Seek Information on Outcomes*

Specialty societies want information on outcomes of care to evaluate the effectiveness of various practices and to set standards for certain procedures and conditions. Such information can then be analyzed in order to promulgate standards for better practice of medicine within the specialty.

*Insurance Companies Want Measures of Outcomes*

HMOs and Preferred Provider Organizations (PPOs) became much more prevalent in the 1970s and 1980s. These types of organizations demanded data on costs, use patterns, and practice patterns because such information was crucial in managing care in these systems. It was also essential to evaluate the costs and quality of care given by the providers with whom these insurance organizations contracted. PPO contracts require the contracting agency to exercise care when designating preferred providers. If these providers were producing poor outcomes, marketing of the plan would be impossible, and the PPO could face legal problems. Insurance companies also need such information in order to market their products successfully in a more competitive environment.

*Regulators Seek Data on Outcomes*

It also became clear that federal and state programs were paying large amounts of money for treatments and for procedures that might not be the most effective means of caring for patients. By the 1980s, the federal government began to allocate research dollars for "effectiveness research" to learn more about the most effective treatments in areas where great variations in medical practice were discovered.

- Regulatory agencies began independent analyses of trends in the use and costs of health care services.
- Federal initiatives, including some at the Veterans Administration, focused increased attention on quality measurement and improvement, including outcomes.
- JCAHO began to examine the possibility of using outcome measurement as part of its accreditation process.
- In order to provide standardized data sets on costs and outcomes, insurance commissioners and state legislators in many parts of the country (California, Florida, Iowa, Maine, Massachusetts, New Hampshire, New York, Vermont, Washington, West Virginia, and others) mandated that hospitals report these data. Several states prescribed the specific data elements that were required. In many

cases, new data elements were mandated beyond the common data set used for billing purposes, at considerable cost to hospitals. Federal regulators (peer review organizations, the Health Care Financing Administration) began to find new uses for data on cost and outcomes of medical care. The federal government used the information for developing changes in payment systems, both for hospitals (Diagnosis Related Groups [DRGs]) and for professionals (relative value scales).

### Employers Want Data on Quality of Care

A broader concern with quality measurement developed in industry. Many industries in the United States became highly concerned with methods of measuring and controlling the quality of the products and services they produced. There was a growing focus on using scientific methods and harnessing the energy and creativity of all levels of personnel in an organization. Total quality management (TQM) principles were adopted by many US industries. In many communities, industries using TQM were represented on hospital boards as well. TQM concepts were introduced into hospital management and eventually began to change the way certain hospitals approached quality.

In addition, unions and industry demanded information on cost, quality, and outcomes as they negotiated contracts. As new benefits were added, it was necessary to analyze whether they were worth what they cost. In some cases, it was necessary to evaluate the performance of providers in order to decide whether to offer certain plans. Companies that self-insured needed to develop information on use, costs, and outcomes in order to better manage their insurance plans. Local providers that used excessive resources or had consistently poor outcomes could pose a real problem for such plans.

### Business Groups/Coalitions Become Interested in Outcomes

Several business coalitions also organized to consider ways to improve health care quality and to control costs. Two examples are The Pacific Business Group on Health (PBGH) and the Leapfrog Group.

The Pacific Business Group on Health was founded in 1989, and represents more than 50 large purchasers of health care, with coverage for more than 3 million employees. The coalition identifies health care and business trends, assesses the impact of those trends and recommends practical steps to advance a common agenda. It works closely with payers, providers, researchers and others to achieve the highest quality and most cost-effective health care. PBGH also works collaboratively with all purchasers in California and with other business coalitions throughout the United States. (http://pbgh.org 2004)

The Leapfrog Group is another example. It represents employers with more than 34 million covered health care consumers in all 50 states. Composed of more than 150 public and private organizations that provide health care benefits, The Leapfrog Group works with medical experts throughout the United States to identify problems and propose solutions that it believes will improve hospital systems that could break down and harm patients. Representing more than 34 million health care consumers in all 50 states, Leapfrog provides important information and solutions for consumers and health care providers. (http://www.leapfroggroup.org 2004)

Table 3–1 illustrates what one set of observers sees as likely uses of performance measures by various stakeholders and the tools that they might apply.

Although comparisons of mortality rates and measures of adverse events across institutions are potentially useful to providers and patients as one way to measure quality of care, such information might be misleading and potentially damaging, if misused. This is particularly important when considering how such "report cards" can be used by the government or the public. Such information must be compiled and interpreted correctly. Several studies have demonstrated that raw death rates, without adjustment for differences in case mix and case complexity, lead to misleading comparisons among hospitals, with those hospitals that treat "riskier" patients appearing to provide poorer care (Moses and Mosteller 1968; Wagner et al. 1986; Pollack et al. 1987; Knaus et al. 1986). Death rates must be risk-adjusted and interpreted carefully along with other indicators of quality.

**Table 3–1** Performance Measures for Improving Quality

| | |
|---|---|
| Consumers | Using performance as selection criteria for providers and plans<br>Using guidelines to evaluate ongoing care<br>Taking a more meaningful role in managing own care |
| Purchasers | Using quality as selection criteria for providers and plans<br>Displaying quality information to employees and families<br>Devising incentives to get employees to choose quality<br>Developing incentive payment systems to reward provider quality |
| Health Plans | Selecting networks based on quality measures<br>Showing quality results to enrollees and physicians<br>Developing incentive payment systems to reward provider quality<br>Submitting quality measures for review by public |
| Regulators | Using evidence-based data to develop regulations<br>Assessing quality impact of proposed regulations |
| Clinicians | Practicing evidence-based medicine<br>Choosing colleagues and services for referrals<br>Submitting quality measures for review by public<br>Using quality methods to improve safety and outcomes |
| Care Delivery<br>Systems | Making quality a strategic factor<br>Developing capacity for quality improvement<br>Developing information systems to support evidence-based<br>    practice and quality improvement efforts<br>Enabling a culture and systems to support quality and safety. |

Source: Galvin, R.S. and E.A. McGlynn. 2003. *Using Performance Measurement to Drive Improvement: A Roadmap for Change. Medical Care.* 41, no.1, Suppl. I48-I60, p.I-51.

## RISK ADJUSTMENT AND BENCHMARKING OF OUTCOME DATA: DATA REQUIREMENTS AND RISK-ADJUSTMENT TECHNIQUES FOR COMPARING HEALTH OUTCOMES ACROSS PROVIDERS AND/OR OVER TIME

### Risk Adjustment

As explained earlier, differences in outcomes across hospitals (patients' responses to treatment) can be viewed as a result of many different factors that may influence health outcomes. Figure 3–2 illustrates that this is a complex situation.

To measure the effect of provider performance on outcomes with accuracy, it is necessary to control for all the other factors. This is clearly not possible, given the existing data sets and measurement tools. However, because "report cards" on providers are going to be produced, it is essential to try to develop as valid an approach as possible for risk adjustment by accounting for as much of the variation that is due to patient characteristics as possible.

Historically, two different approaches have been used to perform risk adjustment of hospital mortality data: hospital-level variables to adjust crude death rates and indirect standardization of patient-level data. Hospital-level data were used in several early studies. In a 1968 study by Roemer *et al.,* hospital-level aggregate measures of patient characteristics, e.g., average age, percentage nonwhite, and percentage of cancer deaths, along with hospital characteristics, e.g., control, occupancy rate, and

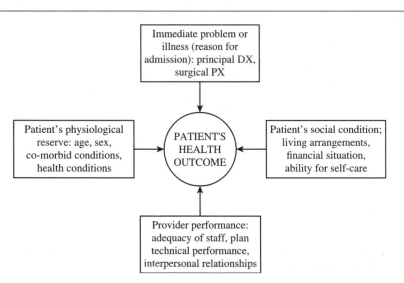

**Figure 3–2** Schematic Diagram of Some Factors Related to Health Outcomes. Source: Reprinted from DesHarnais, S., *et al.,* The Risk-adjusted Mortality Index: A New Measure of Hospital Performance, *Medical Care,* Vol. 26, No. 12, pp. 1129–1148, with permission of J.B. Lippincott, © 1988.

technology level, were modeled in an attempt to understand whether these proxies for case mix and case complexity were related to the observed differences in crude death rates among hospitals. The authors reasoned that if these hospital-level proxy measures were related to the crude death rates, they could be used to adjust the rates to represent more accurately each hospital's performance.

This early risk adjustment, as the authors acknowledged, was rather crude. They justified the approach by pointing out that detailed patient-level data on diagnosis and severity of illness were not yet available. They acknowledged hospital-level proxy measures to be an indirect approach to estimating case mix and case complexity. The authors stated:

> Ideally, one would like to examine the exact diagnosis of each patient admitted and classify it according to a scale of gravity, which might be based on case fatality rates derived from a general literature of clinical investigation. . . . But it is obvious that such a task of calculating average case severity by such an analytic process could present formidable problems of data collection. (p. 98)

It certainly would have been difficult in the 1960s, given the limited availability of computers, to model the risks of death for all types of hospital patients using large data sets, even if such information had been available.

## Using Patient-Level Data for Risk Adjustment

Because hospital-level data are of limited use as proxies for differences in case mix and case complexity across hospitals, there is no apparent justification for using such data for risk adjustment today. Discharge-level data are now available and are much more sensitive for measuring differences in case mix and case complexity across hospitals. The techniques of using adjusted discharge-level outcome data are documented in early studies such as the National Halothane Study in the 1960s (Moses and Mosteller 1968), the Stanford Institutional Differences Study in the 1970s (Flood *et al.* 1982), and work by Luft and Hunt (1986) on the relationship of surgical volume to mortality.

### Risk Adjustment vs. Severity Adjustment

Risk adjustment is an empirical approach, using condition-specific risk factors and outcome-specific models. Severity adjustment is quite different insofar as it makes use of one of any number of standardized indexes to assign a severity score to each case. That score is then used as one of the predictors of the outcome of interest, along with other patient characteristics such as age, gender, etc. The reason severity adjustment is usually inappropriate for adjusting patient health outcomes is really quite simple: most of the severity systems are the results of models designed to predict resource use rather than patient outcomes. Since there is little or no correlation between resource use and patient outcomes, it is not helpful to use severity measures for risk adjustment. Instead, risk adjustment should be done when looking at health outcomes. This means using an empirical approach with condition-specific risk factors and outcome-specific models. Severity adjustment can be relevant, however, when adjusting resource use data such as costs for comparison purposes.

### What Procedures Are Used for Performing Risk Adjustment?

In an article summarizing many of the methodological issues in the risk adjustment of outcome data, Blumberg (1986) described indirect standardization, the principle technique used for risk adjustment of discharge-level data:

> Indirect standardization is the method most widely used for risk-adjusted outcome studies. It requires estimates of the expected outcome in a study population, based on the outcome experience of a standard population. To estimate expected outcome, the numbers of cases in the study population with risk-related attributes are multiplied by the probability of the outcome in a standard population with matching attributes. These expected outcomes in the study population are then compared with the observed number having that outcome in the same study population. . . . The first step involves the development and testing of a risk-prediction model, while the second step is a study of the residuals of the observed less the expected outcomes in the study population. (p. 384.)

## Logistic Regression Models

Typically, logistic regression models are constructed separately for each outcome of interest, using the outcome as the dependent variable and using patient characteristics as the predictor variables. One must take care to avoid using complications of treatment as predictor variables, and one should also avoid using hospital characteristics as predictor variables. Neither of these represent patient risk factors, as one can see in Figure 3–2 on page 82.

Certain interactions resulting from comorbid conditions are undoubtedly more dangerous than others. Ideally, condition-specific risk factors should be used. Moreover, studies that defined a risk factor simply as the presence of any secondary diagnosis often included iatrogenic events as patient risk factors. This was clearly not intended, because the purpose was to measure the patient's risk factors at the time of admission, not to confound risk factors with hospital performance. Although it is not always possible to separate preexisting comorbidity from complications that occurred during the hospital stay, some attempt should be made to exclude the more obvious complications, e.g., postoperative wound infections or a foreign object left in a surgical wound, when these conditions appear as secondary diagnoses.

It is essential to use risk-adjusted measures for outcome variables to allow valid comparisons across hospitals. In order to measure the effect of provider performance on patient outcomes, we must control for all of the other factors that may affect patient outcomes, to the extent that it is possible to do so. Given our existing data sets and measurement tools, it is clearly not possible to control for all of these other factors, especially those risk factors related to the patient's social condition or health behavior. It is possible, however, to use the information contained in existing databases to develop some reasonable proxies for some of the risk factors other than provider performance that are related to patient outcomes. One can use the information readily available in hospital discharge abstract data to assess the risk of various adverse outcomes associated with patients' diagnoses (principal and secondary), ages, and surgical procedures. Once we control for these risk factors, we can obtain much better (although not perfect) comparisons of hospital performance (DesHarnais *et al.* 1990, 1991, 1997).

## USES OF RISK-ADJUSTED DATA: WHAT IS BENCHMARKING, AND WHY MIGHT WE WANT TO DO IT?

Benchmarking is simply the use of external comparisons to understand how one is doing compared to one's peers and/or one's competitors. Usually one works not at the hospital level, but at the service level, or even the diagnosis or DRG level, when doing benchmarking of outcomes. To make meaningful comparisons, the data must first be risk-adjusted, since hospitals differ in the "riskiness" of the patients whom they treat.

External comparisons allow one to identify areas of strength and weakness. These external comparisons are useful when trying to understand how to prioritize problems within one's own hospital, i.e., to decide which quality issues to address first. Benchmarking of risk-adjusted data can also be used to do self-comparisons over time, to see if quality improvement efforts are successful.

### What Standard Should We Use?

Benchmarking requires a decision regarding the type of standard that should be used when comparing outcomes across facilities or within a facility over time.

Such standards may be developed in three different ways:

1. Absolute (Normative): determined by clinical trials and/or consensus conferences. Standards developed in this manner by academic health centers reflect the ideal practice of medicine, or the best possible outcomes that can be achieved under optimal circumstances, i.e., the most skilled surgeon, the best possible equipment, and the best trained team assisting. Although it is useful to know the theoretical "efficacy" of a treatment, or the best possible result one could achieve, such standards may not be realistic under ordinary circumstances of practice. That is why they are often called "best practices." Clinical trials are the basis of "evidence-based" medicine, but they may be better executed than normally because extra resources are put into execution and control. "Consensus conferences" rest on leading expert opinion but still result from a process that one of our colleagues calls GOBSAT, which stands for "Good Old Boys Sitting Around Talking."

2. Empirical: relative to other institutions treating similar patients. Standards developed by comparing oneself to other institutions treating similar patients may be useful to help identify problem areas. If, for example, a hospital is experiencing 20% more unanticipated readmissions than other hospitals when treating a specific type of patient, that could be a signal that some correction is needed. On the other hand, it is possible that the "average" care in the community is poor. Such comparisons are only relative to the level of quality in the institutions used for comparison.

3. Institutional: based on self-comparisons over time. Such standards are often used in conjunction with both quality assurance and CQI. One collects observations of the same phenomenon over time to determine if a process is in control (small random variations) or out of control (major fluctuations). This information uses the institution as its own "control," and can be coupled with the goal of continuously raising standards in the institution. Although this approach is useful, some external comparisons are required to understand how to prioritize problems. One needs such external comparisons (benchmarks) to decide which processes to address first.

## How to Benchmark Outcomes

The following steps should be followed:

- Using the risk-adjustment models, assign the predicted probability of each relevant adverse event to each case.

Examples:

82 year old female admitted to hospital with pneumonia, with secondary diagnoses of cancer of the pancreas and diabetes II
- probability of death is                                           .591
- if discharged alive, probability of readmission       .307
  within 30 days is

36 year old female admitted to the hospital with pneumonia with no secondary diagnoses
- probability of death is                                           .008
- if discharged alive, probability of readmission       .001
  within 30 days

- Add all of the predicted probabilities for each hospital product line, and all of the actual events for the same product line. Use these numbers to develop reports for each hospital, comparing predicted frequencies for each category of adverse event to the observed frequencies. (See Table 3–2).

Note that in this example the hospital has mortality that is significantly higher than predicted, both for pneumonia and for all respiratory diseases, given the risk factors of the patients treated. Readmissions within 30 days of discharge, however, are significantly fewer than predicted for the pneumonia patients, and lower than predicted (but not significantly) for all respiratory diseases.

- Perform statistical tests on the differences between predicted and observed frequencies to determine whether the differences are statistically significant or might merely represent random variations.
- Develop systems profiles, comparing hospitals using these multiple risk-adjusted measures, similar to the example in Table 3-3.

We can use these profiles for a "first cut." Hospitals with unusually poor (significant) patterns of adverse occurrences should examine medical records and perform peer reviews, to determine whether there are problems with the process of care, and if so, whether administrative actions may be required at a system level. In the example above, Hospital A might want to examine why their mortality rates for pneumonia and other respiratory

---

**Table 3–2** Predicted and Actual Mortality and Readmissions, and Ratios, for Hospital A

|  | Predicted Mortality | Actual Mortality | Ratio (P:A) | Predicted Readmissions | Actual Readmissions | Ratio (P:A) |
|---|---|---|---|---|---|---|
| Pneumonia | 23.8 | 35 | 0.68 | 46.9 | 42 | 1.12* |
| All Respiratory Diseases | 70.2 | 87 | 0.81 | 123.3 | 116 | 1.06 |

*indicates statistical significance at 0.001

diseases are relatively high; Hospital C might want to look at its readmission rates for respiratory diseases other than pneumonia.

### Recognizing the Limitations of Outcome Measures

- Recognize the limitations of these measures, which are derived from discharge abstracts and billing data. Relevant in-depth clinical information is missing. We cannot always determine time sequences: for example, whether pneumonia or another upper respiratory infection developed while the patient was in the hospital or was already present at the time of admission.
- We cannot take into account patient compliance, an obvious factor for predicting readmissions.
- Do not assume that data quality is good or uniform across hospitals. Problems with data quality will definitely affect hospital scores on these measures. Poor coding of comorbidities can make a hospital look worse; good coding of complications can make a hospital look worse.
- Do not assume that a hospital that does well on one measure is necessarily doing well on the other measures. There is no evidence that this is true.

Many of these same symptoms are evident in attempting comparisons across cities and countries. Marshall *et al.* (2003) report that indicators

---

**Table 3–3** Ratios of Predicted to Actual Values, by Hospital and by Outcome, for Pneumonia and for All Respiratory Diseases in Three Hospitals

|  | *Hospital A* | *Hospital B* | *Hospital C* |
|---|---|---|---|
| **Mortality** | | | |
| Pneumonia | 0.68* | 1.09 | 1.32* |
| All Respiratory Diseases | 0.81* | 0.98 | 1.03 |
| **Readmissions** | | | |
| Pneumonia | 1.12* | 1.01 | 0.99 |
| All Respiratory Diseases | 1.06 | 1.31* | 0.87 |

*indicates statistical significance at .001

compare reasonably well between the United Kingdom and the United States, but that some caution is needed because of differing practice cultures. Hussey *et al.* (2004) compared five industrialized countries on the basis of 21 indicators and found that each country performs best and worst in at least one area of care and that all could show improvement.

## Problems With the Aggregation of Different Measures of Adverse Events

### Are Different Measures Correlated With One Another?

A valid index of hospital performance must encompass the multiple aspects of hospital care. It may not be possible, either conceptually or technically, to construct a single, all-inclusive index of the quality of hospital care. It is possible, however, to construct several indexes that validly measure important aspects of quality and then to examine the relationships among the various measures to see if they are correlated. If the various indicators are highly correlated, we eventually may be able to construct an overall (unidimensional) quality measure. If they are not correlated, we can conclude that the various components measure distinct dimensions of quality and that the separate measures are all necessary in obtaining a valid impression of a hospital's performance.

A 1991 study by DesHarnais *et al.*, for example, analyzed the relationships among three measures that seem to be "intrinsically valid," in that they clearly are outcomes to be avoided. The three indicators—mortality, unscheduled readmissions, and complications—were adjusted for some of the clinical factors that are predictive of the occurrence of deaths, readmissions, and complications. Risk factors were established empirically within each disease category for each index. The authors demonstrated that hospitals' rankings on the three indexes were not correlated. This result provides some evidence that these different indexes appear to be measuring different dimensions of hospital performance. Thus the three indexes should not be combined into a unidimensional measure of quality, at least not at the hospital level of analysis. Neither should any one measure be used to represent all three aspects of quality.

One cannot simply choose one hospital-wide measure such as a "death rate" to validly represent a hospital's performance. Neither can one simply add up occurrences of different types of adverse events and then claim to have a unidimensional measure of hospital performance. Those hospitals that rank well in terms of mortality rates do not necessarily do well on the other measures and may have excessive readmissions or complications.

*Can Different Measures of Adverse Events Be Weighted to Create a Unidimensional Index?*

Can these different types of adverse events be weighted in a meaningful way so that they can be combined and used as a tool to rank hospitals? Probably not. Even after careful risk adjustment and data quality control, one is still left with the problem of how to weight a death in importance relative to a return surgery or an unscheduled readmission. Clearly, they are not of the same importance, and it would not make sense to treat them as if they were.

## PROFESSIONAL AND INSTITUTIONAL RESPONSES FOR ADDRESSING QUALITY ISSUES IN HEALTH CARE

Given that the management of a health care organization understands the history and politics of quality of health care, has an appropriate conceptual model of quality, and develops suitable risk-adjusted quality measures, what does it then do about quality? The first step is to make sure that everyone shares a quality strategy. The second step is to see that the strategy is implemented consistently across all the major programs of the institution: delivery of care, research, and education.

Linder (1991) suggests that there are three basic strategies, which she calls "models," that institutions can adopt on quality of care, specifically outcomes measurement. No one is against quality by definition, and no one is about to argue for unreasonable prices. Therefore, all three models favor cost control and quality. She describes them as:

- Status quo organizations targeting reasonable quality at a reasonable price. They tend to have medical staff as the dominant group, with individual physicians left to provide quality leadership. Outcomes information in these organizations tends to center on routine compliance-oriented data prepared by medical librarians and nurses.

- Administrative control organizations targeting reasonable quality at an excellent (high) price. Administration tends to take predominant responsibility for quality and focuses on outliers of quality and resource utilization (cost). Nurses tend to constitute the quality assurance staff, and reports tend to focus on identifying outliers.
- Professional network organizations targeting for excellent quality at a reasonable price. These organizations tend to have strong medical leadership and a partnership with the administrative leadership to provide excellent service. The emphasis is on ad hoc studies to inform consensus conferences using the skills of both clinical researchers and information analysts. (p. 24)

About the latter group, Linder (1991) writes:

> Twenty percent of the hospitals had begun to take a very different approach. The administrative and medical staffs joined forces to form an organization that held quality as its first purpose. In contrast to Model 2 (Administrative Control), they believed that financial success would follow from medical effectiveness. Their intent was not to manage the external image of quality, but to continuously assess and improve the organization's actual quality. They believed that the way to achieve this goal was through the free and open discussion of medical effectiveness among professionals. In other words, they used an informed, professional peer network, rather than an authority structure, to manage the organization's performance. The network included administrators, nurses, and physicians, and it addressed both financial and clinical issues. (pp. 27–28)

It would be foolish to attempt to try to classify an entire health care organization into any one of the three categories. That is one of the handicaps of big institutions in attempting to adapt to environmental pressures. They are loosely coupled organizations that seldom respond as a whole, but rather piece by piece (Weick 1976). One department, or even a division of a department, may be in the status quo stage while another is in the professional network stage. For example, at a large academic medical center, one teaching hospital may be in the administrative control stage and another working toward professional networking.

We believe that a forward-thinking health care organization is best served by moving toward the professional networking approach as rapidly as its leadership can take it there. The administrative control approach will not be acceptable to patients or to professionals over time. It does not fit with their concepts of professional autonomy or governance or leadership. Sooner or later, it will lead to a revolution on the part of the staff. The status quo approach, however, appears at worst to set the institution's sights too low for long-run survival and at best to become vulnerable to unpleasant regulatory interventions. That leaves the professional network approach as the only viable alternative for the long run. Getting there, however, will take real medical leadership. There are leaders in medicine who argue that the status quo approach is the prevailing set of professional norms (Cotton 1991).

One fear often expressed by members of the medical profession is that those focusing on health care guidelines are developing protocol-oriented medical automatons or, in other words, promoting "cookbook medicine." Reed and Evans (1987, p. 3280) warn that

> . . . as bureaucratic protocols based on cost containment seek to homogenize heterogeneous conditions and events, and the organizational penalties for being wrong or not conforming to the uniformity in the system multiply, there will be a devalua-tion of concepts such as initiative, innovation, or the utiliza-tion of experientially-based clinical hunches. (p. 3280)

This, however, is hardly necessary. Instead, clinicians need to adapt to the changed environment in several ways:

- They need to overcome some of their resistance to accountability to nonphysicians (administrators, government, consumers), and form working alliances with these powerful groups.
- To cooperate, they need to develop the behavioral skills required to function in interdisciplinary teams.
- They need to develop a reasonable degree of sophistication with the methods and tools used to assess quality and a critical appreciation of their strengths and weaknesses.

If these changes occur, it is even possible that physicians can be empowered to actively participate with others in improving the quality of care (Headrick *et al.* 1991). There can be a change in role and function, but potentially a gain in the ability of physicians to work with others to produce better results. Reed and Evans (1987) point out that the alternatives are either a situation where professionalism inevitably disappears as our society follows its course of economic and organizational evolution, or a situation where "physicians can be much less the prisoners of history." Physicians can choose to "either act creatively, quickly, and decisively in the interests of their profession and their society, or acquiesce to changes planned by others" (p. 3282).

## CONCLUSIONS

Quality is something that all health care providers favor, but it is not, as many would like to believe, something that happens without planning and conscientious effort. The outside world is demanding that health care organizations provide care of the highest quality at a reasonable price. Information with which to make assessments of outcome performance in health care is becoming widely available. Providers can fight to maintain professional autonomy by trying to push the lay assessors back, or they can take the lead by becoming experts on quality assessment, and applying their newfound skills to ongoing operations. They can then educate the public in how to interpret the impact of age, comorbidity, and other risk factors on outcomes measures. The profession can educate its members in how to participate in the process of quality improvement, to cooperate with other disciplines and professional groups, to lead the way in analysis and process improvement, and to help develop consensus about what is currently known and what warrants further study. It can go much further in empowering all of its constituents to follow the scientific method at a pragmatic level in all aspects of medicine and in all settings, to the benefit of its consumers. It can move from being on the defensive about consumer-oriented quality and how it is measured toward being its primary advocate.

# CHAPTER 4

# Measurement and Statistical Analysis in CQI

*Diane L. Kelly and Susan Paul Johnson*

*"In God we trust, all others send data."*

Measurement is a central element of any continuous quality improvement (CQI) effort. Health care institutions are full of data, but they are also full of factoids, opinions, and anecdotes masquerading as facts and as data. An analytical approach requires using data to evaluate the current situation, analyze and improve processes, and track progress. The methods used to analyze data include both those originally developed for industrial models of quality management and those developed in the specialties of biostatistics, economics, epidemiology, and health services research. It is important to understand that analytical tools must not be isolated according to their source; rather, tools from these various disciplines should be considered as an integrated portfolio to draw from depending on the needs of the problem at hand.

Since the initial National Demonstration Project in Quality Improvement in Health Care (see discussion in Chapter 2) concluded that industrial statistical tools may be transferable and meaningful to quality improvement efforts in health care, health care organizations have increasingly adopted these tools. They are easy to understand and simple to use. Many valuable "how to" texts are available that explain the mechanics of the CQI approaches, methods and tools (Brassard 1996; Breyfogle 2003; Carey and Lloyd 2001; Kelly 2003; Langley *et al.* 1996; Lighter and Fair 2004; Streibel *et al.* 2003). This chapter will not duplicate the information provided in those texts. Rather, the purpose of this chapter is to assist in understanding—the role of variation in quality improvement; why measurement and statistical analysis are vital to quality improvement efforts, and how several fundamental continuous quality improvement tools are used to provide improvement in health care.

## THE ROLE OF VARIATION IN QUALITY IMPROVEMENT

This section introduces the general concept of variation, discusses variation in relation to organizational processes, and begins to describe why measurement and analysis are vital to understanding and monitoring process variation.

### Variation: What Is It and Why Study It?

Variation is the extent to which a process differs from the norm. It is related to the statistical concepts of variance and standard deviation, familiar to most medical professionals. One can think of variation as a band of output around the central measure of a process. For example, on *average,* it may takes 10 minutes to complete an X-ray exam on a patient; however, the exam may take as few as 8 minutes or as long as 15 minutes. This range indicates the extent of the variation of the process.

The concept of variation in health care may be viewed from several different levels. Studying variation at the national level highlights health care quality issues relative to access, medical errors, patient outcomes, and resource allocation and may best be summed up by Leatherman and McCarthy (2002):

> The unique organization and financing of health care in American explains why the World Health Organization (WHO) rates the United States, as having the most individually responsive health care system in the world, while it ranks the U.S. in 37th place overall (among 191 countries) because of the significant disparities that exist between those who have predictable access to health care when needed and those who do not. . . . In the U.S., studies published in leading medical journals consistently report findings that people with acute and chronic medical conditions receive only about two-thirds of the health care that they need while 20 percent to 30 percent of the tests and procedures provided to patients are not needed or beneficial. . . . The last several decades have produced a large amount of evidence that there are significant variations in the use of medical treatments and procedures, even for patients whose. . . . symptoms

and illness are similar. . . . This quality problem of unjustified variation reflects a failure to consistently practice in accordance with the scientific evidence and professional expert consensus, as well as a lack of clear evidence in some situations on what approach works best. Unjustified variation not only has potential implications for patient outcomes, but also constitutes mismanagement of resources. (pp. 11–12)

Studying variation from the organizational management perspective provides insights on the links between variation and organization effectiveness and results. Health care organizations are increasingly facing the need to meet requirements for regulatory, public, and payer reporting; to remain competitive through demonstrated improvements in organizational outcomes; and to reduce medical errors through creating a culture free from blame and fear. However, without a clear understanding of variation and its implications, managers may unintentionally undermine their ability to meet these requirements. Attempting improvement efforts in the absence of an understanding of variation puts the manager at risk to (Carey and Lloyd 2001):

1. See trends where there are not trends
2. Blame and give credit to others for things over which they have no control
3. Build barriers, decrease morale, and create an atmosphere of fear
4. Never be able to fully understand past performance, make predictions about the future, nor make significant improvements in the processes

Studying variation on the individual perspective may be considered from practitioner, employee, and customer points of view. With respect to medical management of patients, James (1989) notes the role of individual practitioner variation relative to productivity, risk management, cost-effectiveness, and professional competency:

. . . . variation that increases costs but does not lead to improved medical outcomes is a hallmark of low productivity. When differences in the process that lead to apparently identical medical outcomes are identified, three possibilities exist: 1) some practitioners are under-utilizing and run an increased risk of quality failures, 2) some practitioners are over-utilizing and use resources that aren't really required, or 3) there are differences in skills and clinical acumen among the practitioners. (p. 22)

To ensure quality outcomes, care providers and other employees must be able to effectively, efficiently, and safely execute their responsibilities. Berwick (1991) describes the role of variation in processes carried out daily in health care organizations.

Those who prepare [patients] for [cardiac] surgery rely . . . upon the predictability of the systems. . . . that affect [their] care and outcome. The surgeon knows that coagulation test reports will be returned within 20 and 25 minutes of their being sent; the anesthesiologist knows that blood gas values will be back in 4 to 8 minutes; the pump technician knows that tubing connections will tolerate pressures within a certain range. Each makes plans in accordance with those predictions, and each bases those predictions on prior experience, which is judged to be informative. Sudden, unpredicted variation is experienced as trouble. (p. 1217)

The influence of variation on patients' clinical outcomes may not be discernable to them; however, predictability and consistency in the care they receive will be reflected in their perceptions about their experiences with the health care system. Patients are often asked to rate their experiences in the following areas that reflect predictability and consistency, such as the ones below taken from two widely-used patient satisfaction instruments:

- Sometimes in a hospital, a member of staff will say one thing and another will say something quite different. Did this happen to you? (Picker Institute Europe 2003)
- Following arrival at the hospital, how long did you wait before admission to a room or ward and bed? (Picker Institute Europe 2003)
- How well staff worked together to care for you (Press, Gainey Assoc. 2001)
- Speed of admissions process (Press, Gainey Assoc. 2001)
- Waiting time for tests or treatments (Press, Gainey Assoc. 2001)

From the national, organizational or individual perspective, one cannot escape the role and influence of variation on health care quality (Gold 2004). Identifying, managing, and reducing variation where appropriate is the goal of continuous quality improvement.

## Nature of Process Variation

The innate nature of variation in processes makes us distinguish between two general categories of variation: (1) common cause; and (2) special cause. Common cause variation is that inherent variance in the process that is a result of how the process is performed. It is often referred to as systemic or internal variation. This type of variation is usually random in nature. Special cause (or externally caused) variations are those that can be attributed to a particular source. This type of variation is, therefore, nonrandom. While special cause variation may be traced to the source eliminated, common cause variation can only be reduced by improving the underlying process.

Understanding the difference between common cause variation and special cause variation helps to differentiate between traditional quality assurance (QA) and continuous quality improvement (CQI). QA emphasizes eliminating the defective result or output resulting from the special cause variation. CQI on the other hand emphasizes improving a defective process to reduce the range in which the common cause variation occurs.

As mentioned in the previous examples, one way to think about variation is to think about the predictability of a process. Can anyone tell a patient entering a health care process what to expect with a high degree of certainty? Can anyone tell the patient how long it will take, whom they are likely to see, or how much it will cost? These are the questions that managers will increasingly be expected to answer with a "yes." The amount of certainty in the answer will depend on the amount of variation that has been observed in a process. The less variation that exists, the more certain management can be about answers and vice versa. Reducing inappropriate variation in the process increases the certainty with which managers may expect or predict performance results.

An important characteristic in the health care environment is that no two patients—a key input to the health care system—are exactly alike. Any approach to quality in health care must accept and deal with this variability in the human condition. While managers and clinicians may have little influence on the human variation, they have much influence on the variation in the clinical and work processes. Though variation exists in every process and always will, understanding and managing variation helps managers and clinicians to better align the capability of health care and organizational processes with desired results (McLaughlin 1996).

## Process Capability

In order to understand the expected output of a process, or the behavior of the process, a process capability study may be used. In such a study the variable or attribute to be studied is measured and characterized. Plotting outputs from the process on a histogram can provide the first clues to the question "Is the process inherently predictable or dependable?" For example, Figure 4–1 shows a histogram plotting the turnaround time for 223 STAT blood tests during a 24-hour period at one large hospital. The x-axis represents the number of minutes from the time the test was ordered until the time the test results were reported to the provider. The y-axis reflects the number of tests. Another way of phrasing this question "Is the process inherently predictable or dependable" is "How likely is it that the results of a laboratory test will be reported to the provider within 15 minutes of

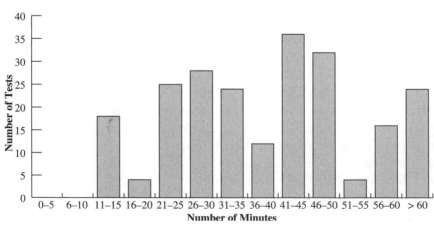

**Figure 4–1** Laboratory Test Turnaround Time

when it was ordered?" The chances are 18 in 223. This type of performance demonstrated by the laboratory process may be considered not predictable or not dependable.

Figure 4–2 shows a histogram of time spent in the dentist's waiting room before being led to the dental chair for the exam to begin. This graph shows data collected for the 35 patients scheduled on a particular date. For this example, the generalized question "Is the process inherently predictable or dependable" is answered by "How likely is it that the patient will be seen within 10 minutes of arrival?" The chances are 29 in 35. This type of performance demonstrated by the dentist's process may be considered predictable or dependable. A process that displays little special cause variation or variation only under predictable circumstances is said to be *under control.*

The shape of the curve formed by the histogram (normal or nonnormal), a measure of central tendency (mean, median, or mode), and its standard deviation all provide valuable information about how the process is performing. The shape of the curve suggests which type of tools should be used for further analysis. Note: this chapter will focus on the normal distribution. The measure of central tendency provides information about the average level of performance while the standard deviation shows the range of performance that may be expected.

In each of these two examples, the time period was a single day. However, the average daily or monthly performance may also be plotted on a chart over time. By plotting the variables over time, managers may

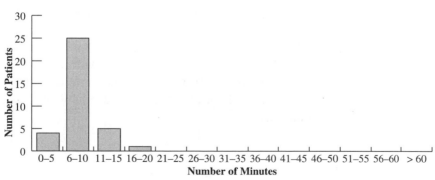

**Figure 4–2** Waiting Time at the Dentist

begin to see patterns or trends in the data that can signal that there is a problem with the process, that it is time to identify the source of the problem, to prompt action to resolve the problem, and to monitor the impact of the solution.

## MEASUREMENT AND STATISTICAL ANALYSIS

While some may assume from the previous discussion on variation that the measurement comes at the end of an improvement effort, measurement and statistical analysis can also be used to measure the capability of an existing process in order to define the need for improvement. This section explores how to interpret and use the information about process capability.

### Interpreting Process Performance

Variation exists in every process and always will. It is the manager's job to determine if the average level of performance and amount of common cause variation is acceptable. But, what is "acceptable"? In both the laboratory and the dentist's office example, it is impossible to determine the acceptable level of performance without first understanding the expectations or requirements for the process. A provider working in the emergency department (ED) would require more rapid turnaround time (TAT) of laboratory results than a provider working in a primary care office. A 30-minute TAT in the ED may be unacceptable, whereas a 24-hour TAT may be acceptable for a primary care office. There may also be specific requirements for analyzing the laboratory specimen. Technology used for one type of test may require 30 minutes to be processed, while a different type of test can be completed within seconds. Customer and technical requirements must both be taken into account in order to interpret if the performance of the process is acceptable or if the process needs to be improved.

### Process Requirements

Process requirements may be thought of as the criteria from which the effectiveness of a process may be evaluated. They function as both inputs

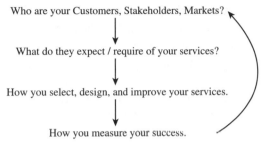

Who are your Customers, Stakeholders, Markets?

What do they expect / require of your services?

How you select, design, and improve your services.

How you measure your success.

**Figure 4–3** Process Requirement Determination Process: Sequence of Questions

to designing a process and outputs from executing a process. In health care organizations, requirements may be considered from three perspectives: the customer, other stakeholders, and the market in general. Figure 4–3 illustrates the sequence of questions that should be asked in order to interpret process performance.

It is essential to first identify the customers, stakeholders, or markets for a process. Chapter 5 provides an in-depth discussion of customers of health care organizations. Brief definitions are provided here. A customer is defined as anyone who has expectations regarding a process operation or outputs. In health care delivery organizations, the primary customer is the patient while the community may be the primary customer for a public health agency. Internal customers are those within the organizations and are sometimes thought of as those departments or co-workers 'downstream' from the process. For example, the recovery room or post-anesthesia care unit (PACU) may be thought of as the customer of the operating room. Patient care units may be thought of as customers of diagnostic departments (i.e., laboratory, radiology). Payers may be considered as external customers, that is, those outside the provider organization. A stakeholder is anyone with an interest in or affected by the work you do. Regulatory bodies such as the Joint Commission on Accreditation of Healthcare Organizations (JCAHO) or the National Commission on Quality Assurance (NCQA) would be considered stakeholders for hospitals and health insurance companies respectively. Professional societies that define practice standards may also be thought of as stakeholders. The market refers to the environment in which you operate and do business and may include socioeconomic, demographic, geographic, and competitive considerations.

Once customers, stakeholders, and markets have been identified, it is essential to identify and understand what they require of your services. For example, patients may require access and competent, courteous providers; payers may require a certain level of clinical results delivered in a cost-effective manner; regulatory bodies require compliance; and markets may require a culturally diverse approach to delivering services.

These requirements are vital to determining how services should be specified and how the processes comprising the services are designed and improved. These requirements also provide the basis for selecting variables or attributes that will measure the process performance. The outputs of the process are then evaluated against these requirements to determine if the process performance is acceptable. Because the health care industry is a dynamic one with customers, stakeholders, markets, and requirements changing over time, the feedback loop illustrates the ongoing nature of this process.

Tables 4–1 and 4–2 illustrate how one health services organization makes operational the link between customer requirements, process design, and measurement. The first column in Table 4–1 summarizes requirements from important stakeholder groups (i.e., regulatory, accreditation, etc.). The next column lists the key organizational processes that address the requirements of these groups. The third column lists the attributes or variables that the organization measures to understand the degree to which their processes are meeting stakeholder requirements and the fourth column indicates the related performance goals. Note that, if the process capability is not aligned with organizational goals as derived from the stakeholder requirements, then the process must be improved.

Table 4–2 illustrates the core processes for each phase of the continuum of care. The patients' interface with this organization follows the following path:

Admission → Assessment → Care Delivery–Treatment → Discharge

The core process(es) for each phase of care are shown in the first column. The second column lists the key requirements for the process, derived from a variety of methods targeted toward understanding requirements of patients, internal customers, stakeholders, as well as the market in which the organization operates. The third column lists the attributes or variables that the organization measures to understand the degree to which their processes are meeting stakeholder requirements.

**Table 4–1**  Links Between Customer Requirements, Process Design, and Measurement

| Requirements | Key Processes | Measures | Goals |
|---|---|---|---|
| Regulatory–Legal | • Corporate Responsibility Process<br>• Contract Review<br>• Licensure | • # Government Investigations<br>• Turnaround Time<br>• Licensure | • 0<br>• 24-48 hours<br>• Licensure |
| Accreditation | • JCAHO Survey | • Scores | • 100% |
| Risk Management | • Public Safety | • Infection Rates<br>• Dangerous Abbreviations<br>• Restraints<br>• Patient Falls | • 0<br>• 0<br>• 0<br>• 0 |
| Community Health | • Charity Care<br>• Healthy Communities Programs | • Cost of Charity Care<br>• Health Status in Selected Populations for Individual Projects | • 25% prior year's operating margin<br>• Project specific |

**Table 4-2** Links Between Process Stages, Requirements, and Measures

| Process | Key Requirements | Key Measures |
|---|---|---|
| **Admit** | | |
| Admitting–Registration | Timeliness | • Time to admit patients to the setting of care<br>• Timeliness in admitting–registration rate on patient satisfaction survey questions |
| **Assess** | | |
| Patient Assessment | Timeliness | • % of histories & physicals charted within 24 hours and/or prior to surgery<br>• Pain assessed at appropriate intervals per hospital policy |
| Clinical Laboratory & Radiology Services | Accuracy & Timeliness | • Quality control results–repeat rates<br>• Turnaround time<br>• Response rate on medical staff satisfaction survey |
| **Care Delivery–Treatment** | | |
| Provision of Clinical Care | Nurse Responsiveness<br>Pain Management<br>Successful Clinical Outcomes | • Response rate on patient satisfaction & medical staff survey questions<br>• Wait time for pain medications<br>• % CHF patients received medication instruction–weighing<br>• % ischemic heart patients discharged on proven therapies<br>• Unplanned readmissions–return to ER or operating room mortality |

| | | |
|---|---|---|
| Pharmacy–Medication Use | Accuracy | • Use of dangerous abbreviations in medication orders<br>• Med error rate of adverse drug events resulting from med errors |
| Surgical Services–Anesthesia | Professional Skill, Competences, Communication | • Clear documentation of informed surgical and anesthesia consent<br>• Peri-operative mortality<br>• Surgical site infection rates |
| **Discharge**<br>Case Management | Appropriate Utilization | • Average length of stay (ALOS)<br>• Payment denials<br>• Unplanned re-admits |
| Discharge from Setting of Care | Assistance and Clear Directions | • Discharge instructions documented and provided to patient<br>• Response rate on patient satisfaction survey |

It is management's job to ensure that the process requirements (also referred to as the Voice of the Customer) and the process performance (also referred to as the Voice of the Process) are aligned (Carey and Lloyd 2001; Wheeler 2000). If the two are not in alignment, then the process must be studied and then improved to improve the process capability.

Figure 4–4 illustrates different process capabilities. Segment a shows the result of a process that is highly unpredictable. Segment b shows the QA approach of looking for outliers. Segment 3 shows the CQI or process

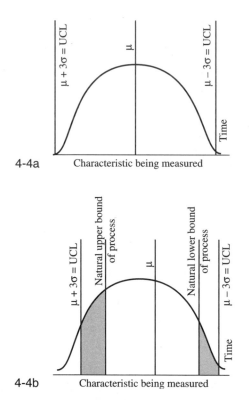

**Figure 4–4** Process Performance vs. Process Limits: (a) A process that does not have difficulty maintaining quality will have normally distributed observations over time. (b) A process that has difficulty maintaining quality may still have normally distributed observations over time but may have control limits outside the natural bounds of the process and a mean that is not at the center of the normal curve. The shaded areas in this diagram represent the areas out of specification.

improvement approach. Notice in the process improvement approach, not only is the average level of performance improved, but the width of the band has narrowed showing a predictable process that will deliver more consistent results.

The graphs in Figure 4–4 are examples of process performance charts, also known as a statistical process control charts. A process performance chart is the most effective way to measure, document, analyze, and understand the capability of a process.

## QUALITY IMPROVEMENT TOOLS

In order to improve a process capability to deliver desired performance results, a systematic, fact-based approach that enables you to implement permanent solutions to root causes of problems should be used. In Chapter 1, Shewhart's Plan, Do, Check, Act (PDCA) cycle was introduced. Many organizations, including health care organizations, have adopted the Shewhart cycle or a tailored version of it as their overall framework for continuous quality improvement. Different tools, techniques, and methods may be used to accomplish the purpose of each phase of the PDCA cycle.

There is not one specified point in the CQI process where one needs to use a given method of measurement and analysis. It should be used on a continuous basis. In the context of the PDCA cycle, data and analytical tools may be used throughout the entire cycle. Different tools will be more helpful in different stages of each improvement project, from the initial analysis to monitoring changes that have already been instituted.

There are numerous tools and techniques available to assist managers, clinicians, and organizational teams in improving processes to deliver desired results. These tools include: activity network diagrams; affinity diagrams; brainstorming; cause & effect (*Fishbone*) diagrams; check sheets; concentration diagrams; control charts; failure mode and effects analysis (FMEA); flowcharts (process, deployment, topdown, opportunity); force field analysis; frequency plots; histograms; interrelationship digraphs (ID); matrix diagrams; Pareto charts; prioritization matrices; process capability charts; radar charts; run charts; scatter diagrams; Suppliers, Process steps, Inputs, Outputs, Customers (SPIOC) diagrams; time plots; tree diagrams; and workflow diagrams; as well as Six Sigma philosophy and methodology.

While space does not permit detailed description of this list of tools, seven fundamental tools that provide a basis for CQI efforts in health care will be explained. These tools are the process flowchart, cause-and-effect diagram, histogram and Pareto chart, regression analysis, run chart, and statistical process control chart. These tools are suitable for any stage of the quality improvement process. However, one can visualize a life cycle of the improvement team's efforts showing how these tools might be applied sequentially at various project stages. How these tools might be utilized over a project life cycle is outlined in Table 4–3.

### Process Flow Chart

One of the most powerful improvement tools is the flowchart to define, describe, and communicate clinical, administrative, and operational processes. Also known as process flow diagrams, these are pictorial representations of how a process works. Simply, they trace the steps that the "object" of a process goes through from start to finish. The object may be a specimen in laboratory tests, a piece of paper in medical records, or a patient in a specialty clinic. Flowcharts are also used to describe the sequence of actions that must be carried out in order to complete a particular task.

To develop a flow diagram, an individual or team may start by:

1. defining the basic stages of a process
2. further defining the process, breaking each stage down into specific steps needed to complete the process
3. following the object through the process a number of times to verify the process by observation
4. discussing the process with the project team or other employees to clarify the process and include any steps that might be missing.

As the steps of a process are described, they may be documented with the symbols customarily used. Figure 4–5 illustrates these various symbols. An activity or action step is represented by a rectangle, a decision step by a diamond, a wait or inventory by a triangle, a document by a symbol that looks like a rectangle with a curve at the bottom, a file by a large circle, and the continuation of the flowchart to another sheet of paper by a small circle.

**Table 4–3** CQI Process Stages and Quality Tools

| Tools | CQI Process Stages | | | |
|---|---|---|---|---|
| | *Describe Process and Identify Sources of Variation* | *Conduct In-Depth Analyses to Clarify Knowledge and Present Results* | *Weigh Alternatives and Make Choices* | *Measure Improvements and Monitor Progress* |
| Flow diagrams or charts | Key tool here | Revisit and update | | Keep current |
| Cause-and-effect diagrams | Key tool here, especially after brain-storming | Stratify for detail | | |
| Pareto diagrams or charts | | Key tool here to stratify causes | Key to deciding on vital few | Use to show change |
| Frequency distributions (histograms) | | Helpful in presentation | | Helpful in monitoring |
| Run charts | | Important to relate data temporally to changes | | Key to knowing whether improvement has been associated with change |
| Regression analysis | | | Useful for testing hypotheses | |
| Control charts | | | | Key to seeing whether the process is or remains under control |

Flow diagrams may be as simple or as complex as you wish. It is important to agree on what level of detail is suitable for the purpose. For example, very detailed flow diagrams may be used in "Standard Operating Procedures" (SOPs) for highly technical procedures. A "high-level" flow diagram may be used to describe a general overview of how the process is

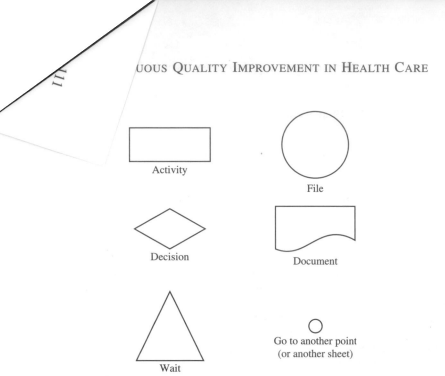

**Figure 4–5** Flowchart Symbols: Arrows are used to connect the symbols indicating sequencing and interrelationship.

carried out. Figure 4–6 shows a high-level flowchart of the medication administration process for the inpatient setting. Once the general process is described, more detail may be added depending on the purpose of the analysis.

Figure 4–7 shows a more detailed flowchart of a similar process. As more detail has been added, the process has evolved from "medication administration" to "medication management" to include additional process stages involving medication inventory management, pharmacy management, and surveillance for adverse drug events. Each step of this process may in turn be charted with finer level of detail, using the decision, documentation, wait and inventory steps and symbols.

Members of a work team or improvement project team are likely to find that there is not a common understanding of how the current process or system works, especially if multiple providers or departments are responsible for carrying out different steps of the process. Quite heated arguments are likely to ensue until they talk it out. With an accurate, shared representation of how the process works, the team is then able to consider how to improve it.

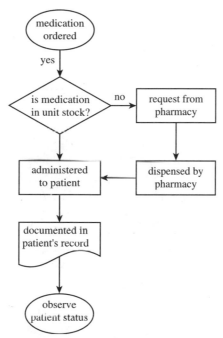

**Figure 4–6** Simple Flowchart of Medication Administration Process.

Once agreement is reached on the representation of the current process, the team may begin to ask questions about that process, including:

1. How effective is the process in meeting customer requirements?
2. Are there performance gaps or perceived opportunities for improvement?
3. Have the relevant stages of the process been represented? Are "owners" of each stage represented on the team? If not, what needs to be done to gather their feedback and ideas?
4. What are the inputs required for the process and where do they come from? Are the inputs constraining the process or not? Which ones?
5. Are there equipment or regulatory constraints forcing this approach?
6. Is this the right problem-process to be working on? To continue working on?

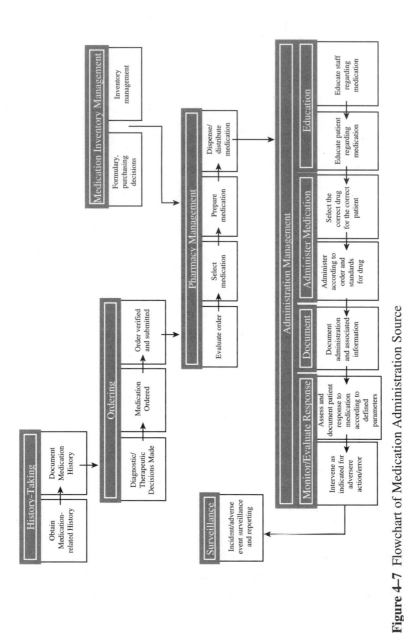

**Figure 4–7** Flowchart of Medication Administration Source

Reprinted with permission by VHA and First Consulting Group from the VHA 2002 Research Series publication, *Surveillance for Adverse Drug Events: History, Methods and Current Issues* by Peter Kilbridge, M.D. and David Classen, M.D. First Consulting Group.

The potential benefits of flowcharting are considerable. Staff come to know the process much better. The results can be used as a training aid. People begin to take ownership of the process by participating in this activity and most important, the possibilities for improvement become clear almost immediately.

## Cause-and-Effect Diagram

Cause-and-effect diagrams, also called Ishikawa or fishbone diagrams, are one of the most widely used tools of CQI. This tool was developed by Kaoru Ishikawa (University of Tokyo) for use at Kawasaki Steel Works in 1943 to sort and interrelate the multiple causes of process variation (Ishikawa 1987).

Cause-and-effect diagrams are most useful to begin to identify sources of variation once the process has already been described and documented using a process flowchart. There is likely to be evidence of variation in the identified problem (either real or anticipated). Additional causes may be revealed either through the flowcharting process or during brainstorming discussions.

Cause-and-effect diagrams are a schematic means of relating the causes of variation to the effect of variation on the process. Another way of thinking about a cause-and-effect diagram is as a schematic drawing to organize the contributing causes to a problem in order to prioritize, select, and improve the source of the problem. The diagram is also referred to as a "fishbone diagram" because the shape resembles the skeleton of a fish.

This tool is especially suited for team situations and is quite useful for focusing a discussion and organizing large amounts of information resulting from a brainstorming session. It can be taught easily and quickly, allowing the group to sort ideas into useful categories for further investigation.

Figure 4–8 shows the multilayered process of making a fishbone diagram. Step 1 of the diagram starts by putting the identified performance gap or problem at the right and a big arrow leading to it that represents the overall causation. Step 2 involves drawing spines from that big arrow to represent main classifications or categories of causes, such as labor, materials, and equipment. Then Step 3 adds along each major spine the specific causes, which also may occur at multiple levels. Sometimes it is useful to draw the diagram in two stages—one showing the main causes and then a separate chart with a spine representing the main cause and its associated levels.

Step 1: Draw spine

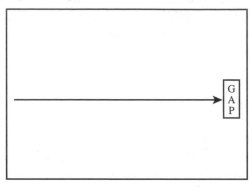

Step 2: Add main causes

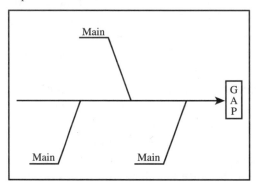

Step 3: Add specific causes

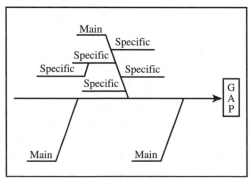

**Figure 4–8** Multilayered Process of Developing a Fishbone Chart

The first pass at a cause-and-effect diagram may not be enough to understand the process, identify the specific cause of an error, and quantify it. Therefore, it may be necessary to stratify cause-and-effect diagrams further to achieve finer gradations of error causes. Increasing the level of detail about causes can help with identifying specific corrective action.

Figure 4–9 illustrates an example of a fishbone diagram that may be used to describe root causes of medication errors in a hospital setting. The problem is "medication errors." The main classifications in this example are: people, policies, procedures, and plant and equipment, each showing a variety of levels of causes.

## Histogram and Pareto Diagram

Once a cause-and-effect diagram is generated, data is collected to quantify how often the different causes occur. These data must then be presented to the study team and later to others. The simplest display is a histogram, a vertical bar chart representing the frequency distribution of set of data. The bars are arrayed on the X-axis representing equal or adjacent data intervals or discrete events. The length of the bar against the Y-axis shows the number of observations falling on that interval or event classification. The histogram displays the nature of underlying statistical distribution. Successive histograms can be used to indicate whether or not there has been a change in the variability of a process. Figure 4–10 shows a histogram of the frequency and causes for the discard of hospital linens.

A Pareto diagram is a vertical bar chart with the bars arranged from the longest first on the left and moving successively toward the shortest. The arrangement of the vertical bars gives a visual indication of the relative frequency of the contributing causes of the problem with each bar representing one cause.

The diagram is named after the seventeenth-century Italian economist, Vilfredo Pareto. When he studied the distribution of wealth, he observed that the majority of the wealth had been distributed among a small proportion of the population (Pareto's law). Juran (1988) applied this concept to quality causes, observing that the "vital few" causes account for most of the defects, while others, the "useful many," account for a much smaller proportion of the defects. He noted that these vital few causes are likely to constitute the areas of highest payback to management.

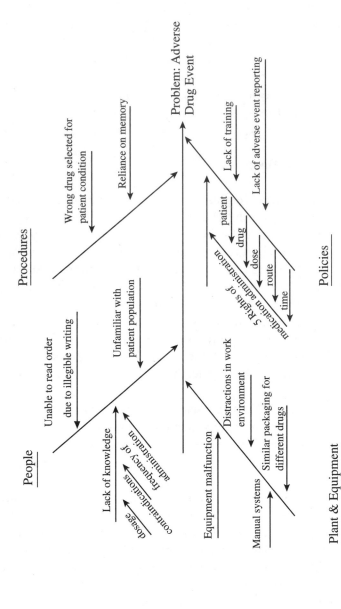

**Figure 4–9** Cause-and-Effect Diagram of Medication Adverse Event: Root Causes of Medication Errors.

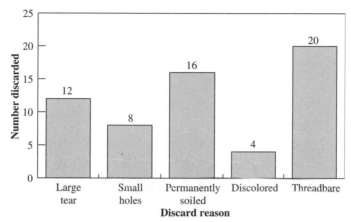

**Figure 4–10** Histogram of Linen Discard Causes

Concentrating on the high-volume causes should have the largest potential for reducing process variation.

On the same Pareto diagram one also develops a cumulative probability distribution incorporating all the proportions of the observations to the left of and including the bar. It is common to display the frequency scale on the left-hand of the Y-axis and the percentage scale on the right-hand edge. Note that there is no X-axis as such, because it is a bar chart.

Just because a cause is identified as having the greatest frequency does not necessarily mean that it should be worked on first. It must also be tractable and not cost more to change than it is worth. It is likely, however, that the first cause to be studied in detail will be among the left-most group. It is important to remember that even though a cause may not be among the most frequent, if it has a devastating result such as causing a patient death, it must be addressed in the course of the improvement effort. Segregating the causes that have large frequencies can help identify potential improvements.

Once the cause-and-effect diagram, such as the one in Figure 4–9 has been described, data would be collected on the frequency of the causes. Figure 4–11 illustrates how a Pareto chart displaying how often the "5 Rights of Medication Administration" contributed to an adverse drug event (ADE). Of 100 ADEs investigated, the Pareto chart shows that "wrong time" occurred most frequently with "wrong patient" next, and so on. This type of Pareto chart is called the Raw Data Format.

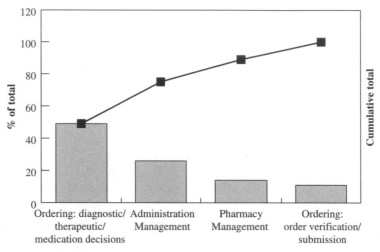

**Figure 4–11** Pareto Chart: Root Causes of Adverse Drug Events

Once data is collected on the various causes, other natural groupings of the causes may be evident. For example, Kilbridge and Classen (2002) describe how ADE's may be quantified according to the steps and phases of the Inpatient Patient Medication Management Process shown in Figure 4–7. A Pareto chart of the data could be displayed as in Figure 4–12. Displaying the data in this manner provides a quick visual picture showing that the "ordering" phases of the process are the source for the largest proportion of ADEs. This type of Pareto chart is called the Percentage Format.

Through these examples, one can begin to see how the tools begin to fit together to both describe the problem and to promote identifying solutions. Since the Institute of Medicine report *To Err is Human* (2000) was published, the topic of medical errors and adverse events has become a priority area for customers and stakeholders of health care organizations. The JCAHO review process now includes accreditation standards around patient safety, medical errors and adverse events. Based on the above findings regarding root causes and other similar studies, consortiums of business organizations, such as the Leapfrog Group, are calling for Computerized Physician Order Entry (CPOE) as a requisite for contracting with health care service providers (Leapfrog Group 2004).

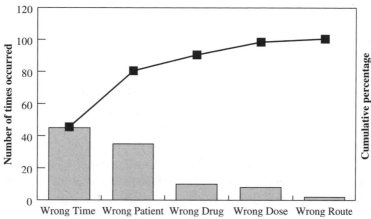

**Figure 4–12** Pareto Chart: 5 Rights of Medication Administration: Cause of ADE's

Referring back to the questions in Figure 4–3, a hospital might answer them in this way relative to Adverse Drug Events:

> *Who are our customers, stakeholders, and other markets?* Patients, JCAHO, and the businesses who buy health insurance that use our hospital.
>
> *What do they expect of our services?* Safe, accurate, cost-effective care.
>
> *How do we select, design, and improve our medication management process?* By understanding and defining the process through using flowcharts; by identifying those places in the process where breakdowns occur; by quantifying the contributing causes to adverse drug events; by prioritizing the causes according to frequency; and by improving the process (or by a new process) or by how we execute the process (i.e., integrate technology).
>
> *How do we measure success?* By ensuring that we have an incident/adverse event surveillance and reporting system in place. The resulting data is reviewed on a regular basis by leaders in the organization, compared against customer, stakeholder, and market requirements; problem areas are identified and processes or execution targeted for improvement as needed.

**Regression Analysis**

One frequent conclusion that observers reach is that one event is temporally or causally related to another. However, individuals are notoriously likely to see associations where they do not exist, so hypotheses suggested by the cause-and-effect analysis or by observation of the distribution of the data have to be tested statistically by some form of correlational modeling. For example, in 1980 Gardner and McLaughlin developed a regression model to forecast the utilization of perishable blood products in a large teaching hospital. They developed a forecasting model that predicted demand quite effectively based on hospital census and some seasonal patterns. The staff reported, however, that one of the attending (faculty) physicians utilized these products much more than the other three attendings on that service. Since the attending physicians rotated on a monthly basis, it was possible to assign a 0–1 dummy variable to each physician to account for which one was on duty during a given month. The model that was augmented to include the physicians indicated that there was not a significant difference in utilization among the four physicians. What the staff had to say about the one physician was not borne out by the data analysis.

Negative findings about cause-and-effect relationships are not a bad outcome in CQI. They help reduce the complexity of the set of cause-and-effect hypotheses to be studied and focus on other alternative causes. Teams report that they frequently started out with erroneous impressions about the causes of poor performance. This isn't surprising—otherwise, they might already have corrected it. If the CQI team had not conducted experiments and analyses to check out those hypotheses early, they would have continued to work in unfruitful areas. This is one advantage of the CQI approach. The team is empowered to use scientific methods of analysis to verify and support any changes that they would like to make, instead of guessing what to do next. Regression analyses or other statistical techniques provide a way of looking for unknown or underrated associations.

**Run Charts and Process Performance Charts**

Continuous quality improvement requires that performance data be monitored on an ongoing basis to identify trends or other characteristics of the phenomenon being observed that change over time. This allows the experienced observer to (1) see what the temporal behavior of the process is; and (2) establish the time of process performance changes so that they

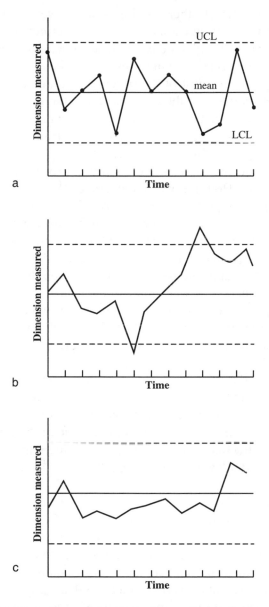

**Figure 4–13** Three Examples of Run Charts. In (a), the data are considered to be under control—the points are apparently randomly distributed on either side of the mean, and do not go outside of the control limits. In (b), there are extreme values (outside the control limits), and thus the process is not in control. Another thing to beware is too many observations on one side of the mean. In (c), there are too many values in a row (>8) below the mean.

can be linked to the time of other possibly related events. Figure 4–13 shows a series of run charts and some diagnostic interpretations of those data. Since the effects of health care errors tend to be asymmetrical, it is best to look at one-sided rules of thumb for process control. A process is considered under control if most of the observations are near the center-line, if there are few points near the extreme values (above the mean plus or minus three standard deviations), and there are no runs (more than eight consecutive observations to one side of the mean). Run charts are very easy to generate using spreadsheet software.

Run charts are frequently used in the quality improvement process to answer the questions, "How are we doing?" and "Are we doing better since implementing the improvement intervention?" To answer the second question, one must be able to compare where one has been with where one is. There are numerous examples of run charts in this book, even though all are labeled as control charts. This is due to the fact that most software packages take a data set and automatically calculate and display the three standard deviation upper and lower limits on the chart.

The industrial quality control literature talks about two types of measures that can be used to develop run charts and their cousins—control charts. Measures can be either attributes or variables.

> Attribute data arise from (1) classification of items, such as products or services, into categories; from (2) counts of the number of items or the proportion in a given category; and from (3) counts of the number of occurrences per unit. . . . Important attributes (are): fraction defective, number of defects, number of defects per unit (Gitlow *et al.* 1989, pp. 78, 79, 144).

Variables are measured directly or based on direct measures only and do not result from a classification scheme. Variable charts are a key part of continuous improvement as the manager or team seeks to reduce variation, come up with a more robust design process, or make the process conform more closely to customer, stakeholder, and market requirements and preferences. Charts often present the variable mean (X-bar), process range (R), and/or standard deviation (s) for a specific process parameter. Unless run charts of key parameters are reviewed on a regular basis, it is difficult to institutionalize a continuous improvement culture within the organization.

A run chart that includes notations indicating the control limits of plus or minus three standard deviations may be referred to as a control chart or a process performance chart. The control limits are referred to as the upper control limit (UCL), which is three standard deviations above the mean, and the lower control limit (LCL), which is three standard deviations below the mean. To use a control chart, the manager or team would have to ensure that the process is free of special causes of variation at the time the control limits were set. They would then follow the charts to see (1) whether special causes were again creeping in; or (2) whether the underlying processes has changed. Because these charts are actually run charts, the most common form is the X-bar chart. This is a plot of the sample mean (X-bar) of the observations. In the run chart most often used in health care, the sample size per observation is usually one. This assumes that there is no sampling error and that all observations are accurate. This can become an important issue in health care where observations can vary so much. Taking blood pressure is a good example. A given patient's blood pressure will vary slightly depending on who is taking it. It will vary even more if different cuffs and measuring equipment are used. It will vary even further depending on the emotional state of the patient at the time of the measurement. All these sampling variations would have to be taken into account, if a study of the effectiveness of the intervention could be quantified.

Control charts can be configured using the simple statistics calculated for the data collected, such as mean, standard deviation, and range. There are control charts used for variable data such as time or distance, and control charts used for attribute data such as mortality rate or whether or not treatment is adequate or timely. For variable data, we will consider X-bar charts and R-charts. For attribute date we consider the p-chart.

Consider a major stakeholder for many health services organization the Centers for Medicare and Medicaid Services (CMS). The CMS has defined required quality indicators for the key inpatient diagnoses of acute myocardial infarction, heart failure, stroke, pneumonia, breast cancer, and diabetes (Jencks *et al.* 2000, 2003). One of the quality indicators for acute myocardial infarction (AMI) is the time to thrombolytic therapy, measured in minutes from time of admission, sometimes referred to as "door-to-needle time." Here we consider how a hospital might configure their data in control charts order to track performance around the care of patients admitted to the emergency department (ED) with the diagnosis of AMI. The tabular data are presented in Table 4–4.

The first example is an X-bar chart shown in Figure 4–14. Suppose that each day for one month, the hospital observed five randomly selected cases of AMI. The "door-to-needle" time would represent the difference

**Table 4–4** Acute Myocardial Infarction: Door-to-Needle Time

| n=5 | MEAN | Range | UCL | $\overline{X}$ Chart Center | LCL | UCL | R Chart Center | LCL |
|---|---|---|---|---|---|---|---|---|
| 1 | 52.1 | 29.32 | 65.56 | 56.13 | 46.70 | 61.99 | 16.34 | 0.00 |
| 2 | 47.7 | 29.73 | 65.56 | 56.13 | 46.70 | 61.99 | 17.21 | 0.00 |
| 3 | 62.7 | 2.77 | 65.56 | 56.13 | 46.70 | 61.99 | 17.21 | 0.00 |
| 4 | 42.2 | 19.00 | 65.56 | 56.13 | 46.70 | 61.99 | 17.21 | 0.00 |
| 5 | 63.1 | 10.33 | 65.56 | 56.13 | 46.70 | 61.99 | 17.21 | 0.00 |
| 6 | 60.2 | 18.40 | 65.56 | 56.13 | 46.70 | 61.99 | 17.21 | 0.00 |
| 7 | 57.7 | 9.38 | 65.56 | 56.13 | 46.70 | 61.99 | 17.21 | 0.00 |
| 8 | 56.4 | 25.43 | 65.56 | 56.13 | 46.70 | 61.99 | 17.21 | 0.00 |
| 9 | 43.9 | 15.89 | 65.56 | 56.13 | 46.70 | 61.99 | 17.21 | 0.00 |
| 10 | 54.8 | 18.74 | 65.56 | 56.13 | 46.70 | 61.99 | 17.21 | 0.00 |
| 11 | 59.4 | 27.65 | 65.56 | 56.13 | 46.70 | 61.99 | 17.21 | 0.00 |
| 12 | 62.6 | 2.96 | 65.56 | 56.13 | 46.70 | 61.99 | 17.21 | 0.00 |
| 13 | 57.7 | 15.76 | 65.56 | 56.13 | 46.70 | 61.99 | 17.21 | 0.00 |
| 14 | 54.8 | 9.12 | 65.56 | 56.13 | 46.70 | 61.99 | 17.21 | 0.00 |
| 15 | 59.4 | 23.88 | 65.56 | 56.13 | 46.70 | 61.99 | 17.21 | 0.00 |
| 16 | 42.6 | 3.61 | 65.56 | 56.13 | 46.70 | 61.99 | 17.21 | 0.00 |
| 17 | 41.5 | 10.13 | 65.56 | 56.13 | 46.70 | 61.99 | 17.21 | 0.00 |
| 18 | 59.8 | 15.84 | 65.56 | 56.13 | 46.70 | 61.99 | 17.21 | 0.00 |
| 19 | 60.2 | 18.40 | 65.56 | 56.13 | 46.70 | 61.99 | 17.21 | 0.00 |
| 20 | 57.2 | 9.38 | 65.56 | 56.13 | 46.70 | 61.99 | 17.21 | 0.00 |
| 21 | 47.8 | 25.43 | 65.56 | 56.13 | 46.70 | 61.99 | 17.21 | 0.00 |
| 22 | 57.7 | 7.22 | 65.56 | 56.13 | 46.70 | 61.99 | 17.21 | 0.00 |
| 23 | 58.1 | 24.43 | 65.56 | 56.13 | 46.70 | 61.99 | 17.21 | 0.00 |
| 24 | 60.2 | 15.97 | 65.56 | 56.13 | 46.70 | 61.99 | 17.21 | 0.00 |
| 25 | 51.4 | 13.86 | 65.56 | 56.13 | 46.70 | 61.99 | 17.21 | 0.00 |
| 26 | 49.8 | 7.34 | 65.56 | 56.13 | 46.70 | 61.99 | 17.21 | 0.00 |
| 27 | 60.2 | 2.28 | 65.56 | 56.13 | 46.70 | 61.99 | 17.21 | 0.00 |
| 28 | 63.1 | 28.82 | 65.56 | 56.13 | 46.70 | 61.99 | 17.21 | 0.00 |
| 29 | 59.2 | 29.98 | 65.56 | 56.13 | 46.70 | 61.99 | 17.21 | 0.00 |
| 30 | 80.2 | 19.24 | 65.56 | 56.13 | 46.70 | 61.99 | 17.21 | 0.00 |
| Sample Mean | 56.1 | 16.34 | | | | | | |

between the time the medications was administered and the time the patient was admitted. Electronic medical records (EMR) facilitates gathering the data, however, in the absence of EMR, the data may be gathered through manual chart abstraction. The data would include the mean time for each of the 30 days that were sampled and the range of the times for

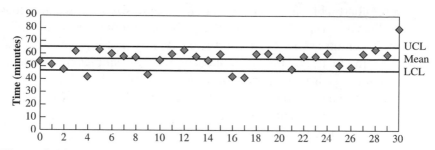

**Figure 4–14** X-Bar Chart—Door to Needle Time
© S.P. Johnson, F. Alemi et al: "Rapid Improvement Teams." *Joint Commission Journal on Quality Improvement*, Vol. 24, No. 3, pp. 119-129, 1998. Reprinted with permission.

**Table 4–5** Factors to Determine Control Chart Limits

| Sample Size | $A_2$ | $D_2$ | $D_4$ |
|---|---|---|---|
| 4 | 0.729 | 0 | 2.282 |
| 5 | 0.577 | 0 | 2.115 |
| 6 | 0.483 | 0 | 2.004 |
| 7 | 0.419 | 0.076 | 1.924 |
| 8 | 0.373 | 0.136 | 1.864 |
| 9 | 0.337 | 0.184 | 1.816 |
| 10 | 0.309 | 0.223 | 1.777 |
| 15 | 0.246 | 0.347 | 1.647 |
| 20 | 0.180 | 0.414 | 1.586 |

each day. Armed with this information, the manager or team could create a control chart using the following formulas:

UCL: $\overline{\overline{X}} + A_2 \times \overline{R}$
Center Line: $\overline{\overline{X}}$
LCL: $\overline{\overline{X}} - A_2 \times \overline{R}$

Where X double bar is the mean of all the sample means, R-bar is the mean of all the sample ranges, and $A_2$ is an estimate of three standard deviations that is dependent upon the sample size and can be looked up in a control chart table. (See Table 4–5.)

For our example, the mean of all the sample means (X-double bar) is 56.1 minutes and the mean of the ranges (R-bar) is 16.34 minutes. Using the control chart table, and considering our sample size of 5, we note that $A_2$ is 0.577. Thus, we calculate the UCL to be 65.56 minutes and the LCL to be 45.70 minutes. The X-bar chart is created by plotting the UCL, the center line, the LCL, and the mean of each group of samples on the chart. The completed control chart is given in Figure 4–14.

R-charts can be used to observe and control. Similar to the X-chart, the R-chart uses a formula and a table to look up the associated factors given the sample size. The formulas for an R-chart are:

UCL:           $\bar{R} \times D_4$
Center Line:   $\bar{R}$
LCL:           $R \times D_3$

Using the same illustrative data, with an R-bar of 16.34 and a sample size of 5, we can look up $D_4$ and $D_3$ to be 2.114 and 0.0, respectively. The calculations indicate that the UCL is 61.99 and the LCL is 0. The R-chart is created in the same manner as the X-chart, by plotting the UCL, the center line, the LCL, and the range of each group of observations. It is common to display this type of control chart directly under the X-bar control chart so the mean values and the dispersion can be viewed simultaneously. Figure 4–15 displays an R-chart corresponding to the X-bar chart in Figure 4–14.

The other frequently used control chart is the p-chart, an attribute chart that shows the proportion of cases in which a given defect or set of defects occurs. A mortality rate would be a natural set of data for a p-chart. To illustrate the p-chart, we consider how one hospital investigated sedation during

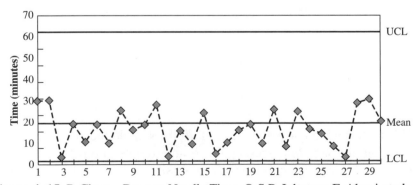

**Figure 4–15** R Chart—Door to Needle Time. © S.P. Johnson, F. Alemi et al: "Rapid Improvement Teams." *Joint Commission Journal on Quality Improvement*, Vol. 24, No. 3, pp. 119-129, 1998. Reprinted with permission.

surgery, an area that plays an important role in both clinical outcomes and patient satisfaction. Pain management and comfort have been identified as an important patient expectation in the hospital setting (Gerteis *et al.* 1993). In this hospital, a grading scheme was used by the clinicians to record their impressions of the effect of the conscious sedation intervention on the patient (5 = in pain, 4 = talking, 3 = awake, 2 = asleep, 1 = not breathing). They considered that levels 1, 4, and 5 were not acceptable and could and should be avoided. One way to monitor the effect of sedation management is to use a p-chart that combines the adequate (level 2,3) and inadequate (levels 1,4,5) sedation levels into two groups. Then, the proportion of inadequate sedation could be monitored and assessed using control charts.

As an example, consider that they recorded the sedation levels of nine persons each day for 30 days. On average, inadequate sedation was seen in 4.8% of patients. This is all the information that is needed to create the control chart. The distribution of p, the proportion defective, is binomial and easy to use. The corresponding control charts are easy to develop. The standard deviation can be easily calculated using a spread sheet or manually once you know the average proportion in all the samples, $\bar{p}$, and the sample size, n, using the following equation:

Standard deviation $= S_p = \sqrt{(\bar{p}(1-\bar{p})/n)}$.

Then, we calculate three standard deviation control limits by using these equations:

UCL: $\quad \bar{p} + 3*S_p$
Mean: $\quad \bar{p}$
LCL: $\quad \bar{p} - 3*S_p$

In the same manner as the X-chart and the R-chart, the UCL center line, LCL, and the individual data points are plotted to create the control chart. Figure 4–16 shows such a p-chart.

The major difference between the p-chart and the others is that the plot is done using attribute data rather that causal variables (and thus simple statistics cannot be calculated, only proportions). It is important in setting up these charts to start with a historical proportion, such as the previous mortality rates. Then you can keep track of the proportion dying over the intervention period and after and compare results.

The p-chart plots the proportion that is measured for each group of observations on the Y-axis with a midline indicating the historical proportion.

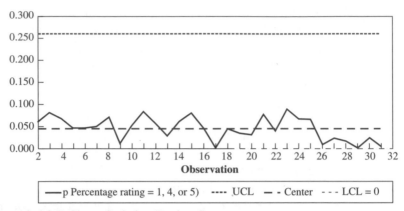

**Figure 4–16** P Chart: Sedation During Surgery

At the very least, the proportion may be monitored for patterns and trends over time. The goals of improvement efforts are to improve the average level of performance and reduce the variable as defined by control limits. One goal of continuous improvement is to monitor the performance over time to ensure the process is performing in a consistent manner within the control limits. The goal of management is to ensure that the process performance is aligned with the customer, stakeholder, and market requirements.

## CONCLUSION

This chapter has described the set of tools that are typically used to identify, measure and interpret the data collection efforts of TQM/CQI teams. Many of the seven tools outlined are used by teams as they move along with their task. Health care CQI participants often encounter measurement and analysis tools very early in their training programs and may assume that they are the essence of the approach. Management must continue to argue that measurement is but one of the core elements of the CQI philosophy, while still remaining flexible about which tools to use when in the process. These tools are not sophisticated, although some team members may be put off by the ones that use statistical methods. Used appropriately, under appropriate managerial and technical leadership, they will help teams implement the CQI philosophy with maximum effectiveness and a minimum of interpersonal conflict. Many of them are illustrated in one or more of the case studies in Part V.

# CHAPTER 5

# Measuring Consumer Satisfaction

*Shulamit L. Bernard and Lucy A. Savitz*

Measures of consumer satisfaction can serve an important role in monitoring quality and improving health care. Oftentimes overshadowed by measures of clinical process and outcomes in monitoring health care quality, consumer satisfaction is emerging as an important indicator of quality. At one time relegated to service improvement efforts by hospitals, measures of patient, or consumer, satisfaction are recognized as the provider's best source of information about "communication, education, and pain-management process, and they (patients) are the only source of information about whether they were treated with dignity and respect" (Cleary 2003). Consumers' experiences can stimulate important insights into how a provider is operating and suggest changes that may "close the chasm between the care provided and that care that should be provided" (Cleary 2003). Furthermore, the marketplace in which the providers operate is demanding that data on patient satisfaction be used to empower consumers and foster provider accountability and consumer choice. Measuring consumer satisfaction provides a comprehensive, systematic, and patient-centered approach for analysis, implementation, monitoring, and improving both the perceived and clinical quality aspects of care (Ford *et al.* 1997).

This chapter provides an overview of key issues and methods related to the measurement of consumer satisfaction. The rationale for measurement is discussed and followed by a series of issues: measurement, data capture, timing, and functional responsibility. An example applying patient satisfaction measures as part of the Balanced Score Card (a measurement system that adds customer and other dimensions to the customary financial measures [Kaplan and Norton 1996]) is presented; and finally, we conclude with a brief overview of the special issue of case-mix adjustment of reported consumer satisfaction measures.

## DEFINING CONSUMER SATISFACTION

Obtaining the views of customers has been a key feature of many modern business practices, however, only in the past ten to fifteen years has the health care sector considered the patient a consumer and developed methods for assessing patient views (Wensing and Elwyn 2002). The idea of patients as consumers stems from a market perspective on health care in which the providers are assumed to be responsive to competition and in which competition can drive increased quality and lower cost. In the context of satisfaction measures patients are considered as parties to an exchange of goods and/or services. Health consumers' views can be divided into three types: measures of preferences, evaluations by users, and reports of health care. Preferences are ideas about what should occur in the health care encounter. Evaluations are patient reactions to their experiences of health care, or whether the process or outcome of their care was good or bad (Pascoe 1983) and reports are objective observations of organization or process of care regardless of their preferences or evaluation; for example, waiting time for an appointment or response from a nurse (Wensing and Elwyn 2002, 2003).

The model used to explain post-purchase satisfaction suggests that consumer satisfaction can be defined simply as:

> . . . the evaluation rendered that the experience was at least as good as it was supposed to be.  (H. K. Hunt 1977)

Post-purchase satisfaction is classically derived by the relationship between the consumer's expectations and the product's (or service's) perceived performance (LaBarbara and Mazursky 1983). If the rendered service or product meets or exceeds expectations, then the consumer is satisfied; if the rendered service or product does not meet expectations, then the consumer is dissatisfied. Kotler and Armstrong (1993) depict the Buyer-Decision Process as a series of five sequential steps, moving from left to right. This is graphically displayed in Figure 5–1.

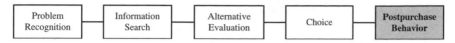

**Figure 5–1** Buyer-Decision Process
Kotler, Philip, Armstrong, Gary, *Marketing: An Introduction, 4th Edition,* © 1997.
Reprinted by permission of Pearson Education, Inc., Upper Saddle River, NJ.

Here post-purchase behavior is directly preceded by four steps that shape expectations against the level of satisfaction that will ultimately be reported. Further, the extent to which consumers spend time moving through these steps is largely associated with the nature of the health care problem being addressed. In the model the key attributes of the health care concern are complexity, amount of patient discomfort, degree of patient involvement, and urgency. For instance, a mother recognizing that a healthy child is in immediate need of a routine sports physical to comply with a school requirement might skip the information search step, and turn to the telephone directory to identify the closest walk-in clinic for a quick appointment. Once the most convenient and timely provider is identified, the purchase decision is made with relatively little investment in the choice. Walking out of the physician's office within 30 minutes and having paid a minimal fee to secure a completed form so that her son could sign up for a team sport may leave both mother and son quite satisfied with the medical encounter. This example can contrast sharply with patients seeking higher order services or services where the doctor-patient relationship is extended over a protracted period of time and where the patient perceives a need to make critical choices (e.g., organ transplantation, cancer treatment, prenatal care and delivery, nursing home care, etc.).

Application of this marketing model to health care is further complicated by the fact that choices and preferences may be severely limited as a result of health insurance limitations, constraining patient choice and/or physician referral options. The complexity of patient perceptions and attitudes together with sometimes limited cognitive ability to process the nature of their own health care situation serves to further complicate the decision process beyond attributes of the patient's immediate health concern. Expectations and preferences are also shaped by a variety of inputs such as personal experiences, those of family and friends, physician recommendations, and directed advertising campaigns.

## WHO IS THE CONSUMER?

The consumer, in general, can be viewed as the party using the provided service and/or product of the exchange. From a health care perspective, the consumer is typically assumed to be the patient in a clinical setting or the enrollee in a health plan. The consumer is the recipient of a direct exchange of health care services, and it is this perspective that serves as the basis for the majority of discussion in this chapter. Nevertheless, measures of consumer satisfaction may broadly target measures for family members, practitioner, staff, and contract service administrators. Examples of other consumers beyond the basic patient-provider exchange are illustrated below:

### Physicians as Consumers:
- Community doctors referring patients to a tertiary care center are consumers of that center.
- Physicians sending specimens to labs for testing and/or ordering scans from radiology centers are consumers of that ancillary service.

### Facilities as Consumers:
- Hospitals purchasing information systems to monitor the quality process are consumers of these vendors.

### Insurers–Managed Care Organizations (MCOs) as Consumers:
- Insurers outsourcing claims processing functions are consumers of the third party administers.
- MCOs contracting with physicians, pharmacies, clinics, hospitals, and home health agencies to provide a continuum of care for their health insurance benefits are consumers for the providers and facilities.

### Government Agencies as Consumers:
- Centers for Medicare and Medicaid Services (CMS) contracting with insurers to provide Medicare and Medicaid risk coverage for eligible beneficiaries is a consumer for the MCOs.
- State and/or federal prisons contracting with health care facilities and providers for services of the incarcerated population are consumers of these facilities and providers.

Beyond these parties to an exchange of health care services, it is also important to note the role of others such as health care workers, suppliers, communities, and families. In particular, families often act as a key agent in the market exchange for health care services, e.g., for minors and frail elderly family members, and have often reported either directly or indirectly as proxies concerning patient satisfaction (Schweikhart *et al.* 1993). However, their perspective, while valuable, must be distinguished from that of the individual experiencing the health care service first hand. In considering the various consumers of health care, it is important to recognize that patients, providers, and payers all define quality differently. These differences result in different expectations of the health care system and, thus, differing measures of satisfaction in evaluation of quality (McGlynn 1997).

## WHY MEASURE CONSUMER SATISFACTION?

We are in an era when health care consumers want to assert more control over dollars and many are willing to pay out-of-pocket for quality. Technologically savvy patients and families are surfing the web and demanding information about health care problems and provider performance. In addition, as hospitals are under pressure to increase the quality of care, insure the safety of their patients, and lower operating costs, greater attention and scrutiny is being given to the accountability function of consumer satisfaction scores. In this competitive health care environment, consumers want and expect better health care services and hospital systems are concerned about maintaining their overall image. There is also attention to ways in which patient satisfaction measurement can be integrated into an overall measure of clinical quality. Consumer satisfaction provides a useful outcome measure for quality of care offered by a health care organization. Ford *et al.* (1997) review the literature that reports benefits of measuring patient-enrollee satisfaction attributable to: increased profitability, increased market share, improved patient retention, improved collections, increased patient referrals, improved patient compliance, continuity of care, reduced hospitalization and length of stay, increased willingness to recommend the organization to family and friends, and reduced risk of malpractice. Satisfaction measures together with clinical outcomes and cost data are increasingly used by employers as part of their value-based purchasing of health care benefits, by insurers in contracting for network services, and by potential partners in establishing health care alliances and systems (Woodbury *et al.* 1997).

The two major sources of future utilization of health care are new customers and repeat customers. Intercorrelations of quality, satisfaction, and loyalty based on a study by Steiber (1988) are depicted in Figure 5–2.

While the direct link between patient satisfaction and market share driven by repeat utilization can be most readily made, positive intermediary influences on compliance and provider change are key with respect to health care behaviors and loyalty and word-of-mouth advertising are related to reputation. For instance, word-of-mouth advertising has been shown to account for a significant proportion of future encounters whereby satisfied customers tell others about their experiences and refer them accordingly (Savitz 1994; Kotler and Armstrong 1993; Davies and Ware 1988).

External reporting and accreditation requirements made by the Joint Commission on Accreditation of Health Care Organization (JCAHO's required reporting and later Oryx-Oryx Plus indicators, current Web site: jcaho.org) and the National Committee on Quality Assurance (NCQA's HEDIS measures, current Web site: ncqa.org) have heightened the importance of patient satisfaction measures, moving them from internal to external performance monitoring and quality indicators. Patient perspectives on their health care experience have been included in the recent NCQA annual State of Health Care Quality Reports (2003) along with the clinical HEDIS measures.

Finally, application of CQI principles in health care organizations has led to the integration of patient-enrollee satisfaction measures that can be used in identifying improvement opportunities in the key components of care—structure, process, and outcome—as described by Donabedian (1982).

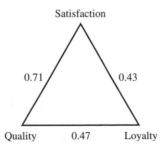

**Figure 5–2** Relationship Between Quality, Satisfaction, and Loyalty.
Note: Numbers represent correlation coefficients for listed elements where 1.0 is a perfect positive correlation and 0.0 represents no correlation.
"How Consumers Perceive Health Care Quality" Reprinted from *Hospitals*, by permission, April 5, 1988, Copyright 1988, by Health Forum, Inc.

## MEASURING SATISFACTION

While patient satisfaction surveys are increasingly used by hospitals, and many questionnaires are available, little evidence exists to guide the choice of the most suitable instrument (Perneger *et al.* 2003). Sitzia (1999) analyzed 195 studies that used instruments to assess the satisfaction levels of health service users and found that, with few exceptions, the survey instruments examined demonstrated little evidence of reliability or validity. However, currently there is an effort to standardize questionnaire items and methods of data collection to obtain survey data to measure patient satisfaction and experience with hospital care. The Centers for Medicare and Medicaid Services (CMS) have been making a significant effort to increase the uniformity of patient satisfaction data and to make it a more integral part of health care quality measurement. Through its hospital report card initiative, CMS piloted a newly developed survey measuring patient experience and satisfaction. Called HCAHPS, the survey was piloted in three states (New York, Maryland, and Arizona), with the goal of collecting data that permits valid comparisons among hospitals to help consumers select a hospital and to create incentives for hospitals to improve the care they provide. A 27-question draft version of this instrument appears at the end of this chapter as Appendix 5A. A national implementation strategy is being developed which is expected to result in hospital satisfaction data available on the CMS Web site.

The term CAHPS refers to a comprehensive and evolving family of surveys, funded by a collaborative effort of public and private research organizations, that ask health care consumers and patients to evaluate the interpersonal aspects of health care. CAHPS initially stood for Consumer Assessment of Health Plans Study, however, as surveys have evolved beyond health plans, the acronym now stands alone as a registered brand name (for further information see www.cahps-sun.org). CAHPS is intended to probe aspects of care that consumers and patients have identified as important and for which they are the best source of information.

The primary purpose of HCAHPS was "to provide information to consumers about the quality of care from the patients' perspective so that hospitals can be reliably compared (www.cahps-sun.org)." Hospitals and physician practices have access to multiple surveys through vendor services. The purposes of many of the satisfaction surveys available through vendors include providing providers with information to improve quality of care, contribute information for performance incentives, and gauge how well customers' expectations are being met. The HCAHPS and vendor surveys differ in the way questions are asked highlighting the difference between subjective ratings of satisfaction, patient service ratings, and more objective reporting of event occurrences. For example:

Patient Satisfaction:
How well did your physicians keep you informed?
    a) Excellent
    b) Very Good
    c) Good
    d) Fair
    e) Poor

Patient Ratings:
How well did doctors explain things in a way you could understand? (On a scale of 0–10 with 0 being the worse and 10 being the best)

Patient Experience:
During your hospital stay, how often did doctors explain things in a way you could understand?
    a) Never
    b) Sometimes
    c) Usually
    d) Always

Measuring patient experience, rather than satisfaction, is gaining leverage with employers, payers, clinicians, and the government (Scalise 2003; Liang et al. 2002). The HCAHPS effort emphasized experience in its development. Researchers who used multiple strategies in the development of the HCAHPS surveys, including a call for measures; review of existing literature; cognitive interviews with patients; testing of the draft instrument in a CMS three-state pilot in Arizona, Maryland, and New York; consumer focus groups; public input in response to Federal Register notices; and multiple opportunities for stakeholder input (see www.cms.hhs.gov/quality/hospital/3StatePilot Analysis Final.pdf). After reviewing questions from multiple sources, analyzing focus group results, and analyzing pilot test results for item validity and reliability, eight domains of questions were included in the HCAHPS survey. They are:

1. Nurse Communication
2. Nursing Service
3. Doctor Communication
4. Physical Environment
5. Pain Control
6. Communication about Medicines
7. Discharge Information
8. Overall Rating of Care/Recommendation of Hospital to Others

In an earlier effort at measuring consumer satisfaction, Zifko-Baliga and Kampf (1997) found that patients used more than 500 criteria to evaluate hospital quality. Personal choice emerged as a significant factor in predicting enrollee satisfaction. In a study done by researchers at Kaiser Permanente, 10,000 adults enrolled in a large group-model HMO in northern California in 1995 and 1996 were surveyed. For each of nine satisfaction measures (i.e., time usually spent with physician, explanation of diagnosis and treatment, technical skill of physician, personal manner of physician, use of latest technology, focus on prevention, concern for emotional well being, your overall satisfaction, recommendation of your physician to others), respondents who had chosen their own physician were 16% to 26% more likely than those who had been assigned a personal physician to report their health care as very good or excellent (Schmittdiel et al. 1997). Findings such as these are important to communicate to practitioners an understanding of the exchange process that they are involved in and to evaluate appropriate satisfaction measures.

A follow-up study (based on Fletcher et al. 1983) conducted by the American College of Physicians (ACP) in 1993 continues to be relevant today. The study included a series of focus groups with patients and physicians to understand the relative importance of measures of satisfaction in office-based medical care as part of the Patient Centered-Care Project. The critical steps suggested in this study are depicted in Figure 5–3.

A comparative analysis of physicians' and patients' importance rankings for 125 attributes of the medical care encounter was completed by

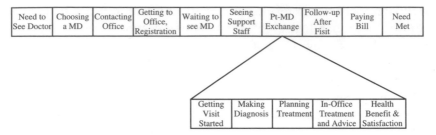

| Need to See Doctor | Choosing a MD | Contacting Office | Getting to Office, Registration | Waiting to see MD | Seeing Support Staff | Pt-MD Exchange | Follow-up After Fisit | Paying Bill | Need Met |
|---|---|---|---|---|---|---|---|---|---|

| Getting Visit Started | Making Diagnosis | Planning Treatment | In-Office Treatment and Advice | Health Benefit & Satisfaction |
|---|---|---|---|---|

**Figure 5–3** ACP, The Patient-Centered Care Project, Steps in Office-Based Medical Care.

ACP researchers. Major discrepancies were found throughout the list and examples of these are provided in the partial list below:

| Patient Rank | MD Rank | Difference | Questions How important is it that: |
|---|---|---|---|
| 26 | 113 | (87) | the doctor explains the results of any evaluation by a consulting specialist to the patients? |
| 80 | 10 | (70) | the doctor discusses important information about patients' health in a private place? |
| 12 | 81 | (69) | the doctor explains the purpose of each medicine prescribed in a way patients understand? |
| 23 | 79 | (56) | the doctor clearly explains the possible side effects of medicines? |
| 5 | 58 | (53) | the doctor gives patients solid facts about the likely benefits and risks of treatment? |
| 11 | 64 | (53) | the doctor tells patients how to take medicines in a way that patients understand? |

The ACP study underscores the critical need to measure consumer satisfaction using data from those who utilize the services rather than simply assuming that as providers we understand what patients want and what will ultimately satisfy their expectations. Clearly, practitioner understanding of patient expectations is incomplete. More recent studies confirm that, while there is some overlap between clinicians and patients in crucial elements of quality, there is also disagreement about the relative importance of elements such as access to care, coordination of care, and provision of information. Patients place greater value on these domains than do physicians (Kaya et al. 2003).

## Data Capture

In general, patient-enrollee satisfaction measures are among the most readily available outcome measures. Accreditation requirements and marketing efforts have already been established to collect these measures without the burden of purchasing new and/or reprogramming existing systems to generate such quality measures as is the experience with clinical quality measures. It is also important, however, to address issues involved in data capture with respect to how the data will be collected, when it should be collected, and which functional area will responsibility for data capture and reporting.

## Alternative Modalities

There are multiple modalities available to health service researchers and health care organizations in collecting patient satisfaction data, which can then be translated into information for CQI purposes. Alternative modalities have important advantages and disadvantages that must be considered together with the data needed in determining how to proceed.

Ford *et al.* (1997) provide a comprehensive comparison of advantages and disadvantages associated with various qualitative and quantitative modalities for measuring consumer satisfaction. While a detailed specification of how to capture satisfaction measures using these alternative modalities exceeds the scope of this particular chapter, an itemized listing of these methods with a brief description is presented below. There is an extensive literature on each modality that the reader is encouraged to consult as needed.

*Qualitative Modalities*

- Management Observation—formal observation and documentation of the patient care process
- Employee Feedback Programs—formal employee feedback on all aspects of the patient care process
- Work Teams and Quality Circles—continuous employee input through teams
- Focus Groups—homogeneous groups of consumers are brought together and input is facilitated in an open-ended forum
- Mystery Shoppers—an observational technique that provides a snapshot of the service experience from a user perspective

*Quantitative Modalities*

- Comment Cards—voluntary patient–enrollee ratings of service quality
- Mail Surveys—questionnaires mailed to users for completion and return (Appendix 5–A shows one such questionnaire which would be used for many government-financed programs when finally approved)
- Point-of-Service Interviews—self-administered or interviewer administered questionnaires completed usually following service delivery at the delivery site
- Telephone Interviews—personal interviews with users over the telephone by trained interviewers

Critical considerations when comparing these optional measurement modalities involve expense, timeliness of feedback, required staff competencies to develop and administer the measurement instrument, desired depth of understanding, and complexity of the data capture effort. Work teams and quality circles have become a well established part of CQI efforts, providing useful and timely consumer satisfaction information that is non-episodic. However, this particular method does not offer information that is necessarily generalizable or comprehensive. Comment cards are the least expensive and complex service evaluation technique, however, the results are often biased with respect to the type of consumers who are inclined to respond and the type of information typically provided.

A qualitative approach is particularly useful for exploring patients' views in areas that have not been previously studied (Wensing and Elwyn 2003). In general, any modality offers only a snapshot of the service experience and must be replicated over time in order to provide feedback useful to the CQI process.

A clear understanding of organizational capabilities and commitment together with the intended purpose of satisfaction measures is necessary in order to select the modality to be used. Selection of the appropriate data capture modality involves learning more about information-gathering techniques and choosing the right technique for the target group and desired depth of information sought. Trade-offs between budgetary constraints and methodological rigor are often central selection criteria.

## Timing

Little attention has been paid to the appropriate timing of patient-enrollee survey administration and/or interviewing in the data collection process. Most marketing efforts have done collecting at either point of service and/or a short-term non-service-specific follow-up following discharge or encounter via mail or telephone. As we begin to use such data as part of the CQI process, more consideration should be given to the appropriate timing of such data collection. For instance, it may make sense to query emergency room visits at point of service; however, follow-up of services with extended recovery periods may be more meaningful if they are conducted at clinically reasonable points in the recovery process (e.g., 6 weeks following care for hip replacements). However, considerations of the recovery process must be balanced with the ability for the patient to provide accurate recall. Survey vendors provide a data collection protocol as part of their service; the HCAHPS methodology also specifies data collection protocols and timing of survey implementation.

## Validity and Psychometric Properties

Patient satisfaction survey instruments should be validated to ensure that the questions measure what they are intended to measure. The science has much improved since 1994 when a review of 195 studies of patient satisfaction showed that only 46% reported some validity or reliability data and only 6% reported evidence of measuring the intended domain (Sitzia 1999). Cognitive testing of the survey items with the intended audience should be reviewed as part of an evaluation of a survey instrument under consideration. Survey instruments should also have adequate psychometric features (Streiner and Norman 1989). For example, high response rate to an item usually indicates that the question is relevant and understandable while a low item response rate may suggest confusion with the item or response categories (Wensing and Elwyn 2003). Questionnaires that are designed to measure different aspects of quality should demonstrate variation across patients (ability to discriminate) as well as variation between measurements at different points in time (e.g., responsiveness to change and interventions). Once valid and reliable consumer satisfaction measures have been produced, they become a valuable component of the feedback loop in the CQI process. Only through dissemination of this information that it can actually be used for performance improvement.

## Satisfaction and the Balanced Score Card

The Balanced Score Card (BSC) is not a new tool. Kaplan and Norton developed the premise for this approach through a series of articles that were published in the Harvard Business Review in the early 1990s and later compiled this work together with a more in-depth discussion of examples from the field in a book (1996). In addition to strict financial outcomes, health care financial managers need to consider and monitor intangible assets that have an impact on the organization's bottom line. These include clinical processes, staff skills, and patient satisfaction and loyalty. The balanced scorecard is an integrative approach to performance evaluation that examines performance related to finance, human resources, internal processes, and customers (Oliveira 2001). BSC is more than a measurement tool; it is a management system used to achieve long-term strategic goals by linking performance to outcomes and can be used to: (1) guide current performance through feedback; and (2) target future performance improvement. The instrumentation of BSC focuses on a single strategy where multiple, relevant measures are linked together in a cause-effect network. Measures transcend the traditional financial accounting framework used to assess organizational performance, seeking to build internal assets and capabilities together with forging the integration of strategic alliances. Leading (structure and process) and lagging (outcomes) measures are identified in four categories: financial performance, customer knowledge, internal business processes, and staff learning and growth. Customer satisfaction is typically included in the customer knowledge category. Indicators are selected by a designated group within an organization and periodic reports are disseminated for monitoring and evaluative purposes.

Application of this innovative tool is occurring with greater frequency in health care (Hall et al. 2003; Pink et al. 2001; Pineno 2002). Several major integrated delivery and hospital systems are currently implementing BSCs and a national conference has been organized to demonstrate the value added of this approach in the health care industry.

Macdonald (1998) reported on the application of the BSC in aligning strategy and performance in long-term care at the Sisters of Charity of Ottawa Health Service. The section of their developed BSC addressing customer satisfaction is shown in Table 5–1.

## Case-mix Adjustment: Addressing a Special Issue in Measuring Consumer Satisfaction

Using performance measures to suggest improvement opportunities as part of CQI often results in internal staff criticism such as "my patients are sicker" or "my patients are different." Case-mix adjustment methodologies have been used to control for explainable differences in subpopulations of patients-enrollees so that valid comparisons may be made with adjusted performance measures. Case-mix and risk adjustment techniques are a common feature of the computer macros that estimate CAHPS measures and are used to adjust consumer ratings and composites to allow for cross plan comparisons (Landon et al. 2004). The CAHPS comparisons case mix adjusts for consumer characteristics such as age, gender, education, self-reported health status, and proxy respondent. Hargraves and colleagues (2001) examined patient characteristics thought to be associated with reports and ratings of hospital care and considered these as adjusters to hospital ratings and reports. Demographic and health status variables were evaluated by exploring how adjusting reports and ratings for hospital differences in such variables affects comparison of performance among hospitals. Their findings suggest that the demographic variables with the strongest and most consistent associations with patient-reported problems

**Table 5-1** A Balanced Scorecard Example

| Strategic Objective | Lag Indicators | Lead Indicators |
| --- | --- | --- |
| Meet clients' needs, priorities, and expectations in a manner that exemplifies the SCOHS values of respect, compassion, social justice and community spirit. | • Overall Satisfaction"—clients and families (all programs)<br>• Satisfaction with physical, social, emotional and spiritual care (all programs)<br>• % of patients satisfied with service in the language of their choice (all programs)<br>• % of patients who feel they are treated with respect; participate in decisions about their own care (all programs) | • Volunteer hours per patient day (% variance) (Human Resources)<br>• Direct care hours worked per patient day (% variance) (Finance)<br>• Staff stability ratio (Human Resources)<br>• # and nature of projects which focus on "increasing patient, resident, or client quality of life (all programs and departments) |

Excerpted from Macdonald, M.: "Using the Balanced Scorecard to Align Strategy and Performance in Long Term Care," *Healthcare Management Forum*, 11(3):36, 1998.

were age and reported health status. Patient gender and education sometimes predicted reports and ratings but not as consistently as the other two variables. However, overall, the impact of adjusting for patient characteristics on hospital rankings was small. Nevertheless, the authors recommend adjusting for the most important predictors, such as age and health status to help alleviate concerns about bias. As with the earlier study, the authors also recommend that data be presented stratified by groups of patients (ie, medical, surgical, obstetrics) to facilitate interpretation and target quality improvement efforts.

## CONCLUSIONS

Patient satisfaction surveys are used increasingly to gauge consumer experience with health care. However, efforts to adequately measure consumer satisfaction are complex. As with any evaluative (whether formative or summative) effort, the consideration must be given to the ultimate end use of the generated satisfaction measures. In doing so, key measures should be selected given the context of the particular health care service and/or procedure. Relevant consumers should next be identified and their input solicited. Assessment should be made of alternative modalities for gathering data from consumers. It is important that this choice be aligned with the intended use of this information in light of organizational constraints on resources, time, and internal capabilities. Then the collected satisfaction measures should be applied as part of the CQI process.

# Hospital CAHPS®

## SURVEY INSTRUCTIONS

- You should only fill out this survey if you were the patient during the hospital stay named in the cover letter. Do not fill out this survey if you were not the patient.
- Answer *all* the questions by checking the box to the left of your answer.
- You are sometimes told to skip over some questions in this survey. When this happens you will see an arrow with a note that tells you what question to answer next, like this:

  ❑ Yes
  ❑ No  →  **If No, Go to Question 1 on Page 1**

---

**All information that would let someone identify you or your family will be kept private.**

**You may notice a number on the cover of this survey. This number is ONLY used to let us know if you returned your survey so we don't have to send you reminders.**

---

**Please answer the questions in this survey about your stay at the hospital named on the cover. Do not include any other hospital stay in your answers.**

## YOUR CARE FROM NURSES

1. **During this hospital stay, how often did nurses treat you with *courtesy* and *respect*?**
   1 ❑ Never
   2 ❑ Sometimes
   3 ❑ Usually
   4 ❑ Always

---

Draft HCAHPS 27-Item Survey

**2. During this hospital stay, how often did nurses *listen carefully to you?***

1 ❑ Never
2 ❑ Sometimes
3 ❑ Usually
4 ❑ Always

**3. During this hospital stay, how often did nurses *explain things* in a way you could understand?**

1 ❑ Never
2 ❑ Sometimes
3 ❑ Usually
4 ❑ Always

**4. During this hospital stay, after you pressed the call button, how often did you get help as soon as you wanted it?**

1 ❑ Never
2 ❑ Sometimes
3 ❑ Usually
4 ❑ Always
5 ❑ I never pressed the call button

## YOUR CARE FROM DOCTORS

**5. During this hospital stay, how often did doctors treat you with *courtesy* and *respect?***

1 ❑ Never
2 ❑ Sometimes
3 ❑ Usually
4 ❑ Always

**6. During this hospital stay, how often did doctors *listen carefully to you?***

1 ❑ Never
2 ❑ Sometimes
3 ❑ Usually
4 ❑ Always

**7. During this hospital stay, how often did doctors *explain things* in a way you could understand?**

1 ❑ Never
2 ❑ Sometimes
3 ❑ Usually
4 ❑ Always

## THE HOSPITAL ENVIRONMENT

8. **During this hospital stay, how often were your room and bathroom kept clean?**
   1 ❑ Never
   2 ❑ Sometimes
   3 ❑ Usually
   4 ❑ Always

9. **During this hospital stay, how often was the area around your room quiet at night?**
   1 ❑ Never
   2 ❑ Sometimes
   3 ❑ Usually
   4 ❑ Always

## YOUR EXPERIENCES IN THIS HOSPITAL

10. **During this hospital stay, did you need help from nurses or other hospital staff in getting to the bathroom or in using a bedpan?**
    1 ❑ Yes
    2 ❑ No  → **If No, Go to Question 12**

11. **How often did you get help in getting to the bathroom or in using a bedpan as soon as you wanted?**
    1 ❑ Never
    2 ❑ Sometimes
    3 ❑ Usually
    4 ❑ Always

12. **During this hospital stay, did you need medicine for pain?**
    1 ❑ Yes
    2 ❑ No  → **If No, Go to Question 15 on page 3**

13. **During this hospital stay, how often was your pain well controlled?**
    1 ❑ Never
    2 ❑ Sometimes
    3 ❑ Usually
    4 ❑ Always

14. **During this hospital stay, how often did the hospital staff do everything they could to help you with your pain?**
    1 ❑ Never
    2 ❑ Sometimes
    3 ❑ Usually
    4 ❑ Always

15. **During this hospital stay, were you given any medicine that you had not taken before?**
    1 ❑ Yes
    2 ❑ No  → **If No, Go to Question 18**

16. **Before giving you any new medicine, how often did hospital staff tell you what the medicine was for?**
    1 ❑ Never
    2 ❑ Sometimes
    3 ❑ Usually
    4 ❑ Always

17. **Before giving you any new medicine, how often did hospital staff describe possible side effects in a way you could understand?**
    1 ❑ Never
    2 ❑ Sometimes
    3 ❑ Usually
    4 ❑ Always

## WHEN YOU LEFT THE HOSPITAL

18. **After you left the hospital, did you go directly to your own home, to someone else's home, or to another health facility?**
    1 ❑ Own home
    2 ❑ Someone else's home
    3 ❑ Another health facility  → **If Another, Go to Question 21**

19. **During this hospital stay, did doctors, nurses or other hospital staff talk with you about whether you would have the help you needed when you left the hospital?**
    1 ❑ Yes
    2 ❑ No

20. **During this hospital stay, did you get information in writing about what symptoms or health problems to look out for after you left the hospital?**
    1 ❑ Yes
    2 ❑ No

## OVERALL RATING OF HOSPITAL

Please answer the following questions about your stay at the hospital named on the cover. Do not include any other hospital stays in your answer.

21. **Using any number from 0 to 10, where 0 is the worst hospital possible and 10 is the best hospital possible, what number would you use to rate this hospital?**
    - 0 ❑ 0 Worst hospital possible
    - 1 ❑ 1
    - 2 ❑ 2
    - 3 ❑ 3
    - 4 ❑ 4
    - 5 ❑ 5
    - 6 ❑ 6
    - 7 ❑ 7
    - 8 ❑ 8
    - 9 ❑ 9
    - 10 ❑ 10 Best hospital possible

22. **Would you recommend this hospital to your friends and family?**
    - 1 ❑ Definitely no
    - 2 ❑ Probably no
    - 3 ❑ Probably yes
    - 4 ❑ Definitely yes

## ABOUT YOU

**There are only a few remaining items left.**

23. **In general, how would you rate your overall health?**
    - 1 ❑ Excellent
    - 2 ❑ Very good
    - 3 ❑ Good
    - 4 ❑ Fair
    - 5 ❑ Poor

**24. What is the highest grade or level of school that you have *completed?***

1 ❑ 8th grade or less
2 ❑ Some high school, but did not graduate
3 ❑ High school graduate or GED
4 ❑ Some college or 2-year degree
5 ❑ 4-year college graduate
6 ❑ More than 4-year college degree

**25. Are you of Hispanic or Latino origin or descent?**

1 ❑ Yes, Hispanic or Latino
2 ❑ No, not Hispanic or Latino

**26. What is your race? Please choose one or more.**

1 ❑ White
2 ❑ Black or African American
3 ❑ Asian
4 ❑ Native Hawaiian or other Pacific Islander
5 ❑ American Indian or Alaska Native

**27. What language do you *mainly* speak at home?**

1 ❑ English
2 ❑ Spanish
3 ❑ Some other language (please print):_____

**THANK YOU**

Please return the completed survey in the postage-paid envelope.

# CHAPTER 6

# Understanding and Improving Team Effectiveness in Quality Improvement[1]

*Bruce Fried and William R. Carpenter*

Teams play a major part in all aspects of health care. In the area of quality improvement, the team is the primary vehicle through which problems are analyzed, solutions are generated and change is evaluated. In this chapter, brief in-practice cases are used to illustrate the potential of teams for fostering improvement in organizations, and the problems encountered when teams are poorly organized. In-Practice 6–1, illustrates both the positive and negative potential of teams. State University Hospital (SUH) sought to assemble an integrated, multi-departmental team to address a complex problem involving many organizational components that rarely interacted in a concerted, coordinated manner. Each department had developed systems addressing end-of-life records and documentation for its own processes, but because these were not integrated with the others' systems, all departments—indeed, the organization as a whole—experienced problems that were badly compounded by an unpredicted environmental change brought to light by State Donor Services (SDS). In its initial attempt to address the organ donation problem, the team was given inadequate time to get organized, leading to a production schedule that was unrealistic. The tight time frame did not provide adequate time to determine the composition of the team. Several members were inexperienced, and while they were supportive of the team's goals, they could not contribute in a significant way to the team's

---

[1]The In-Practice caselets are reprinted with permission from a chapter by these authors in S.M. Shortell and A.D. Kaluzny, *Health Care Management: Organization Design and Behavior,* 5th Ed. Albany, NY: Thomson Delmar Learning, 2006.

work. Senior management provided inadequate support to the team, neglecting to extend the authority of organization leaders to the team and its chair. This led some key team members to dismiss the team as inconsequential and to an overall lack of commitment.

These events at SUH exemplify the violation of many of the central tenets of building a successful, high-performing team. The situation was improved, however, as senior management became more involved, setting an appropriate timeline, changing membership, and articulating the importance of the team to the organization. As team composition and size were restructured to include the proper participants, senior management also granted the team visible and legitimate authority to undertake its tasks, and an environment of psychological safety was created where open communication was encouraged and individual team members could contribute with no risk of rebuke by others.

---

**In-Practice 6–1**  State University Hospital and State Donor Services

State Donor Services (SDS) centrally manages the state's organ procurement and donation process. There had been a trend of declining organ availability for transplant, despite efforts to increase awareness and success in registering donors through the Division of Motor Vehicles. To help solve the problem, SDS approached State University Hospital (SUH), one of the biggest sources of and utilizers of donated organs through its renowned organ transplant programs. Initial exploration of the problem quickly indicated a consistent demand for organs, but organ donations at SUH were down, matching the pattern seen by SDS.

Chris Carter—the new administrator for SUH's Emergency Department—was asked to build a team to solve this problem for SUH. The hospital COO told Chris that this was a top priority because of the high visibility of the transplant programs, the revenues it brought to the institution, and the fact that the Chairman of Surgery had just threatened to leave the institution if SUH "didn't fix this problem it had obviously created." The COO gave Chris two weeks to get a team together and develop a solution, which Chris would present at SUH's monthly Executive Meeting. Chris asked the

---

*continues*

**In-Practice 6–1** continued

COO for advice regarding whom to have on the team, and the COO referred him to the Chief Nursing Officer (CNO).

Chris went immediately to the CNO, but the first available meeting time she had was in three days. In the meantime, Chris gathered as much information as possible. On the third day, the CNO's secretary called to cancel the meeting, but suggested that he talk with the Nursing Division Director for Medicine. She met with Chris that afternoon, and together they formulated a list of people whom they thought would be able to address the issue. SUH was a functionally-structured organization, so they built a team with nursing directors from each of the transplant services and the emergency department, the Director of Patient Care Services, a clerk and a physician from the Emergency Room, the State Medical Examiner—whose office was located at SUH and was responsible for autopsies—and a clerk from his office.

The earliest possible meeting time for this group was in three weeks—well beyond the COO's deadline. Nonetheless, Chris set up a meeting with as many team members as possible, and met with the others individually. Members from this team would be able to meet only once, or perhaps twice at most given the aggressive deadline and members' schedules.

Fearing the approaching deadline and wanting to waste no time, Chris got right to business when the group met. He told the group his goals and invited an open discussion of each team member's experiences with organ procurement. It quickly became evident that several members of the team were too new or too junior to be helpful, with a few of Chris's invitees having asked more junior colleagues to be a part of the team in their stead. The Medical Examiner immediately called into question the validity of the group and the authority by which he had been called to this meeting. When Chris told him this was a high-priority project for the COO and CNO—stating only their names and not their titles—the Medical Examiner indignantly replied that he had never heard of these people, and that this was a waste of his time. When Chris clarified their titles, the Medical Examiner became less vocal, but remained indignant. He had been focused on solving a problem of declining autopsies, which placed SUH at risk of violating a state regulation. He was angry to have been diverted

*continues*

**In-Practice 6–1** continued

from this pressing problem and felt that Chris's group would draw organizational focus and energies away from his own needs. His sourness spread to others in the group, which, coupled with their inexperience and a lack of appropriate representation, rendered the meeting—and the group—effectively useless.

In an effort to avoid a public display of this disaster, Chris reported his lack of success to the COO prior to the Executive Committee meeting. The COO realized the impossibility of the goals he had set for Chris. He extended the deadline three months and also extended the weight of his authority by agreeing to attend the next team meeting. These two key factors allowed Chris to rebuild a more appropriate, representative, and experienced team.

Ultimately, the organ donation problem was traced to a series of new federal regulations and SUH's fragmented approach to processing end-of-life paperwork. In summary, each operational unit had set in place their own processes for responding to the regulatory requirements, none of which were integrated with the other operational units, thus creating hours of work for the clinical staff, most of whom gave up trying to secure organ donations. Interestingly, the Medical Examiner's problem of a declining autopsy rate was also a result of this same paperwork-processing

---

Teams exist everywhere in health care. Teams are used for virtually every activity carried out in health care organizations, including both clinical and management-focused activities. While medical knowledge is growing exponentially, the application of that knowledge to clinical service delivery is limited by the effectiveness and efficiency of teams charged with putting that knowledge into practice. Similarly, as new management techniques and technologies are developed, including quality improvement methods, successful use of these approaches is dependent upon appropriately staffed, well-functioning teams. Clearly, we have moved well beyond the era of the autonomous heroic clinician (or manager, for that matter): behind every successful clinician or manager is a high functioning team. And, given what we know about the effectiveness of teams in most organizations, it can safely be said that the performance of virtually all clinicians and managers could be markedly improved by improvements in team effectiveness.

Teams also play a critical role in improving the performance of health care systems, whether a medical group practice, a hospital inpatient unit, or a long-term care facility. While effective patient care certainly requires that physicians possess current clinical knowledge, patient outcomes are dependent upon how well a patient care team works—whether team members understand and agree on patient care goals, how members communicate with each other, and the effectiveness of team leadership. In sum, teams are the building blocks of health care organizations and are absolutely essential to implementing an organizational strategy, caring for individual patients, designing and implementing a new information system, or identifying and solving quality problems. Teams are not an option but a necessity. As such, it makes great sense to examine these building blocks and see how they can be strengthened.

In this chapter, we use the concept of team very broadly, and borrow from the concept of the microsystem (Nelson *et al.* 2002). A microsystem is one of several subsystems of a larger system that is integral to system performance. This perspective, drawn from systems theory, is not a new concept, but clearly helps us understand how the human body, an automobile, or an organization operates. When examining the performance or health of any system, it is essential to examine (among other factors) the effectiveness of each component subsystem (e.g., the respiratory system), how these subsystems communicate with each other and work together (e.g., the nature and adequacy of coordination between a hospital pharmacy and an inpatient unit), and the adequacy of information about system and subsystem performance (e.g., the extent to which the driver of an automobile is provided with information about the automobile's performance).

According to this view, a health system is composed of many subsystems. In the patient care arena, these may be referred to as *clinical microsystems,* or front-line systems or teams charged with meeting the needs of the patient population. It is these smaller microsystems that actually provide those services that result in positive patient outcomes, provider and patient safety, system efficiency, and patient satisfaction. And, as is true with any large system, the effectiveness of any large health care system can be no better than the microsystems of which it is composed (Nelson *et al.* 2002).

Using the terminology of the microsystem, it is apparent how a microsystem is in fact one type of team, as defined by Nelson *et al.* (2002):

> A clinical microsystem is a small group of people who work together on a regular basis to provide care to discrete subpopulations of patients. It has clinical and business aims, linked processes, and a shared information environment, and it produces performance outcomes. Microsystems evolve over time and are often embedded in larger organizations. They are complex adaptive systems, and as such they must do the primary work associated with core aims, meet the needs of internal staff, and maintain themselves over time as clinical units. (p. 474)

This definition may be slightly altered to apply to all other types of teams in health care. The key concepts in relation to teams are:

- People working together towards specific goals,
- using multiple interconnected processes,
- producing performance outcomes, and
- having access to information about the team's performance.

In addition, such teams must adapt to changing circumstances, ensure the satisfaction of team members, and maintain and improve their performance over time.

In this chapter, we bring together classical research and theory about teams with recent work on clinical microsystems. We demonstrate how our knowledge of teams informs our understanding of team performance and the role of teams in quality improvement efforts.

## TEAMS IN HEALTH CARE

As medical knowledge grows increasingly complex and the medical specialties continue to develop around specific focus areas of that knowledge, there is a risk that health care organizations will lose their patient-centered orientation. There is a paradox in relation to the adoption of new medical technologies and procedures. On the one hand, increasingly specific diagnostic and treatment procedures imply a narrowing of focus. This is desirable because we all support the discovery and implementation of procedures to improve the accuracy and specificity of diagnoses and the development of pharmaceuticals, technology, and procedures that treat a disease in a manner that is most specific to the individual and the disease state. However, to diagnose, treat, and follow up with a patient requires information from multiple sources, and, very often, the involvement of multiple individuals. For example, psychopharmacology is becoming increasingly specific and sophisticated. However, better utilization of new pharmaceuticals for the benefit of the patient requires that psychiatrists have an understanding of patients' home environments. Moreover, a team of individuals (e.g., social worker, psychiatric nurse) is likely required to ensure that patients are compliant and that home support and respite services are available to caregivers. Thus, the need for patient-centered multi-specialty teams becomes ever more important as health care providers and organizations strive to deliver the best care possible.

Health care system complexity extends beyond the clinical care arena and into administrative areas. Teams fill an organizational need of helping to identify and respond to such changes, as health care organizations continue to operate in environments with increased regulation and oversight, ever more complex payer contracts, and increasing pressure for cost-effective and efficient operations.

At the most basic level, clinical health care teams are comprised of health care providers—and in some cases, nonclinical personnel—from multiple disciplines, focusing on a patient or a group of patients with similar health care needs. This patient-centeredness has extended upward and outward to all aspects of many health care organizations. Indeed, the industry has seen a trend away from organizational structures based on functional areas of technical expertise (e.g., nursing, environmental services, registration, medicine, surgery) and towards functionally integrated organizational structures with clinical care teams based on patient needs (e.g., children's services, women's services, cancer care services). The individual clinical specialists serving on these teams report not only to their disciplinary head (e.g., chief of nursing, chair of medicine), but also to team leaders associated with specific patient-centered service areas.

While the multidisciplinary team model has been adopted by patient-centered healthcare organizations, these teams and supporting organizational structures do not spontaneously form, nor are they easily managed.

Given the functional nature of most health care organizations, there are clear forces working against the formation and maintenance of teams. As discussed later in this chapter, reward systems are typically designed around performance of one's particular discipline, rather than a team focus. Where teams do exist, performance is, more often than not, suboptimal. A substantial body of research demonstrates that key elements are necessary for teams to perform to their maximum potential (Hackman 2002). If these elements are not attended to, teams can easily exhibit poor communication, member dissatisfaction, patient dissatisfaction, disjointed care provision, and inefficient and ineffective operations nested in a cumbersome bureaucracy.

## HIGH PERFORMANCE TEAMS AND QUALITY IMPROVEMENT

The focus of this chapter is on the importance of high-performing teams to quality improvement efforts, and on approaches to improve the outcomes produced by teams. Teams are critical to success in quality improvement for a number of reasons.

1. Quality problems are often not visible to individuals at senior management levels, but the impact of problems can be experienced by the entire organization, as seen in the organ donation case. Hospital staff nurses, for example, may see repeated examples of poor communications between shifts that result in a myriad of problems for patients and families, physicians, and other hospital staff. Each occurrence of a problem may be dealt with, but in aggregate, communication problems become costly in terms of time, quality, and continuity of care. It is the individuals doing the work, or those within the clinical microsystem that are most aware of problems that have become systemic in nature, and that require systematic solutions. The farther one is from the front line of care, the more removed one is from seeing day-to-day problems. Thus, if we wish to identify quality problems, we need individuals on our teams who are close to the problem and understand its manifestation and nuances.
2. Individuals involved in a dysfunctional process are usually those who are most knowledgeable about the process and its context. Much of quality improvement involves process analysis and process

improvement. To understand a process, it is essential to have participation from individuals who have the best, most detailed understanding of the process. What appears on paper as a theoretical process flowchart may be quite inaccurate when compared to how a process actually operates.

3. Individuals at the front lines often have the most feasible suggestions for improvement. It has long been known that individuals at relatively low levels of the organization often acquire considerable expertise, and in some cases, power. A receptionist in a pediatric group practice, for example, may have a very clear understanding of why waiting times are unacceptably long at certain times. Because of this individual's many years of experience in this position, he or she may also have developed an understanding of how the practice operates and may have valuable suggestions about how scheduling and staffing may be altered to help ameliorate the waiting time problem. If we are interested in solving such a problem, it is important to have individuals on a team who both understand the problem and can suggest interventions that are both effective and feasible.

4. Addressing quality problems requires the support of all individuals in the organization, not simply those at a senior level. Identifying and proposing solutions to quality problems is key to quality improvement efforts, but unless those involved in solution implementation understand fully the rationale for the effort, implementation is likely to fall short. Quality improvement initiatives cannot simply be handed off to a team for implementation. Those involved in implementing the solution must be involved so that they understand the quality improvement strategy and can identify possible obstacles to effective implementation.

5. High-functioning teams empower people by providing opportunities for meaningful participation in problem identification and problem solving. Participants feel they are contributing in a positive way to the success of the organization, and more than simply through their particular discipline. Among the consequences of empowerment is that people feel greater commitment to the organization and exhibit a sense of ownership. Together these promote in people a greater willingness to identify quality problems and participate in developing and implementing solutions.

As seen in the introductory organ-donation case, the well-intentioned manager tasked with solving an institution-wide problem was unable to compose his team of the most appropriate members, the team was unable to realize these benefits, was unable to become a high-performing team, and was unable to reach its goals. The manager's inability to build an appropriate team was, in turn, a function of an unrealistic timeline and a lack of initial support by senior management. Given a second chance, and provided with a more appropriate timeline and sufficient authority, the manager built a team of individuals with appropriate experience and organizational diversity, which was able to develop, perform, and reach its goals. Such well-designed and managed teams can maximize communication, collaboration, patient and staff satisfaction, and effective and efficient clinical care provision in an organization that is continually able to adapt and improve in the changing environment.

How do we develop and sustain high-performing quality improvement teams? There is much that we know about successful teams, and while there is no guarantee that using all of the concepts and recommendations in this chapter will bring success, it provides a framework to use to assess the likelihood of team success and guide intervention in specific areas to improve performance.

## UNDERSTANDING AND IMPROVING THE PERFORMANCE OF QUALITY IMPROVEMENT TEAMS

In this section we present information about teams and their management, relate the information specifically to the area of quality improvement teams, and use our case examples to illustrate selective concepts and principles.

### The Task

The particular task given a group affects many other aspects of team management, such as team size, and team composition, and the manner in which decisions are made. Most quality improvement teams are faced with the task, generally speaking, of engaging in the PDCA cycle: Planning, Doing, Checking, Acting. They are typically also involved in problem analysis, and often in identifying alternative courses of action.

The clarity of the task as well as the authority of the team to carry out the PDCA cycle is very important. Related to this, the team must have a shared understanding of the goals of the team.

Although certain types of teams have clear and self-evident goals, quality improvement teams may face ambiguity. Most commonly, teams are unclear about their authority to implement change. Does a team have the authority to make decisions about change or simply to make recommendations? There is no magic answer to this question; many highly variable factors ranging from organizational priorities to intraorganizational dynamics to environmental changes may drive such a decision. What is most important is that teams have a clear understanding of their goals and their authority, whatever those goals and that authority may be. It is disheartening and demoralizing for a team to *think* it has the authority to implement a change only to face the reality that the team is intended only to suggest or recommend. Goals do sometimes change in quality improvement efforts, particularly as more fundamental problems are identified that underlay the presenting problems.

As illustrated in the Greenwood Family Practice (see In-Practice 6–2), goal definition presents a problem. The initial goal in this situation was to improve the provision of preventive services. However, little analytic effort was spent trying to understand the important causes of this problem. The team adopted a premature solution, and the goal drifted away from improving preventive service rates to constructing and implementing a Preventive Services Chart (PSC). While such a chart may have been useful as part of the solution to the performance gap in preventive services, the team became fixated on this as *the solution,* at the expense of generating other additional alternatives. Implementing a solution became the goal, losing the initial focus on the problem of low preventive services rates. Team member time was spent constructing a tool instead of trying to understand the fundamental causes of the problem. Basically a "solution" presented itself, and the solution became the goal in itself. A key problem faced as a result of this is that the team did not work on what seemed to be a very major problem facing the practice, namely the variation in protocols for preventive services. The team also did not sufficiently examine the problem of recordkeeping, and never did come to an understanding of whether their rates were really low, or if the problem was an artifact of poor record keeping. As discussed later, effective leadership may have kept the team on task and focused on its primary goal.

**In-Practice 6–2:** Preventive Services at Greenwood Family
Medicine

Greenwood Family Practice is a five-clinician family medicine
practice serving a largely middle class suburban population. In addition to the medical staff, the practice employs four nurses, one receptionist, and three medical records and insurance technicians.

The practice recently held a one-day retreat and identified two priority areas: attention to family concerns, and greater emphasis on ensuring the provision of timely preventive services. One of the physicians recently attended a continuing medical education program on
preventive services. Upon her return, she decided to assess the practice's provision of preventive services.

With a nurse and one of the medical records technicians, a sample
of children's patient charts was reviewed. She and the other physicians were surprised when she distributed the results:

- Half of the children were behind schedule in at least one
  immunization
- Vision screening was noted on no patient charts.
- Fifty percent of children had had anemia screening
- Twenty-five percent of children had their blood pressure
  recorded in chart
- Fifteen percent had had tuberculosis screening
- Thirteen percent of child were screened for lead

The medical staff was surprised by these findings, but medical
records personnel and nursing staff found this information consistent
with their impressions. The review indicated that even children who
were seen for an annual physical were often not updated on preventive services—or this information was not recorded in the patient
chart. It was felt that high patient volume made it impossible to ensure that appropriate preventive services were provided to all children. In addition, the practice saw many drop-in patients. The nurses
felt that while these drop-ins caused added tension from the increased workload, they also presented an opportunity to check on
preventive services needs.

*continues*

**In-Practice 6–2** continued

The findings were discussed at the monthly meeting for all staff, and it was decided to form a team to address the problem. A medical records technician was asked to schedule a meeting. It was decided that two nurses and four physicians would participate on this team.

The first meeting was scheduled over the noon hour (12:00 to 1:00). One physician arrived at 12:20 while another had to leave early, at 12:45. Virtually the entire meeting was spent attempting to find an appropriate date and time for follow-up meetings.

At the next meeting, the physicians stated that during an acute visit, physicians simply didn't have time to go through the chart to determine if a patient needed updating on preventive services. It was decided, therefore, that the nurses would review each chart for the day's patients and fasten a form listing all preventive services. Services needing updating would be circled. The medical records staff was asked to design this form.

When the physicians saw the resulting form, they felt it was poorly designed. Some services were not included, and immunization schedule information was not included. The physicians asked the medical records technician to redesign the form. The technician and a nurse to added the immunization schedule and other information. When presented to the physicians, they discovered disagreements in several areas. Immunization schedules differed, and practices varied on lead and TB screening. They decided that the form should include separate columns for each physician, each column specifying a physician's preventive services preferences. A form was created reflecting each physician's preventive service preferences.

After the new preventive services chart (PSC) was developed, the nurses expressed concern about the lack of time available to record preventive services needs, but agreed reluctantly to start reviewing charts and entering preventive service information on each chart. After six weeks of working with this system, the following events unfolded:

- Nurses complained that medical records staff were not making charts available in time to do the preventive services review.
- Physicians complained among themselves that preventive service information was incomplete or inaccurate in over 50% of the cases.

*continues*

**In-Practice 6–2** continued

- Nurses were spending an additional 1 to 2 hours in the office preparing the next day's files and complained that the charts were very hard to decipher. The nurses requested, and were denied, overtime pay. One nurse left the practice.
- Confusion was rampant when charts were prepared for one physician, but another physician actually saw the patient. This caused increased patient waiting time. An even more difficult problem was caused by drop-ins for whom the record review was not prepared. Nurses spent up to 30 minutes reviewing drop-in charts and recording relevant information. Backlogs resulted and nurses neglected their other roles.
- The system was eliminated and physicians decided to independently deal with preventive services.

## Team Characteristics

Team characteristics refer to basic physical and psychological aspects of a team and include team composition and size, team relationships and status differences, psychological safety, team norms, and the stage of team development. Each is discussed below.

## Team Composition and Size

What is the optimal team size? This obviously depends upon the nature of the team, its goals, and tasks. In some cases, team size and composition are mandated. Examples of this include sports teams and accreditation teams. Teams must be sufficiently large to have the requisite expertise, but not so large that they are cumbersome and difficult to manage. A team size of seven is a general rule of thumb, although this number is derived from experience rather than scientific evidence. In Greenwood Family Medicine, the team faced multiple problems because of its large size: scheduling meetings, keeping order during meetings, establishing a protocol for discussion, and decision making.

Interestingly, although the team was too large, it in fact did not have all of the expertise required to address the preventive services problem. Specifically, the medical records staff, which foresaw the difficulties with the new system, were not included on the team—even to selectively provide input or react to proposed solutions. When deciding upon team composition, one needs to consider the tasks facing the team. For example, if information is required about information technology, it would naturally be helpful to have someone knowledgeable in this area. In the Greenwood Family Medicine case, abstracting information from medical records was a key aspect of the intervention. Medical records staff familiar with the structure of the medical record could have contributed substantially to the design of this intervention.

Team size therefore goes hand-in-hand with group composition. The team must have adequate diversity and expertise to inform all necessary aspects of the team's tasks and goals. Yet the team must not be so large that reaching consensus or following an appropriate timeline is impossible. In Greenwood Family Practice, it would have been advisable to cut the team size by 50%, and ask team members to consult and obtain input from their constituencies about the team's work.

### Team Relationships and Status

A central tenet of quality improvement is participation of all team members. We often learn of quality problems and solutions from individuals without formal authority in the team or organization. In fact, it is often those on the front lines—people working within the clinical microsystem—who have a unique perspective on a situation. Involving appropriate people is only the first step, however. In any team, people bring with them their roles and status from regular organizational life. Physicians working on a team with nurses bring with them their higher professional status and authority. The physician-nurse relationship is thus "imported" into the team. And these preformed relationships and status systems influence the effectiveness of a team. The most obvious example is that of status differences stifling participation. Individuals from a lower status group are less likely to contribute than those of higher status. They may feel condescended to, intimidated, or may simply feel that their input is not valued. For quality improvement teams, such status differences are dysfunctional. Quality improvement team leaders need to find a way to diminish the impact of status differences.

Team members also bring with them other aspects of interrelationships from outside of the team. We may find two individuals with a history of interpersonal problems serving on the same team. Unfortunately, relationship problems and dysfunctional status differences can dramatically affect the work of a team. It is truly the remarkable team that can dispose of status differences and interpersonal animosities in the interest of team goals. At the very least, team leaders need to be aware of the presence of status differences and the impact of those differences on communication and team effectiveness. One way to avoid the problems of status difference and interpersonal conflict is to have a team leader with sufficient authority and respect to be a moderator, encouraging lower status members to participate, keeping higher status members in check, and defusing tension driven by team member conflict.

Quality improvement teams often come together amidst great enthusiasm about tackling a difficult problem. However, the work of a group may create frictions and bring to the surface latent conflicts or reignite old disputes. Interprofessional rivalries may also surface in quality improvement teams, and multidisciplinary teams should explicitly agree to put aside such conflicts. Otherwise, a substantial amount of work time will likely be spent managing these conflicts. Quality improvement teams, like other teams, are also prone to personality clashes that may be very destructive to the work of a team. Health care is particularly prone to difficulties posed by status differences because of the traditional professional hierarchy that is still maintained in most organizations.

In Greenwood Family Practice, status differences were destructive to the work of the group. First, medical records staff were not included, likely because they were considered nonprofessional staff and thus their perspectives and opinions discounted. Status differences, with likely elements of intimidation, also prevented both nurses and medical records staff from voicing their reservations about the use of the Preventive Services Chart. There was also tension and status differences between the two "high-volume" physicians and others in the practice. These differences were not beneficial to the work of the team.

## Psychological Safety

Team psychological safety is defined as a shared belief that the team is safe for interpersonal risk taking (Edmonson 1999). A central tenet of quality improvement is the belief that people must be forthcoming and honest about quality problems. Individuals involved in improvement efforts must feel that their suggestions will be heard without fear of intimidation, condescension, or castigation. Where people feel this safety, there is a greater likelihood of their participating effectively in quality improvement efforts. Further, psychological safety is an important prerequisite for implementing organizational change. People need to feel psychologically safe if they are to feel secure and capable of changing (Schein & Bennis 1965).

Status differences certainly affect psychological safety. Where status differences have an oppressive presence, it is very unlikely that team participants will feel the willingness to participate in discussions of quality. In the Greenwood Family Practice case, the medical records staff had a clear sense that the Preventive Services Chart plan was doomed to failure, but felt uninvited. Although they voiced reservations about the plan privately, they did not feel psychologically safe to voice their concerns. More than likely, they would have been criticized by others in the practice for being negative, resistant to change, or perhaps lazy. This is similar to the Donor Services case (In-Practice 6–1), where many of the lower status team members were reluctant to participate actively or positively given the negative and highly vocal nature of the Medical Examiner, a higher status individual with whom many of the team members had to work on a daily basis. They felt that if they didn't follow his lead in the team meetings, they would incur repercussions later.

Team leaders need to consider questions of psychological safety: do participants feel safe in making recommendations, participating in discussions, and perhaps of greatest importance, expressing skepticism and disagreement? It is only by creating such a climate that team members will not become "yes-men and yes-women."

## Team Norms

A norm is a standard of behavior that is shared by team members. Norms have a strong impact on individuals in organizations, essentially establishing the "rules" under which people function. Norms set expectations and establish standards of behavior and performance. Behavioral norms consist of the rules that govern the work of individuals. In a team context, behavioral norms might designate how people are expected to participate on a team, attendance at meetings, the type of language and dress that are acceptable, and the use of formal procedures (e.g., Robert's Rules of Order). Norms are different in every team. In Greenwood Family Medicine we see the interaction between status differences and norms. Although there was likely a superficial belief in the desirability of a democratic and participative climate, it was clear that among the behavioral norms of the team was that of hierarchy. For example, nurses were directed to produce a form (and then several versions), and physicians declared the termination of the quality improvement initiative. Norms about attendance at meetings were very loose—at least for the medical staff. One meeting, in which arguments ensued about whether the preventive services issue was office-wide or specific to the physicians, ended with no conclusion, summary, or future plans. Evidently, norms were never established for how meetings would be conducted or expectations for attendance. Collectively, these were dysfunctional norms. Participation was inhibited, full discussion of issues was repressed, and meetings were inefficient and ineffective.

In contrast to behavioral norms, performance norms govern the amount and quality of work expected of team members. In the Greenwood Family Practice case, performance norms were broken, leading to difficulties for the practice. While there were expectations about working hours for nurses, the new Preventive Services Chart system caused them to work up to three hours after regular working hours. This change in work demand was not anticipated, and breaking this performance norm caused morale problems and the departure of at least one nurse.

## Stage of Team Development

Teams go through various life cycle stages, and different tasks and levels of productivity characterize each stage. We can conveniently think of teams going through four stages: forming, storming, norming, and performing. A team begins in the forming stage when goals and tasks are established. It is characterized by generally polite behavior among team members, which may mask underlying conflicts. Individuals often do not feel psychologically safe at this time, and may be reluctant to contribute and disagree. Team members, still unclear about the norms of the team, may stand back until they get a sense of the team.

When team members begin to feel more comfortable, there is usually a period of "storming," which may be mild or severe. Team members may compete for roles, may argue about team goals and processes, or may simply attempt to stake out their ground.

If the team resolves its storming stage (and this is not necessarily the case), a norming stages emerges in which there is agreement on team norms and expectations. Team member roles are clarified, although these may change during the life of a team. Following the norming stage is a performing stage in which the team is in the best position to accomplish its goals. Conflicts have been resolved, roles are clear, norms are established, and team time can be spent on the substantive work of the team rather than on resolving issues of process.

Teams can and do function at all stages of their development. However, at earlier stages, much energy is lost to "process loss," that is, focusing the team's energies and time on team maintenance functions rather than on the substantive work of the team. Teams are most effective when they have matured, that is, they have successfully progressed through the first three stages and are able to focus upon team goals and tasks.

What stage of development was the Greenwood Family Practice team? The team assembled for the preventive services improvement project included virtually all members of the practice. This team did not show evidence of maturity. Norms of behavior were unclear (for example, attendance at meetings), decision making and rules for discussion were not well developed, and perhaps most importantly, role relationships among participants still reflected their roles in the practice. Physicians assumed a rather superior role in the practice, which may or may not have been appropriate. On the improvement team, however, such a role was clearly inappropriate and blocked the team from accessing information needed to address the preventive services problem. It is likely that the events that transpired in this case could have been predicted from observing the team in its normal operations.

## RESOURCES AND SUPPORT

As open systems, teams require resources in order to survive and flourish. Resources come in a number of forms, including financial resources, intellectual resources, information, people with the necessary knowledge, skills and abilities, equipment, communication systems, and moral support and credibility. Further, individual team members require support, including recognition for their work on the team and rewards for their performance. At the most fundamental level, a team functions best when ensconced within an organization that supports the concept of teamwork, and more specifically, respects the work done by the team. We begin our discussion of resources and support at this level, which we refer to as organizational culture.

## Organizational Culture

Many definitions have been suggested for organizational culture. Broadly speaking, organizational culture refers to the fabric of values, beliefs, assumptions, myths, norms, goals, and visions that are widely shared in the organization (French 1998). An organization can have a single culture, although there are often subcultures within the organization. Among health care organizations, for example, we would expect to see cultural differences between a large teaching hospital and a small rural medical practice. Within an organization, teams themselves can develop their own culture, which may include (like ethnic cultures) rituals, a specific language, particular modes of communication, and unique systems of rewards and sanctions.

Organizational culture has a number of implications for teams. First, effective teams are usually characterized by strong cultures that are supportive of the work of the team. In a quality improvement team, for example, we would hope to see a culture characterized by interdisciplinary respect, open communication, and a collective spirit. It would be very difficult to imagine a successful quality improvement team that does not share these and other cultural characteristics. However, a team can have an appropriate culture but be enmeshed within an organization with a contrary culture. Kiassi *et al.* (2004) report that organizations select those quality improvement programs that fit with their existing cultures.

Consider an organization characterized by intense and dysfunctional competition, low staff participation in decision making, and interprofessional rivalries and antagonism. We can consider this type of organization as having a dissonant culture (Fleeger 1993). Notwithstanding the skills of an effective team leader, can we really expect team members drawn from such an environment to perform effectively on a multidisciplinary team? More than likely team member attitudes would mirror their attitudes and behaviors outside of the team. Team members would probably exhibit distrust, a "them versus us" norm, and skepticism about their role in decision making. Consider the behavior and attitudes of team members drawn from a positive or consonant culture. We would expect team members to bring with them the very supportive cultural attributes of the larger organization; this would contribute to team growth and performance. We can see how the larger organizational culture can be viewed as a resource: the larger culture can be highly supportive, unsupportive, or in fact destructive to the work of the team.

Cultures are very difficult to change, so team leaders and participants must understand the impact of the culture of the larger organization on the work and culture of the team. Team members' negative or dysfunctional attitudes may simply reflect how they are treated in the larger organization. Team leaders should acknowledge the difficulty of leading a participative improvement team within a larger organizational culture that is nonparticipative and autocratic. Staff who work in a rigid, overbearing culture are likely to become skeptical when suddenly asked to participate in decision making, wondering whether their opinions will be valued, and so forth. Continuous quality improvement efforts in health care often confront this contradictory culture issue, experiencing the difficulties of attempting to introduce a culture that is inconsistent with the dominant organizational culture.

In the State Regulatory Agency case (see In-Practice 6–3), there was a culture that stressed the importance of customer relations. Great value was placed on the need to provide accurate and timely information. The team that was formed to analyze and make recommendations about the problem of providing inaccurate information motivated by the same belief in the importance of its service mission. Complaints from customers about poor information were greeted with sincere concern. In no case were attempts made to discount the truthfulness of these complaints.

---

**In-Practice 6–3:** Erroneous Information at a State Regulatory Agency

The Department of Health and Emergency Services is a state regulatory agency dealing with a variety of health care professional issues. Its roles include credentialing emergency medical service (EMS) personnel, providers and educational institutions; developing and enforcing administrative code; and serving as a primary collection point for statewide EMS data. Among its most important roles

*continues*

**In-Practice 6–3** continued

is responding to requests for information about credentialing requirements for health and EMS personnel. These requests come from physicians, hospitals, EMS providers, city and county governments, and other organizations.

The agency has one main office and three regional offices. The main office has thirty staff; each regional office is staffed by five to seven staff. Each regional office has a regional manager reporting to the Operations Section Chief. Since each regional office serves approximately one-third of the state the volume of requests can be overwhelming. Each staff member is responsible for serving as primary contact for 8 to 14 counties.

The agency recently learned that a significant amount of inaccurate information has been distributed by regional staff. The agency learned about this problem from complaints that inaccurate and contradictory information had been given out. For example, a hospital requested information about how nurses could challenge the EMS exam. The hospital was informed that nurses could challenge the EMS exam when in fact agency policy prohibits any healthcare provider from challenging a credentialing exam

In response to this problem, the agency Director formed an Education/Credentialing Team with one liaison in each regional office and the team leader in the main office. The team's goals included improving consistency among the three regional offices, ensuring accurate information distribution, and educating regional staff on agency policy. In addition to the team leader and regional office liaisons, the team also included members representing each specialty within the agency. These specialists would provide technical information about their particular specialty and serve as primary contact for regional offices in their area of expertise.

The team met monthly for twelve months to discuss issues and develop policy. One of its first tasks was to determine the underlying reason(s) for its information dissemination problem. The team obtained information from its membership and through discussions with other staff in the state and regional offices, EMS providers, physicians and educational institutions. Information was obtained through formal and informal discussions, surveys, and through a web-based forum.

*continues*

**In-Practice 6–3** continued

Among the team's discoveries was that staff did not have clear channels of communication with senior management, and were not informed about changes in regulatory requirements. The team also learned that regional office staff were trying to be "experts" in too many different fields.

The team suggested a number of changes, including:

- Assigning each regional staff member an area of specialization where they would serve the entire region instead of 8 to 14 counties. For example, a provider specialist that would be the primary point of contact for all provider issues for the entire regional office.
- Each of these specialist will serve as the regional office representative on all statewide and intra-agency committees that focus on that area of specialization
- Each regional manager will serve on a committee with senior management that will meet monthly to ensure that up-to-date information is distributed to each regional office

These changes were implemented at the state and regional offices. Mandatory committee attendance was difficult because of statewide travel restrictions and budget shortfalls. These obstacles were overcome by using advanced computer technology and telecommunications. Other obstacles included changes in job descriptions that were resisted by several "old timers." Their fears were eased by giving them an opportunity to assist with writing their job description.

Six months after these changes were put in place, the distribution of incorrect credentialing information dramatically decreased. Specialists in the regional offices actively consulted other specialists to learn about current policy in their area. An informal telephone survey found consistent information dissemination from each regional office. Among the most successful strategies was formation of teams. This promoted consistency in information exchange and developed interagency communication between all regional offices and the main office. It was also felt that success was attributed in large part to the manner in which team members were selected and how it functioned.

*continues*

**In-Practice 6–3** continued

The team concept has continued to grow within the agency and-currently every staff member within the agency serves on at least one team. Some members serve on several teams and have taken on additional work responsibilities because the team approach has provided them the opportunity to have a strong voice within the agency. Senior leadership was careful not to push the team approach too fast and did not force anyone to join a team right away. Since the education team was formed first, management emphasized the work that team performed and allowed the education team to provide monthly updates to staff. This helped show that voice is important within the agency and that if staff work together as a team the team will have a significant influence on agency policy as well as administrative code.

## Material and Nonmaterial Support and Recognition

Regardless of their function, effective teams require material resources. As noted above, material resources come in a number of forms and vary depending upon the purposes and needs of the team. Provision of necessary material and nonmaterial support to a team is a reflection of the moral support and encouragement given a team by the larger organization and, in particular, senior management or other authority. Consider a team that is given appropriate space and time to meet, where senior managers on occasion voluntarily drop in on team meetings to provide information or simply to reinforce the importance of a team's task, and where support staff are assigned to the team to assist in its work. Further, while the team is given a specific mandate and set of goals, the team decides the manner in which it carries out most of its work. Finally, upon presenting a preliminary report, detailed feedback and questions are provided the team. In all likelihood, team members will feel as if their work is valued and that the team's work is indeed making a contribution to the larger organization. Consistent with the motivational and satisfying qualities of jobs defined in the Job Characteristics Model, such a team provides teams and team members with autonomy, feedback, a sense of meaningfulness, and a belief that their work is having a broad impact (Hackman and Oldham 1980). In sum, teams given appropriate support can be highly motivating. Where this support is absent or ambiguous, teams will be starved for support and will be unlikely to produce at an optimal level.

The State Regulatory Agency case provides a good example of how a team was provided with adequate support. Perhaps the most important resource provided this time was the time and energy of various individuals internal and external to the agency. Time was provided for team meetings and team members felt that the work they were doing was worthwhile and valued by others in the larger organization. Where travel restrictions posed obstacles to team members meeting, computer technology—telecommunications and teleconferencing—was used. This again reinforced the importance, not only of the team's work but also of the importance of each team member's contributions.

## Rewards

Related to support and recognition is the need for team and individual rewards. From the perspective of the team, rewards typically come in the form of recognition and commendation for the team's work. In quality improvement, team rewards usually consist of the intrinsic satisfaction of achieving results. Rewards may also consist of the positive feelings created by a successful team effort.

In addition to team rewards, individuals on teams need to be rewarded. Participation on teams is often thought of as something of a voluntary effort, that it is really not a part of a staff member's "real job." Job descriptions themselves may indicate little about team participation. Performance appraisals may not include team participation criteria, and compensation and promotion decisions may not take into consideration a staff member's contribution to the work of a team.

It is likely that an organization that is team-oriented will be more likely to recognize individual contributions on teams. Performance appraisal and incentive pay programs will explicitly consider team member contributions. Such systems may actually elicit performance feedback from team members and leaders. If team meetings are to be held after normal work hours, appropriate compensation is provided.

Rewards are therefore important from the perspective of both the team and its individual members. Like individuals, teams are motivated by appropriate recognition and rewards. Individuals working on teams should receive the message that their participation on teams is important, necessary, and a key part of their jobs.

Members of the State Regulatory Agency team were able to see the consequences of their work, namely a substantial decrease in the amount of erroneous information provided and better relations with their customers. Team members also saw their recommendations put into action, which communicated to team members the value of the team's work. This set the stage for a more team-focused agency and the likelihood that future team efforts would meet with success.

## TEAM PROCESSES

Team processes refer to those aspects of the team dealing with leadership, communication, decision making, and member and team learning. Each of these factors can have an important effect on the effectiveness of a team.

### Leadership

Leadership in teams refers to the ability of individuals to influence other members toward the achievement of the team's goals. Note the use of the word *individuals* rather than leader; as discussed below, an individual with no formal authority may emerge as a leader and influence member behavior.

There is no single model of leadership that is appropriate for all teams. Depending upon the team's purpose, leadership may be focused on one individual, while in others leadership may be shared or rotated among team members. Teams also have formal and informal leaders. A sports team, for example, may have a coach or manager, but there clearly can be informal leaders, usually not specifically appointed as such, but nevertheless assuming a leadership function. A multidisciplinary healthcare team may have a nominal team leader, but typically power and authority flow to that person or persons with specialized expertise. There are therefore numerous sources of leadership and power. This can be seen in the case of Jones Hospital (see In-Practice 6–4), which has many different, unique programs and program leaders with specific clinical expertise. These providers sometimes work independently, but more often than not work in

**In-Practice 6–4:** Formation of A Medical Center Service Line to Address Needs for Communication and Quality Improvement Service Lines within a Service Line

In 1998, Jones Hospital decided to develop service lines in an effort to better coordinate administrative, clinical, and business development needs of the institution. Jones Hospital is an academic medical center with 850 beds and an operating budget of over $1 billion, The objectives of this initiative were to integrate hospital and physician practice operations and bring together support services in an effort to develop more efficient and effective operational planning, market development, and patient care quality improvement. To accomplish this, the hospital divided all functional areas into thirteen service lines, one of which was the Oncology Clinical Service Unit (CSU). This CSU encompassed, among others, inpatient medical oncology units, radiation oncology, and the adult bone marrow transplant program.

A few of the organization's goals were realized in the four years after the creation of the CSU structure: communication among functional areas was enhanced, identification of strategic opportunities was improved, and day-to-day management was stronger. However, expectations were not met regarding strategic plan development, collaborative business plan development, resource allocation, and revenue management. It was noted that the challenges of meeting organizational goals were in part due to the continuing decentralized management of several critical areas. Even with the creation of the CSU, other oncology areas remained independent of the service line: the Jones Oncology Network, the NCI-designated Comprehensive Cancer Center, the Tumor Registry, the Cancer Protocol Coordination Team, the medical school clinical departments, and the faculty practice plan's outpatient clinics. These, in addition to various support functions such as Management Engineering and Medical Center Finance, were critical to success with oncology strategy and operations. Yet, there was no structure that pulled the various constituencies together to work toward improving cancer patient care.

To address this problem, the medical center conducted a review of all oncology service areas and related support functions, including

*continues*

**In-Practice 6–4** continued

an assessment of specific challenges attributable to the current infrastructure. The review and assessment revealed operational fragmentation due to a lack of coordination and communication, independent priority setting among areas, few change-implementation efforts, and a misalignment of incentives regarding both compensation and patient flow. Further, the review pointed to the near impossibility of developing strategic and business plans for growing patient populations since there was not an agreed-upon process for developing and approving such plans among the many stakeholders.

To address these difficulties, the CSU developed an internal program model to enhance efficiency and effectiveness by taking a patient-centered, quality improvement approach. Based on the major cancer patient populations, specific programs were created inside the CSU, including the Adult Bone Marrow Transplant Program, the Breast Oncology Program, the GI Oncology Program, and the GYN Oncology Program, among others. Each program operated using a matrix model centered on the cancer patient experience. This structure allows the CSU and others to focus on the needs of specific patient populations regardless of location or type of service. It reduces the organizational unit to a more manageable size in which problems can more easily be identified, analyzed, and solved by the people who are (a) the most familiar with the specific needs of each type of patient; and (b) the most capable of developing a solution.

Two groups provide the leadership for this new structure: the Strategic Governance Council and the Program Meeting. Both comprise representatives from all areas of oncology. The Strategic Governance Council addresses issues of strategic direction and includes the most senior physician from each of the major areas of oncology in addition to the senior administrator from the service line, physician practice plan, oncology clinics, and oncology outreach program. This Council sets the strategic direction and approves all plans in a well-defined planning process. The Program Meeting leads the operational implementation of the strategies and plans created by the Strategic Governance Council, and further serves as the central forum for communication of strategic priorities and progress

*continues*

---

**In-Practice 6–4** continued

reports on major projects and issues for all oncology operations, health system-wide.

Critical factors contributing to the successful creation of this new structure included agreement on planning processes and sufficient resourcing by centralized services such as informatics, finance, clinical laboratories, pharmacy, and radiology. The creation of the new model has resulted in significant improvements in communication, planning, and resource management; cooperation among the many stakeholders; shared decision-making regarding strategic and operational plans; expedited operational problem resolution; and a dramatic financial improvement in the service line overall.

---

concert to collaboratively provide multidisciplinary care for a heterogeneous oncology patient population. While these individuals guide their individual programs' operations on a daily basis, these program leaders are unified under the constructs of the Strategic Governance Council and Program Meetings, where the roles and influence of each are formalized, and they are each able to communicate in a fairly respectful and egalitarian environment. These forums provide information to the Oncology Leadership Group, which distills the information of the larger forums into guiding principals and strategies for Oncology Services as a whole. While the Leadership Group has a physician head that holds authority within the Group, it is not possible to say that this position holds unilaterally directive authority over all the programs. The position and indeed the Group serve to integrate the perspectives and needs of the multidisciplinary programs, and as such provide continuity and uniformity of vision, strategy, and upward and outward communication for the Oncology Service Line as they seek to continuously improve clinical care and the health care experience for the oncology patient population.

Where a team task is clear and unambiguous, a top-down leadership style may be justified, although even in such settings, input from team members may be valuable. In essence, the role of a leader in such a situation is to see that the job is done and that team members communicate and coordinate their work. In the quality improvement area, however, leadership must take on a different look. Quality improvement is by definition ambiguous; quality improvement is largely a problem-solving process. Team members participate on a quality improvement team because they have expertise that needs to be brought to bear on the problem. Team members do not need to be told what to do, but rather to participate actively in identifying problems, analyzing causation, developing interventions, evaluating the impact of change, and so forth. Team members are brought onto a quality improvement team because no single person has the expertise to solve a particular problem. Team member passivity is most definitely not an appropriate strategy.

So we can see that the style of leadership most appropriate in quality improvement is one that emphasizes participation and that builds trust among team members. It is a style that encourages members to express their views and to take risks, and that develops the team and helps it to become mature and more effective. All of these traits can be seen in the Jones Hospital Oncology Service line. Leadership must also focus on keeping people engaged, motivated, and stimulated to creativity and innovation. Quality improvement teams are, if not voluntary, dependent upon the good will of participants for their success. Some successful teams encourage [WRC9] shared leadership by allowing specific individuals on a team to take on leadership roles for particular phases of the quality improvement process. The overall leader therefore also assumes a training role, helping to develop team members' skills in team leadership and project management.

This participative style is appropriate not because it is humane and fosters a happy workforce (although it is likely to do these things), but because team members' active participation is absolutely essential to success. Because quality improvement teams often do not exist within the formal hierarchical structure of the organization, leaders must certainly attend to issues of motivation and commitment as well.

## Communication Networks and Interaction Patterns

A key maintenance task in any team is the exchange of information. Methods of communication are essential and central in any team activity, whether it is an operating room team, a string quartet, a sports team, or a quality improvement team. Communication is necessary not only within the team, but also between the team and the larger external environment, including other teams. Communication is critical and cannot be left to chance. Consider the consequences, for example, of there being no formal means of communication between attending physicians and nursing staff in a hospital—or if there was no forum for communication among the 30 or more oncology programs at Jones Hospital? This was actually what drove Jones Hospital to completely restructure its organization to a service line format. Communication and coordination deficiencies were identified as the underpinning factors contributing to less than optimal performance, declining patient care coordination and patient satisfaction, and a perception of reduced quality of care.

In any team, information must be conveyed and a key question is how and how effectively and accurately information is exchanged. Like all other teams, quality improvement teams require a communication structure. Interestingly, a substantial proportion of health care quality problems reside in communication structure problems in the organization.

Communication networks come in several varieties, and each situation demands a different type of communication structure. Where the team task is simple, it may be most efficient to use a centralized structure in which information passes from the team leader to other team members. Alternatively, information can be passed from the team leader to another team member who, in a hierarchical manner, passes it down to the next individual. Neither of these models allows for upward communication. In other teams, one individual assumes the role of network hub and communicates with other members. Information from team members must pass through the hub in order to reach other team members. An all-channel communication structure is dense; communication lines are open and encouraged between all members of the team. Such a structure is most useful for complex situations where the work of each team member is interdependent with others' work. In such situations, formal lines of authority are blurred or meaningless. In teams focused on patient care, quality improvement, research, or management, it is important for team members to have ready access to other team members, as is seen in the Oncology Service Line's new structure that provides such access through their formalized communication forums. Information is passed not only from the team leader, but also among team members, making centralized models inappropriate. Similarly, going through an intermediary is inefficient and may use up valuable time.

Quality improvement teams typify teams requiring such a rich communication structure. The work of a quality improvement team is complex, and communication lines must be open between all members. For example, an intervention aimed at decreasing waiting time in a clinic requires interaction between clinicians on the team, support staff within the clinic, those involved in data collection, and so forth. The leader of such a team would assume the important role of ensuring that communication networks are in fact open, and that team members are able to communicate with each other.

Communication between a team and its external environment is also important. As an open system, teams are often dependent upon other individuals and other teams inside or outside the organization. Leaders here assume boundary-spanning roles, in which they ensure that relationships with critical outside groups are workable. This is particularly important in a hospital setting in which a particular work unit's operations are highly dependent upon their interactions with other units (for example, patient care units are highly dependent upon the pharmacy, dietary department, and so forth). The Oncology Leadership Group fills this role for the Oncology Service Line. The Leadership Group is the broker between Oncology and Medical Center Senior Administration for such needs as major redeployments of resources to support Oncology strategic priorities, redesign and reallocation of clinical space, or needs for changes in the operational interface with independent departments such as Pharmacy Services, which, to fit strategic and political needs, maintains an independent departmental structure in the organization. A quality improvement team likely relies upon information and resources from outside of the immediate team, and just as communication networks among team members is critical, so are strong and reliable networks between the team and other units and teams. An isolated team that neglects its external relations is likely to perform poorly because key relationships are not well managed.

**Decision Making**

Decision making is a task of all teams, and the manner in which decisions are made is critical to team success. Teams may reach decisions by consensus, voting, or team members may simply advise the team leader, leaving the final decision to the leader. There is no single best way for a team to make decisions, and the mode of decision making is often dependent upon the circumstances and goals of the team. The president of a hospital, for example, may charge a team with the task of analyzing an acquisition possibility. The team may return with recommendations and options, but the final decision remains with the president. In a multidisciplinary mental health treatment team, it is likely that decisions will be based on team consensus, although the team leader (who may be the psychiatrist) may reserve the right to override the team's recommendations. In still other teams, particularly those where there is no single person in a position of formal authority, the team as a whole may make decisions. In such situations, team members should discuss how decisions are to be made—by voting, working towards consensus and compromise, or perhaps by deferring to the individual most knowledgeable about a particular issue to be decided. Indeed, in the Jones Oncology Service Line, the decision making process and the people who make the decisions are highly dependent on the decisions themselves. Depending on the nature and criticality of the issue at hand, there are decisions made by formal vote in the Strategic Governance Council, informal consensus in the Program Meeting, and by mandate in the Leadership Group. The success of such decision making is dependent upon open communication among the members of these groups—all information is shared, and a record is kept through meeting minutes of all bodies of decisions made. When an individual has a problem with a decision made at the Leadership Group, for example, the forum for discussion of such concerns is formally built in to the Service Line structure via the other two groups.

Regardless of the mode of decision making, it is critical that team members understand their role in decision making. Assuming an advising rather than decision making role is acceptable to team members as long as they do not expect to be in the position of making decisions. The decisional authority of the team and that of team members needs to be specific and clear.

Teams often strive for cohesion, and in general cohesion is a positive force. Efforts should be made to develop a team such that members understand each other, are at ease communicating with each other, and feel a unified sense of purpose and solidarity. Taken to an extreme, however, cohesion can develop into conformity and "group think" in which team members become so cohesive that they lose their independence as free thinkers, and may fear expressing views opposed to what they consider to be the team consensus.

## Member and Team Learning

Peter Senge popularized the idea of the learning organization in his book, *The Fifth Discipline* (1994). A learning organization is one that proactively creates, acquires, and transfers knowledge and that changes its behavior on the basis of new knowledge and insights (Garvin 1993). The implication of this definition for teams is clear. First, effective teams continuously look for new information to improve their performance, whether new technology, new organizational processes, or new concepts. They are open to new ideas and in fact seek them out. They do this by including people on teams with new expertise and alternative perspectives, and by ensuring that team members are engaged in continuous training and learning. Effective teams then attempt to use new information, ensuring that new knowledge is transferred to the team. This new knowledge is then used to change the team's behavior in pursuit of higher levels of achievement. Teams may enhance their ability to learn and apply new knowledge through the use of a number of facilitating factors, including scanning the environment for new information; identifying performance gaps within the team; adopting an "experimental mindset," such that team members are open to new approaches; and having leadership supportive of change. (See Moingeon and Edmonson 1996, for a more in-depth discussion of facilitating factors.)

Team and organizational learning are key aspects of continuous quality improvement, and it is no surprise that the capacity to learn is a hallmark of effective teams. A quality improvement team is faced not only with enhancing the learning of the organization, or the organizational subunit with which it is working, but also with improving the learning and performance of itself as a team. Effective quality improvement teams review their own performance, satisfaction of members, and seek to develop strategies and new team management techniques that will enhance their performance. Some teams "debrief" after each meeting to review the progress of their work and the manner in which they worked, and seek to learn from this and improve their capabilities. Learning from experience and learning from the broader external environment are trademarks of effective organizations and teams.

# PART III

# Implementation

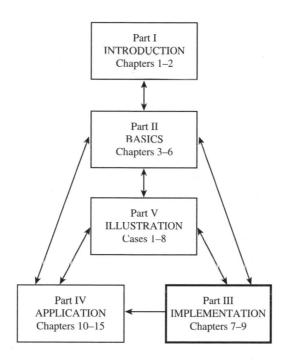

CHAPTER 7

# CQI, Transformation, and the "Learning" Organization[1]

*Vaughn M. Upshaw, Arnold D. Kaluzny,
and Curtis P. McLaughlin*

Managed care has changed how we provide health care and how we manage health care organizations. While the advent of CQI in health care organizations was initially viewed as a panacea for many of the problems associated with quality, the realities of the managed care world have challenged many of these initial expectations of continuous improvement efforts. Consider a few of these realities (Batalden 1996; The Advisory Board Company 1997). "Quality" is not the only criteria by which to judge organizational performance, and cost reduction is the watchword of managerial action.

- Organizations are characterized by "right sizing," "down sizing," and layoffs unprecedented in health services, with declining employee loyalty.
- Improvement initiatives are short-lived, and avoid dealing with the substantive challenges facing the organization.
- "Integration" has not fulfilled expectations and there is increasing interest and experimentation in the "unbundling of provider risk."

Yet managed care and the institutional transformation in the delivery of health care needs its own approach to continuous improvement, a process that goes beyond simply incrementally reducing variance to improve quality, but one that aggressively promotes quality of health services through

---

[1]In part adapted from McLaughlin, C.P. and Kaluzny, A.D. "Total Quality Management Issues in Managed Care," *Journal of Healthcare Financial Management,* 1997:24(1):10–16.

191

organizational learning. The objective of this chapter is to assess the underlying dimensions of the transformation in health services, explore the changing roles for CQI, evaluate new approaches to transformation and organizational learning, and identify strategies for securing physician participation and leadership in organizational learning and change. Organizational learning has been defined as "a process of increasing knowledge and innovating work routines through the interplay of action and reflection that is more extensive than individually focused training and repetition." (Carroll and Edmondson 2002, p. 55) Organizational learning encompasses CQI teams; improvement collaboratives, such as the Institute for Healthcare Improvement's Breakthrough Series; and many health care re-engineering efforts. While this may take on different names, the process is generic. For example, in the United Kingdom, the health system has adopted the term, "clinical governance," a mandated multiprofessional approach to learning and improvement (Heard *et al.* 2001). The aim of clinical governance is to establish a culture of quality improvement through the "10 Cs", which are:

- Clinical performance
- Clinical leadership
- Clinical audit
- Clinical risk management
- Complaints
- Continuing health needs assessments
- Changing practice through evidence
- Continuing education
- Culture of excellence
- Clear accountability

## TRANSFORMING HEALTH CARE

A fundamental change accompanying the transition to managed care is that the locus of control for technological decision making in health services has moved from the individual professional to the organization (Hurley 1997). Managers assume that greater control over costs and quality will be achieved through managed care mechanisms, such as DRG reimbursements, capitation, or prior approvals. However, the dynamic nature of work processes within health care organizations may or may not be consistent with the implementation or use of these managed care approaches. The challenge is to effectively and efficiently provide a continuum of clinical products, each with sufficient variability to adapt to the individual needs of patients and providers.

The practice and management of health services will undergo continued refinements and further codification, however, these changes will be successful only if they are accompanied by organizational learning as a way to speed up the adoption of evidence-based practices and still enable the customization of care to meet the needs and expectations of providers and patients, that is, an institutional commitment to expand the organization's capacity to maintain or improve performance based on its own experience and reflection; utilizing the skill, insights and knowledge of individuals within the organization; and using that knowledge, skill and insight to meet the challenges of new situations (DiBella *et al.* 1996; Carroll and Edmondson 2002). Appropriately practiced in health services, CQI is one of the building blocks for institutional knowledge and learning, but will not succeed without active participation from physicians who bring intellectual capital and can provide key leadership to facilitate learning and innovation.

Traditionally, managers merely consulted or hired a health care professional to determine whether managerial strategies would be in serious conflict with physicians' methods, norms, and values; organizational values; or the patient's interests. Health care managers were neither concerned with, nor technically prepared to evaluate clinical performance. However, the growth of managed care has assumed greater organizational responsibility and control over clinical issues.

Why the change? The continuous and significant introduction of science and technology into the art of medicine over the last fifty years had made possible, perhaps inevitable, a shift from the craft or guild structure of medicine toward an industrial structure As described in Chapter 1, most sectors are in some stage of the transition to mass customization (Boynton *et al.* 1993). Manufacturing industries went through the first step, adopting mass production approaches, in the late 19th and 20th centuries.

Medicine and many other professional services have made this transition much later because of insufficient predictability of cause-and-effect and the natural variability inherent in their work processes, and because of the high degree of autonomy and highly decentralized, local organizational structures (McLaughlin 1996). The historical analogy—the craft guild—was especially applicable to physician practices that were often referred to as a cottage industry. As with most technological change, the transition did not take place until all the factors—technical, economic, and social—were aligned.

In the 1970s and 1980s, hospitals served as the industrializing institutions of health care. They amassed large amounts of capital and absorbed the emerging technologies quickly. Some even experimented with mass production; for example, the surgicenter focused on cataract removal (McLaughlin *et al.* 1995). However, they tended not to employ physicians but rather operated as the physician's workplace. As the hospital became increasingly corporate, an uneasy truce developed between the craft orientation of the physicians and the hospital's industrial model. Health care went through a period of rapid technological change where the increased technical capacity also meant increasing costs. Employer concerns about rising health care costs and the obvious excesses of fee-for-service medicine created a demand for managed care.

## ACCEPTING CONTINUOUS IMPROVEMENT

Hospitals were once considered impersonal at best and, at worst, dangerous. Organizations made little effort to promote institutional learning and the institution had little or no control over the performance of professional personnel. Even today, hospitals find variable needs of individual patients and providers are often poorly accommodated. Information flows are fragmented and unreliable, and glaring differences in costs and outcomes are evident to those paying claims. Because of the craft nature of medicine, best practices are not easily disseminated nor widely adopted. Each provider has considerable autonomy over his or her work, often maintaining practices which are questionable or simply obsolete (Davies and Harrison 2003).

The adoption and institutionalization of continuous improvement provided an opportunity to better manage professional personnel. The alternative is a "culture of entrapment" in which autonomy works against learning and where shallow, but plausible, justifications impede even obviously necessary improvements (Weick and Sutcliffe 2003). Continuous improvement assumes capabilities for process dynamism and institutional learning. Teams within the institution, usually multidisciplinary teams, work cooperatively on the improvement of the institution's processes. Establishing ownership of patient-level processes that integrate professionally-dominated knowledge and skills is one of CQI's objectives. One might even go so far as to classify this as capturing a competitive edge in intellectual capital. This was not a problem when the intellectual capital was assumed to be that of the professionals and not the institution. However, there is evidence that in the future processes improvements may not be shared among the profession, once they are considered to be competitive weapons of organizations (McLaughlin and Johnson 1995).

## CONTINUOUS IMPROVEMENT AND MANAGED CARE

Managed care covers a variety of organizational forms. Some forms of managed care maintain provider autonomy (as in an IPA or PPO) but oversees care delivery processes by monitoring and comparing the results among providers on broad criteria such as cost, readmission rates, etc. Other less open systems, such as a staff model or group model HMOs, give greater attention to the actual process of care applying various CQI innovations initiated by both the clinicians and corporate-level managers and staff.

Fully integrated systems may have multiple internal perspectives seeking to improve a single treatment process. For example, epidemiological research, cost containment, cost analysis, and care delivery units may all undertake CQI activities for a particular disease process. These four perspectives are likely to differ not only in the technology they use, but also with respect to evaluative standards, quality criteria, economic criteria, the relevant time horizon, and the relationship to the enrollee population. Although difficulties can result when these perspectives are at odds with one another, the opportunity for organizational learning greatly improves when these groups communicate with each other and share their respective views.

Continuous improvement is well aligned with many elements of managed care such as DRG reimbursement, capitation, and prior approvals. By continually seeking to reduce errors and improve processes, CQI offers an opportunity to facilitate the larger transformation of health care organizations. Under DRG reimbursement systems, institutions are paid a flat amount for a specific type of admission based on a measure of industry best practices and it is assumed that institutions will exercise sufficient control over their processes to operate within that cost range. Under capitation, providers receive a flat monthly fee for providing a specified set of services to enrolled individuals during that period. Providers are expected to profit on the basis of their ability to appropriately manage the care for people enrolled. Other cost containment procedures such as prior approvals for admissions and surgical procedures assume that employees possess sufficient technical knowledge to accept or countermand the decisions of the clinician. Prior approvals assume institutional knowledge is superior to the professional training and knowledge of providers.

Fundamental to the application of both CQI and managed care is the mutability and dynamic nature of clinical processes and the ability of both institutions and clinicians to improve their performance over time. Both CQI and managed care consistently seek to identify and implement evidence-based best practices, using such tools as clinical guidelines and clinical pathways, and processes like product and case management. Nevertheless, many clinicians perceive both CQI and managed care as a challenge to their personal and professional autonomy and financial security.

Despite physician concerns, CQI allows all personnel, including providers, an opportunity to participate in shaping and transforming how the organization provides heath services. It builds institutional skills needed to analyze processes and it provides a mechanism for providers to retain their sense of autonomy and maintain control over organizational activities that affect clinical outcomes.

The critical issue now facing managers and clinicians working within a managed care is how to accommodate the tradeoffs between quality and cost now that early savings achieved under managed care are diminishing and health care costs are again beginning to rise. Conflicts that must be resolved include balancing quality improvement and cost control processes as well as decision-making power for upper management and operational level professionals. For these and other issues, CQI provides a mechanism by which the organization learns to effectively accommodate the quality/cost trade off facing managers and clinicians.

## GETTING TO MASS CUSTOMIZATION

Patients and providers are quite variable and both expect care that adapts to a range of conditions including differences in anatomy, physiology, cognitive style, psychological status, family setting, and economic resources. Both will evaluate their health care experiences in terms of how those needs are met. One concern is that managed care and health professionals will never agree on the role of variability in an efficient system. Management tends to follow industrial models that focus on the importance of reducing unnecessary variability rather than coping with inherent variability. Health care providers, on the other hand, use medical approaches that focus on inherent variability, often ignoring issues of unnecessary variability. Because insurers have a tendency to manage in the industrial model, they generally ignore or penalize inherent variability creating potential barriers to mass customization.

The tendency of continuous improvement efforts is incrementalism—starting with the existing process and improving it, rather than radically changing the process all together so that it better integrates new technologies, especially information technologies. As well described by Ellen Gaucher (1994):

> Within health care, some of our processes are so bad that we could spend the rest of our professional careers trying to continuously improve them. We need to throw them out and begin with a clean sheet of paper and make sure we understand what the elements of each of these processes are. We need to redesign them to be effective in the long run.

Business, health policy, and political figures have all taken up major change issues. Now with better data in hand about variability in health care and the human cost of medical error, the political and public policy pendulum has swung toward forcing some rationalization of the fragmented health care system. Politicians such as Newt Gingrich (2003) and Patrick Kennedy (Gingrich and Kennedy 2004), and management gurus such as Clayton Christensen (Christensen *et al.* 2000) and Michael Porter (Porter and Teisberg 2004), have joined long-time change advocates such as Regina Herzlinger (2002) and Hillary Rodham Clinton (2004) in this call. Along with these external calls for change at the national level, regulatory and quality monitoring organizations have increasingly mandated institutionalized learning processes for organizations and professions.

## THE TASK AHEAD

Both continuous improvement and managed care need to recognize the inherent transitional nature of health care delivery. Continuous improvement efforts must shift their focus from simply avoiding unnecessary variation to facilitating organizational learning for mass customization as a means of providing health services. Managed care organizations must recognize that their role is just not to minimize costs but to develop the institutional and professional knowledge that will result in the types of coordinated delivery systems that can provide quality and efficient care to a defined population. Increasingly, care is being customized so that it meets and adapts to specific needs without compromising overall standards for cost and quality. The challenge for hospitals, health maintenance organizations and other providers is to demonstrate that services are efficient and that they are improving health outcomes for individuals, enrolled populations, and in some instances, for the larger community.

Merely selecting the lowest cost provider that is unwilling or unable to invest in the information systems that will provide the key to mass customization is not acceptable. All stakeholders, including HMOs, hospitals, insurers, and that professional groups, must see themselves in a transition process that customizes care for the individual, while improving the health status of the population given available resources. Simultaneously, purchasers, consumers, competitors, and regulators will require information to assess the cost, quality, utilization, and availability of health services.

Information systems must be flexible, interoperable, expandable, available, and user-friendly. Information technology must provide information that is accurate, timely, and useful for decision makers at all levels, accessible, and able to accommodate the demands of providers, managers, and employees. Information systems are critical to monitoring and improving the long term performance in an organization. They have to provide feedback that can be integrated back into the system in a timely and functional manner.

Concurrent with the increased need for information, health services are realizing that they must reduce and reorganize staffing within the organization. Large numbers of categorically skilled employees who provide institutionally-based services are no longer required, but rather employees are needed who can perform multiple functions, work in cross-disciplinary teams, and operate in smaller units. Reducing workforces, retraining and reassigning personnel, and requiring new working relationships all contribute to compromises in morale. To make these changes successfully, clinicians and managers must foster quality work, reward loyal and high level performance, secure commitment from employees, and build a spirit of learning while undergoing continuous and fundamental transitions.

## MANAGING TRANSFORMATION AND LEARNING

To succeed in a rapidly changing environment, health care organizations need to smoothly manage the transformation process and take on the challenge of becoming what Peter Senge (1990) described as "learning organizations" places where "people continually expand their capacity to create the results they truly desire, where new and expansive patterns of thinking are nurtured, where collective aspiration is set free and where people are continually learning to learn together."

As presented in Figure 7–1, health services are in the process of transition from a professional model characterized by individual responsibility, professional autonomy and accountability to a transformational model characterized by shared responsibility and collaborative decision making, continuous innovation and learning. Traditional CQI provides important skills needed to make the transition but transformational models provide organizations the opportunity to assure that both incremental and radical learning occur in order to meet the challenges of an uncertain and complex environment. Through organizational learning, health care organizations can better face the reality of managing costs, providing high quality services, and improving outcomes while accommodating individual needs through case management, patient education, phone triage, and supportive patient decision making.

As presented in Figure 7–1, the transformational model has a number of distinguishing characteristics fundamental to CQI.

- *Leaders and employees share overall responsibility, as well as take individual responsibility.* Operating under transformational models, health care managers and clinical leaders share responsibility for accomplishing the organizational mission with other personnel. Everyone understands that they are important to the success of the organization and they know what role they play in that success. Individuals, teams, units, and departments are committed to carrying out their responsibilities.
- *People at multiple levels assume leadership.* Leadership roles for making decisions and guiding change must be afforded to people working in managerial or clinical roles, line staff, and field positions. Changes and decisions designed by people in offices apart from where the work is performed usually have limited effect. For real innovation and improved performance, people working directly with

| Professional | TQM | Transformational |
|---|---|---|
| • Individual responsibility | • Collective responsibility | • Leaders and employees share |
| • Professional leadership | • Managerial leadership | overall responsibility, as |
| • Autonomy | • Accountability | well as take |
| • Administrative authority | • Participation | individual responsibility |
| • Professional authority | • Performance and process | • People at multiple |
| • Goal expectations | expectations | levels assume |
| • Rigid planning | • Flexible planning | leadership |
| • Responses to complaints | • Benchmarking | • Outcome driven |
| • Retrospective | • Concurrent performance | • Shared decision |
| performance | appraisal | making |
| appraisal | • Continuous | • Continuous |
| • Quality assurance | improvement | planning |
| | | • Future orientation |
| | | • Performance enhancement appraisals |
| | | • Continuous innovation |

**Figure 7–1** Emergence of Transformational Models for Organizational Performance.

problems and systems need to be involved in designing and deciding how to improve processes and quality. These are the people on the sharp end of processes.

• *Outcome driven.* People throughout transformative health care organizations demonstrate commitment to achieving outcomes, improving quality and adding value. Employees, providers, and managers recognize that improving outcomes means those individual expectations for quality and clinical services such as disease treatment and management meet and exceed standards.

• *Shared decision making.* It is critically important that people understand the core business, values, and mission of the organization so that they can participate in the decisions that affect it. Straight talk about what is occurring in the environment, how the organization is positioned to respond, and what people need to do to make necessary changes must be modeled and supported by managers and leaders. People need to understand their roles in helping the organization succeed, but they also need to define their roles and how they will contribute.

- *Continuous planning.* People must be motivated to make change, and able to participate meaningfully in the change process. In general, participation will be more effective when the issues and changes are not routine (Schwarz 1989). Transformational change in organizations prepares people to participate in planning and anticipating next steps in an evolutionary change process. When the organization is undergoing regular and dynamic change, people from across the organization must be informed and involved in deciding what changes should be made, in what order, and by what methods. Through functional and cross-functional teams, providers and managers can involve others in mapping strategies and preparing for new challenges (Carroll and Edmondson 2002).

- *Future orientation.* Unlike what has come before, health service organizations must be defining what the future will be and setting their sights on how they will make that happen. A potential danger for the transformative organization is that it might achieve its objectives for the future and turn its attention to categorizing its accomplishments. Such a retrospective orientation will slow the organization and reduce people's motivation to stay ahead of the trends. Transforming leadership continually brings forward the vision of the future organization and indicates how the organization can get from where it is in the present to where it wants to be in the future.

- *Performance enhancement appraisals.* In addition to rewarding and assessing performance improvements for employees, transformational organizations need to commit real resources and support structures to recognizing creativity and innovation. We need to look beyond improving how we get things done, to question and explore new ways of doing what needs to be done. Employees need to know that they will be rewarded for going outside of the traditional structures to redesign and recreate the organization. Such changes will improve more than employee performance, they will increase employee dedication and contributions to the organization's future success. Commitment is greater in organizations that are actively managing change, obviously uncomfortable with the status quo, and creating a new standard for performance (McNeese-Smith 1996; Pascale *et al.* 1997).

- *Continuous innovation.* To excel in the future, health service organizations will need to establish systems that reward people for good work to recognize efforts that surpass expectations. Transformative models provide support for people to demonstrate creativity and innovation that extend beyond standard performance. Clear systems for highlighting outstanding performance and contributions of providers, administrators, and employees can serve to energize others and provide standards against which to assess poor performance (Pascale *et al.* 1997).

## PHYSICIAN LEADERS AND TRANSFORMATION

There are multiple roles for physicians in leading and managing within transforming organizations. Physicians may be designers of change, developing incentives, exploring opportunities, and gathering resources to promote transitions. Physicians may also serve in stewardship roles to assure that there is a broad commitment to organizational learning; or they may contribute by performing in teaching roles where they demonstrate vision and values related to the work of the organization (Barnsley *et al.* 1998).

To secure physician leadership, it is important to identify what will make it attractive for physicians to participate in planning and leading organizational change and then provide them opportunities to exercise leadership within the transformational organization. It will be important, for instance, for physicians see that they have a central role in making and controlling key decisions that affect the provision of health services. It is also important for physicians to help identify where targeted cost savings can occur which will enhance efficiencies without compromising patient care. Physicians and managers will both want to see the organization enhance its performance, but physicians have a particularly important role in designating common measures for preventive care activities and setting targets for meeting primary care goals. Other areas of interest to physician leaders include improving patient satisfaction, utilization rates, and resource consumption.

Physicians have central roles in helping define what the overall goals should be with regard to health status and quality outcomes. To foster participation in the design, planning, and implementation of transformational strategies, physicians need to understand how their participation will contribute to the change process, they should have access to trained facilitators who can support their efforts, and the organization should provide physicians with opportunities to develop their leadership competencies.

Organizational strategies can complement physician roles to improve quality and cost of clinical care if they are well designed. Assuring that the organization's incentive structures and strategies are consistent and complementary can have a significant influence on physician performance. One organization for example, treating both capitated and fee-for-service clients, was successful in controlling costs when the same incentives were provided to physicians regardless of the patient's source of reimbursement (Flood *et al.* 1998).

Beyond the physician's role in the provision of care, there are additional areas in which physicians have an interest. For example, providers are concerned with issues such as market growth, percentage of revenue allocated to medical costs, administrative costs, and financial returns. These factors directly influence organizational decision making and clinical activities. As a result, all participants need to know that their interests are being protected as the organization develops strategies for enhancing growth and reducing costs.

To secure a shared vision around which to align strategies for improving organizational performance, managers, providers and employees must participate in developing a common view of the future, clarifying the values associated with the core business, and articulating shared beliefs about how to achieve high quality health care at reasonable cost. The successful health care organizations will be those able to make the transition from focusing exclusively on standardization of all processes, to reducing instances of *poor* care for individuals (Carroll and Edmondson 2002).

## Strategies for Learning

To develop an organizational culture that promotes learning and teaching, managers and physicians need key strategies that support such activity. Because people generally act as if their beliefs are the "truth," and that this truth is obvious and based upon real data, organizational leaders need techniques that help people learn how to achieve desired results. Figure 7–2 presents the ladder of inference (Argyris 1990) and illustrates why

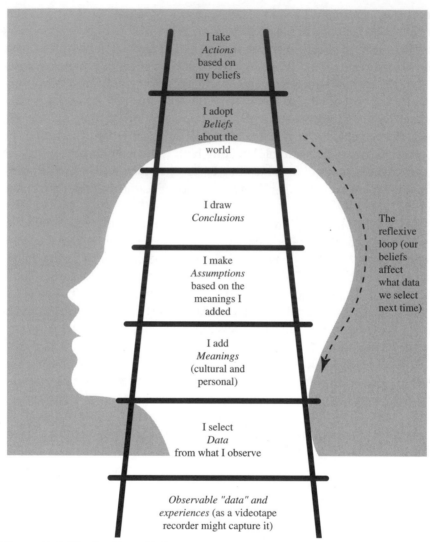

**Figure 7–2** The Ladder of Inference
From *The Fifth Discipline Fieldbook* by Peter M. Senge, Charlotte Roberts et.
al, copyright © 1994 by Peter M. Senge, Charlotte Roberts, Richard B. Ross,
Bryan J. Smith, and Art Kleiner. Used by permission of Doubleday, a division
of Random House, Inc.

most people do not recognize that beliefs and truth are not the same thing.
Further, this model demonstrates why it is important to clarify perceptions, check perceptions against facts, and assess the influence of cultural
beliefs and attitudes (Senge *et al.* 1994).

As you can see from this diagram, the world of observable data is not perceived in the same way by all observers. Individuals independently select the data perceived to be important, add their own cultural and personal meanings, make assumptions and draw independent conclusions, adopt their own beliefs, and then, finally, take action based upon these beliefs. When working in teams, all members may have access to the same data, but every member may act differently in response to the same information.

The ladder of inference can improve communication in three ways:

1. By becoming aware of one's own thinking and reasoning, an individual learns to be more *reflective.*
2. Once a person has reflected upon his or her own thoughts and reasoning, then that individual can better *advocate* his or her position to others. And
3. As individuals better understand how to reflect upon and advocate for their own positions, they are also better able to inquire into the thinking and reasoning of other members of the team.

In combination, the skills of reflection, advocacy, and inquiry are important communication skills that facilitate team and organizational learning. To improve learning within the organization, managers and physician-leaders can stimulate communication in a number of ways.

- *Test assumptions by gathering facts.* Once people describe their beliefs, then others can ask them to provide evidence for their conclusions. Often people have come to conclusions based, in part, on evidence and, in part, on assumptions. Only by having open discussions where people can explain what facts they used and how they reached their conclusions is it possible to learn what data they selected, what data they ignored, and what data are missing.
- *Engage people in discussion of what they assume to be true.* Physicians and other clinicians need to listen to other's views of reality. All people witnessing the same event do not necessarily have the same understanding of what has occurred. Differences emerge based upon our own experiences, biases, and beliefs. Therefore the physician and other clinicians must invite others to share their views of the situation and seek to understand what others believe to be true.
- *Prepare people for teaching and learning.* Not all people are equally able or prepared to learn the same things at the same time. Research has shown that learning occurs more readily when the message is

delivered in a way appropriate to the level of the learner (Hersey and Blanchard 1984). Managers and clinicians must be able to recognize levels of readiness for learners and apply appropriate methods for teaching and coaching.

- *Integrate learning and teaching focus.* Do physicians and other clinicians assure that everyone in the organization is supported in their efforts to teach and learn? To build a learning organization, managers and clinicians must be sure that policies and practices are aligned with incentives for people to acquire, develop and practice their skills. For example, if the policies support learning but incentives only reward work, people will chose to work instead of attending workshops or seminars that enhance their learning. Managers must assure that their expectations for performance are reinforced by the incentives within the system.

- *Develop a teachable point of view.* Physicians and other clinicians need to tell their own stories that illustrate core values, beliefs, and expectations. What are the key experiences that have shaped your own life? How do these experiences continue to guide your own work? When leaders develop a teachable point of view, they engage people's imaginations and encourage commitment. By telling their own stories, leaders provide real and honest examples of success, failure, and learning while communicating values, behaviors, and skills that are important to the organization.

- *Be a role model.* Leaders who demonstrate a positive attitude toward achievement encourage commitment and performance from those around them. Leaders can increase participation in decision making as employees gain familiarity with mission, values, and goals of the organization. As people gain ownership of the organization's mission, leaders must provide them with ongoing opportunities for participation in shaping the future of the organization. Through greater participation and ownership, leaders create an environment where big ideas can lead to big accomplishments.

Central to applying these strategies is assuring that managers and clinicians communicate in ways that others within the organization understand. Through story telling and shared participation, leaders work with others in building mental models that incorporate the vision of the organization that they want to create. Developing common models requires more than creating a desirable vision for the future, however. Before people can build new organizational patterns, they must have a clear understanding of what is not working, why it isn't working, and how it needs to change.

A common understanding depends upon different groups within the organization learning and becoming familiar with complementary values and norms that collectively contribute to the organization's vision. The key is to build a shared mental model while accommodating different viewpoints and expectations that arise based upon people's varying roles and responsibilities. Clinical leaders, for example, need to have the flexibility to develop expectations for the organization that respond to improving care for individuals while management needs mental models that represent improving organizational efficiencies. Using scientific evidence from clinical applications and research, clinicians can accumulate the necessary information they need to motivate changes in the provision of care. Similarly, managers can improve organizational processes by gaining cooperation from clinicians in designing, implementing, and evaluating organizational changes, using relevant evidence and proven methods of improvement.

In health services, rapid change and competitive markets frequently require organizational responses and innovations that are more dramatic than what can be accomplished through incremental quality improvement efforts. Making big changes and fostering a climate of innovation only occurs when people understand their roles, apply CQI tools, have the flexibility to make key decisions that affect their work, and are accountable for their service to customers. Managers and clinicians must articulate expectations for quality and service, but then give people the opportunity to meet these expectations in a manner consistent with the needs of the situation. An individual with multiple complex health problems cannot be successfully managed in a single ten-minute office visit; thus clinicians and managers need to have both the flexibility to develop and tailor cost-efficient options for managing complex patients and incentives that reward appropriate customization.

Learning to provide specific information about what needs to be accomplished, supported by evidence, will facilitate other's acceptance. By communicating how change will be accomplished using concrete and measurable terms, leaders can stimulate others to find ways to make the vision a reality. Leaders must demonstrate the same kind of energy, commitment, high standards, continuous learning, and willingness to share information that they expect from those around them (Adler *et al.* 2003).

By sharing stories, modeling commitment, and listening to others, it is possible to move organizations toward deeper learning. It will not happen without commitment from all participants, however, and pursuing a comprehensive organizational priority on learning, demands a substantial commitment of the leader's time and attention. The reward for such commitment is a greater capacity to grow leadership within the organization (Tichy 1997; Adler *et al.* 2003).

Individuals respond to a crisis by changing their behaviors, yet when there is no perceived crisis, little change occurs. However, Tucker and Edmondson (2003) report that many health care organizations are quick to convert "errors" which are unacceptable and create crises into "problems" which are more tolerable. What is needed is a way for healthcare leaders to communicate a sense of crisis—not to create panic, but to create a sense of urgency, a need to make change in order that the organization, the patient, the community, and the system survive and thrive. Managers, physicians and other key personnel must help others recognize that the traditional treatments will not cure chronic organizational problems. Just as chronic health problems grow more severe the longer they remain undiagnosed and untreated, many of our current organizational problems will not be cured if treated incrementally. The organizations that will survive will be those that institute revolutionary strategies and foster opportunities for quantum ideas to emerge (Tichy 1997).

Managers and clinicians alike need to find ways to expose chronic, underlying organizational issues that are amenable to correction and invite participation in figuring out how to correct these problems. In many instances, changing long-standing problems will need new approaches and greater organizational flexibility. Building an innovative culture will only occur if employees are rewarded and recognized for their contributions to resolving organizational problems. Leaders need to commit themselves and their organizations to employee training and development that promotes innovation and change, learning and teaching (Barnsley *et al.* 1998).

### Strategies for Physician Involvement

Within the healthcare organization, physician participation and involvement in organizational change and transformation is imperative. In order to secure participation from physician leaders, there are multiple strategies managers can employ.

- *Provide information about organizational goals and objectives.* Disseminating information that describes the organization's interest in change and improvement allows physician leaders to consider the impact on their work and patients. Providing explicit information about the goals that are to be accomplished is essential to gaining buy-in and participation from others. In addition, the organization must make sure that incentives for participation are clear and available. Another key component of information sharing is to outline the outcomes that are expected as a result of the effort. People are more likely to participate in planning and implementing strategies when they understand the final impact expected. Edmondson (2003) refers to the way in which the change is presented as "framing." Doing it the right way provides the motivation and the acceptance of changed roles necessary for successful implementation.

- *Align leadership style and task.* By attending departmental meetings, board meetings, intraorganizational meetings, and practice meetings, managers can observe physician interactions and identify clinical leaders who have the skills and recognition needed to persuade others for the need to change. Different leadership styles are needed for different types of issues. By observing how physicians interact with one another and learning who the opinion leaders are for various issues, managers can better match physician leaders to the tasks that need to be accomplished.

- *Use data and partnerships.* Physicians, because of special expertise or commitment, have particular issues upon which they want to focus. By inviting physicians to take leadership on a specific issue, administrators can gain clinical participation in improving key parts of the system. Physicians' medical training prepares them to use scientific evidence as a basis for decision making, thus they are particularly well suited to using data to identify solutions for organizational problems. Physician leaders are also instrumental in gaining the support of their peers in organizational change. The traditional "separate but equal" hierarchies that characterize health care decision making structures persist in keeping medical and administrative decisions apart. To overcome such artificial boundaries, health care leaders must seek out physicians who are willing to partner with administrators at multiple levels in leading organizational change (Edwards *et al.* 2003).

- *Minimizing boundaries.* Physician participation in organizational decision making only occurs if the incentives across the organization are aligned to support their contributions outside of the clinic.

Physicians and administrators need to know that the organization values and rewards participation in activities that foster team decision making. Further, the organization's policies must promote integrating information from multiple sources that collectively contribute to good clinical and management decisions (Barnsley *et al.* 1998)

Ultimately, successful health care organizations will be those that learn to communicate across formal and informal boundaries. Boundaries may be ideological, vertical, horizontal, geographic, external, or a result of time (Barnsley *et al.* 1998). Regardless of the type of boundary, these restrictions create limits on what our health care organizations might become. The goal is to become boundaryless in seeking options to improve health care.

## CONCLUSIONS

This chapter examines some of the underlying changes occurring in the health care industry and an analysis of how these changes are transforming the business of health care. Understanding the nature of the changes in the health care industry serves as a platform for an assessment of the changing roles for CQI within health care organizations. New approaches to transform CQI are presented so that it better attends to both incremental and radical changes that are a necessity for organizational learning. Emphasis is given to the development of organizational structures and processes that promote mass customization and challenges health service providers and organizations to look beyond traditional roles and methods to learn more about how to improve services for individual customers. Professional managers and clinicians are both involved in leading health care organizations, and both must adopt strategies for securing physician participation and leadership in organizational learning and change.

# CHAPTER 8

# Measuring & Assessing Adverse Medical Events to Promote Patient Safety

*Lucy A. Savitz and Shulamit L. Bernard*

Patient safety has become an important focus of quality improvement since publication of the second edition of Continuous Quality Improvement in Health Care. In addition to a series of reports on this topic from the Institute of Medicine, beginning with *To Err Is Human* (2000), a variety of tools (e.g., Agency for Healthcare Research and Quality patient safety indicators) and techniques (failure mode and effects analysis) have become industry standards in our efforts to enhance patient and provider safety. This chapter discusses the evidence, tools, and techniques together with associated accreditation and reporting requirements that influence health service organizations' opportunities for actionable responses.

## DEFINING SAFETY AND ADVERSE EVENTS

Quality of health care has been defined as "the degree to which health services for individuals and populations increase the likelihood of desired health outcomes and are consistent with current professional knowledge" (IOM 1990, page 21). As noted by many (IOM 1990; Chassin 1998; Chassin and Galvin 1998), improving quality requires attention to three sets of problems: (1) overuse of services; (2) under use of services; and (3) misuse of services.

Cutting across these sets of quality problems is the traditional triad of structure, process, and outcomes (Donabedian 1966; Lohr 1997). Structural aspects of health care are not direct measures of quality. They are factors that enable or hinder the provision of high quality care. They include attributes of health care delivery facilities and personnel and the policies and procedures (systems) that influence how they function. Process measures are the things done to and on behalf of patients—in essence, the preventive, diagnostic, therapeutic, rehabilitative, and palliative services provided or made available to individuals and populations. Outcomes are the end results of the provision of those services, denominated across a spectrum from death through serious morbidity to functioning, quality of life, and optimal well-being.

Recently, attention has focused on "medical errors" and patient safety (IOM 2000), which form a significant subset of quality of care problems. Errors in the health care context are seen as the "failure of a planned action to be completed as intended or use of a wrong plan to achieve an aim" (p. 179). Errors can be "active" (readily observed within the practitioner–patient interaction, for example, and leading to immediate consequences) or "latent" (problems in design, organization, training, or other factors that lead to mistakes on the part of practitioners or others but that may be dormant or invisible within the health care system for appreciable amounts of time).

Accident investigators have found that most disasters in complex organizations had long incubation periods characterized by a number of discrete events, signaling danger, that were overlooked or misinterpreted (Vaughan 1996; Dorner 1996). Cultural adaptation to system stressors and deviance from standardized processes (e.g., not double checking patient wristbands per hospital policy) can be attributed to such situations (Spath 2000). System safeguards and abilities of caregivers to identify and correct errors before an adverse medical event (AME) occurs make single-error AMEs highly unlikely such that AMEs "...typically result from a combination of latent failure, active errors, and breach of defenses" (Leape 1994).

Cook and Woods (1994) describe the layering effect of multiple sources of latent error. We have used their conceptualization in framing our systems perspective of AMEs to include:

1. Characteristics of treatment/technology;
2. Characteristics of the patient; and
3. Characteristics of the work environment.

Latent errors are inherent to each layer, but do not result in an adverse event unless checks and balances at the individual levels fail and latent errors across layers occur simultaneously. These observations have

". . . important implications for health care organizations whereby patient safety can be enhanced with the introduction of measures that continually evaluate risk-prone processes" (Spath 2000, p. xxvi). Leape (1994) has suggested that patient safety improvements will only come about when leaders of health care organizations and the professionals providing care accept the notion that AMEs are "an inevitable accompaniment of the human condition, even among conscientious professionals with high standards."

Quality of care problems have tended to move from mechanisms of quality assurance toward quality improvement. This means, briefly, that emphasis on external, regulatory, punitive, and "individual-oriented" tactics has declined; and emphasis on internal, data-driven, and "systems-oriented" approaches has increased concomitantly. Similarly, attention has moved from measuring processes of care (often considered in terms solely of "utilization rates") to assessing outcomes. Clinicians, researchers, and administrators implementing quality improvement programs are encouraged by the current literature to take a more comprehensive view of the environment, procedures and processes, practitioners associated with care delivery, and the interactions of those factors with the patient population served. This evolved conceptualization of quality improvement represents a systems perspective (Jervis 1997). Vaughn, in describing her study of the Challenger disaster (1996), describes a number of elements of complex systems—multiple, interrelated processes, an operating environment with tight resources, and time demands on involved staff. From this perspective, health care organizations can also be clearly characterized as complex systems, having similar risks to the ill-fated Challenger.

These trends—combined with expanding knowledge of appropriate care (through evidence-based practice guidelines, for example), a growing body of tools for measurement and analysis, and the recognition of the significance of latent (not just active) errors—lead inexorably to a need to take a systems approach to understanding quality. Error reduction strategies have been tailored to reduce reliance on memory (e.g., checklists and computerized decision aids), improve information access (e.g., chart flags for patient allergies), and error-proof processes (e.g., when computerized order entry systems are designed to prevent entry of lethal drug doses). Standardized tasks (e.g., care protocols and clinical practice guidelines) and reduction in the number of handoffs (e.g., reengineering care processes to minimize the number of staff involved) have been widely adopted in the hopes of reducing the likelihood of AMEs (Leape 1994,

1998; Cook and Woods 1994; Spath 2000). Focusing on single variables, analyzed linearly, or on individual practitioner-patient interactions, is no longer acceptable. Conceptual frameworks now reflect longitudinal and multifactorial perspectives, both distal ("root") and proximal causes of problems, and the idea of learning organizations.

### EVIDENCE FOR SAFE PRACTICE

The Agency for Healthcare Research and Quality (AHRQ) reported the effects for 79 evidence-based patient safety practices (Shojania *et al.* 2001), which were defined as "a type of process or structure whose application reduces the probability of AMEs resulting from exposure to the health care systems across a range of diseases and procedures." To stimulate the universal implementation of safe practices, the National Quality Forum (NQF) applied a formal consensus development process to its member organizations, refining the AHRQ list to include 30 recommended safe practices. The level of evidence for these practices varies. That has become an issue as health care leaders contemplate whether or not to implement.

The Leapfrog Group has also worked actively to drive the implementation of safe practices; initially with its three leaps—computerized physician order entry, volume thresholds, and intensive care unit staffing. (Sarudi 2001). More recently, the Leapfrog Group developed standards and time frames for implementation of a subset of NQF practices together with a survey process and scoring system for voluntary reporting of progress. The results of this survey are shared with purchasers, health plans, and consumers (Devers and Liu 2004). However, reporting hospitals can envision using this same data for monitoring performance and benchmarking, although there are concerns about the reliability of self-reported data. Devers and Liu (2004) conclude that implementation of these standards is "...a stretch for most hospitals."

Simultaneously, the Joint Commission on Accreditation of Healthcare Organizations (JCAHO), as part of its accreditation process, approved a set of patient safety goals that have been refined on an annual basis. The goals for 2005 will require hospitals to comply with 12 goals consisting of 25 distinct practices (JCAHO 2004).

A comparative study of twelve communities by the Center for Studying Health System Change (Devers *et al.* 2004) found that a quasiregulatory organization such as JCAHO has been the primary driver of hospitals' patient safety initiatives and that professional (e.g., specialty societies) and market initiatives (e.g., Leapfrog Group) have had a lower impact to date. This study also found that employers and health plans did not provide strong incentives to the hospitals (especially financial) to meet the standards or participate in Leapfrog surveys (Devers and Liu 2004). Additionally, this study found that compliance with Leapfrog standards were perceived as restricting physician autonomy and reducing their productivity and income. Finally, the same study has also reported that many hospitals and physicians do not agree with Leapfrog's approach and specific standards, questioning the evidence behind them and its failure to address constraints such as shortage of board certified critical care physicians and differences among hospitals.

Challenges in implementing and reporting patient safety practices reflect issues around the decision to adopt, prioritization of select practices, and methodological difficulties encountered in the identification process. Discussions with experts suggests a consensus in understanding that the decision to adopt in some cases is centralized at the system level, while the majority of such decisions are decentralized to the hospital/unit levels given the diversity of NQF/Leapfrog safe practices. The common circumstances of low volume, resource constraints, and capacity limitations in small and/or rural hospitals is also challenging for implementation in these types of facilities. We found nothing in the literature explicitly reporting on a macroscopic perspective for prioritizing and rationally clustering the implementation of safe practices. While the AHRQ report used the ease of implementation (including costs, logistical barriers, and policy issues) as criteria for inclusion, difficulties in capturing all relevant outcomes such as near misses, inability to demonstrate conclusive evidence due to low frequency of some events, and difficulties with sorting out specific parts of interventions from complex, multidimensional practices and environments are few of the challenges shared by those who identified the reported list of safe practices (Shojania *et al.* 2001).

Additionally, the number of organizations collecting the evidence for safe practices as well as variation in actual identified practices and their domains bring further challenges. In fact, the NQF recognized that the lack of standardization of safe practices might mitigate some of their benefits. In a report of *Safe Practices for Better Healthcare,* the NQF recognizes that the choice of practices implemented by different providers will depend on individual circumstances such as practices that are already implemented, availability of resources, environmental constraints, and patient mix (NQF 2003). However, information technology (IT) based safe practices that offer event monitoring and detection are believed to hold great promise in AME prevention and are being widely encouraged.

## ADVERSE MEDICAL EVENT MONITORING AND DETECTION

Event monitoring systems are intended to identify critical events based on clinical rules as data enter a data repository and generate alerts. Hypothetically, trigger alerts (or flags) are consequently routed to appropriate providers for more detailed examination of patient records. Clinical triggers are flags to clinicians that identify the potential for error; these can be retrospective (i.e., voluntary reporting, code- or criteria-based case finding), concurrent, or prospective. Such flags are often incorporated into computerized physician order entry or electronic medical records systems. Braithwaite *et al.* (2004), for example, used the involvement of a hospital's Medical Emergency Team as a trigger to see whether the patient's deterioration was possibly related to an adverse event. Over an eight-month period, 31% of the team responses were considered attributable to medical errors.

A set of triggers related to a single adverse event class are then viewed together as an adverse event detection system, which can be manual or supported by IT. Prospective trigger surveillance methodology was originally developed at LDS Hospital (the flagship hospital of Intermountain Health Care) to detect adverse drug events (ADEs) by integrating computer programs with hospital information system (Classen *et al.* 1991). Retrospective trigger tools such as AHRQ's Patient Safety Indicators (PSIs) use administrative data that can be used to compare performance across similar inpatient facilities and/or monitor trends in measures over time. Prospective trigger tools are intended to provide rapid, real-time identification of adverse events and enable timely opportunities for intervention. Examination of trends in prospective and retrospective trigger tool results can also be used to identify patterns that are likely to generate adverse events. While both retrospective and prospective error detection systems have relied on manual and IT systems, future efforts are aimed at providing IT solutions that enhance the impact of such systems. Most effectively, an IT-based error detection system integrates data from multiple IT system sources (i.e., ICD code data from the billing or case mix system and clinical data from pharmacy, lab, and/or electronic medical records systems).

Patient safety systems have evolved with the increased use of automated systems using advanced IT architectures. One advantage of these systems is the identification of greater numbers of events than possible with methods relying solely on individual reporting or sampling techniques. Our study will examine reported event monitoring systems. The initial review of the literature on error detection systems shows that available tools are predominantly retrospective or prospective ADE systems. This is summarized in Figure 8–1.

A recent IOM patient safety report, *Patient Safety: Achieving a New Standard for Care* (2004), describes "state of the art" injury tracking. Figure 8–2 shows the four parallel elements that the report describes— prospective clinical triggers, ICD code-based case finding, criteria-based case finding, and voluntary reporting.

Retrospective efforts are more common and include such criteria-based case finding initiatives as Quality Assurance Royal North Shore Case Finding (QARNS from Royal North Shore Hospital, Sydney, Australia), JCAHO Sentinel Events, and NQF Never Events initiatives. The JCAHO Sentinel Event criteria, the NQF Never Event criteria, and QARNS are the best examples of criteria-based chart review. Nevertheless, these combined with voluntary reporting in a culture of safety have resulted in relatively poor case finding. Thus efforts have pushed onward to ICD code-based, case finding with more positive results, like reports from the AHRQ-funded, patient safety demonstration grant to Utah–Missouri. As the field advances and our IT systems evolve, we are striving to move closer to detection either concurrently or, more desirably, on a prospective basis before an error occurs. Cutting-edge work done at LDS Hospital (part of Intermountain Health Care) and Brigham & Women's (B&W) is indicated in the exhibit; these noteworthy efforts provide a strong foundation for encouraging the direction of our proposed work. An "x" represents a gap in these efforts where quality improvement researchers are working.

Compared to traditional voluntary incident reporting systems, such a comprehensive system that involves multiple "triggers" may increase detection of injury rates by more than 100 times. It may also detect large numbers of "near misses." Such injury detection and tracking is an essential first step in consolidating professional opinion about reducing injury

| Type of Error | Author(s)/Year Published | Data Sources | Detection Timing | Brief Description |
|---|---|---|---|---|
| ADEs | Jha et al. 1998 | Laboratory and pharmacy | Prospective | Event monitor based on 52 rules |
| | Rachke et al. 1998 | Patient demographics, radiology orders, pharmacy, and lab results | Prospective | Targeted 37 drug-specific ADEs |
| | Levy et al. 1999 | Lab results | Prospective | Monitored for 25 laboratory abnormalities |
| | Classen et al. 1991 | Lab and pharmacy data | Prospective | Multiple sources of detection based on potential ADE signals |
| | Honigman et al. 2001 | Lab, pharmacy, administrative data, and free-text searches of outpatient records | Retrospective | Rules based on ICD-9, free search and 29 drug-laboratory and allergies rules |
| Nosocomial Infections | Evans et al. 1986 | Microbiology, laboratory, and pharmacy | Prospective | Monitors antibiotic use in relation to infectious disease |
| | Rocha et al. 1994 | Microbiology | Retrospective | Boolean logic activated by positive microbiology results |
| Surgery | Iezzoni et al. 1994 | California discharge abstract data | Retrospective | Screening program identifying 27 preventable in-hospital complications |
| | Weingart et al. 2000 | Administrative | Retrospective | Computer algorithm that screens potential medical and surgical complications |
| General Hospital | Bates et al. 1995 | Administrative | Retrospective | 15 screening criteria and multiple screen strategies |
| Anesthetic Procedures | Benson et al. 2000 | Data from all anesthesia procedures | Retrospective | Screened for hypotension, hypertension, bradycardia, tachycardia and hypovolemia |

**Figure 8–1** Reported Electronic Trigger Tool Applications in Identifying Adverse Events

**Retrospective Chart Review**

| Common events | Prospective Clinical Triggers | ICD Code-Based Case Finding (Utah-Missouri (AHRQ)) | Criteria-based Case Finding | Voluntary Reporting |
|---|---|---|---|---|
| | LDS/B&W | | | |
| | CDC infection control | | | |
| Adverse drug events | x | x | Relatively poor case finding | Relatively poor case finding |
| Iatrogenic infections | | | | |
| Pressure injury | x | x | | |
| Mechanical device failures | LDS | LDS | | |
| Venous lines | x | x | | |
| VTE | x | x | | |
| Transfusions | | x | | |
| Patient falls | B&W | x | | |
| Patient transitions | x | x | | |
| **Rare events** | | | | |
| "Wrong" surgery | | | Current most effective method | Current most effective method |
| "Kidnapping" | | | | |
| Suicide | | | | |
| - etc. - | | | | |

**Figure 8–2** A Comprehensive System for Finding Potential Patient Injuries.

rates significantly (i.e., keep the pressure on). It is also an essential component in understanding the epidemiology of injury, in testing possible solutions, and in establishing transparent accountability for health care delivery. The IOM report describes injury detection and tracking as happening through a three-step process: (1) case finding, (2) evaluation, and (3) classification. In the next section, we provide a detailed discussion of a tool developed by AHRQ for retrospective injury detection and tracking.

## TOOLS FOR DRIVING EVIDENCE-BASED QUALITY IMPROVEMENT: THE AHRQ PSIS

In response to industry need, AHRQ created a user-friendly tool to use in quality monitoring and surveillance activities by health care decision makers—the AHRQ quality indicators (QIs). The QIs are currently organized into three groups:

- **Prevention Quality Indicators (PQIs),** ambulatory care sensitive conditions that evidence suggests may have been avoided through high quality outpatient care,
- **Inpatient Quality Indicators (IQIs),** reflect quality of care inside hospitals and include mortality for medical conditions and surgical procedures; utilization of procedures for which there are questions of overuse, underuse or misuse; and volume of procedures for which there is evidence that a higher volume is associated with lower mortality,
- **Patient Safety Indicators (PSIs),** focus on surgical complications and other iatrogenic events reflective of hospital quality of care. A detailed explanation of the AHRQ QIs can currently be found at: http://www.qualityindicators.ahrq.gov.

The QIs were created to inform health care planning, support evidence-based policy development, and facilitate quality monitoring and surveillance activities. These QIs are constructed using existing hospital discharge data and can be integrated into existing information infrastructures. AHRQ has developed software, which can be used in conjunction with SAS or SPSS, to calculate QI rates from inpatient discharge data derived from the Nationwide Inpatient Sample (NIS), the State Inpatient Database (SID) that are part of AHRQ's Healthcare Cost and Utilization Project

(HCUP)[1], or any hospital administrative data. Required programs to generate these indicators are available from the AHRQ web site and RTI International has developed a QI Training session to support adoption of these tools. Finally, AHRQ is planning to release a more user-friendly software version in early 2005 to further assist users.

The IOM report, *To Err is Human: Building a Safer Health System,* crystallized widespread public concern about the need to take action to reduce the occurrence of apparently common, serious medical errors. (2000) Achieving this goal involves identifying errors in practice and initiatives to avoid and prevent them. It also requires national and regional attention to monitor and report to the public about patient safety. This can be accomplished by using measures that screen for potential problems that patients experience resulting from exposure to the health care system and that are likely amenable to prevention by changes at the level of the system. The key intent of PSIs (see Figure 8–3) is as a "screening tool" or "starting point" for further analysis to reduce "potentially preventable errors" through system or process changes.

These indicators use standardized data routinely available to hospital quality improvement teams. Because these data are standardized, results are comparable across facilities. For this reason, AHRQ PSIs have been incorporated into the National Health Quality Report, an annual report first released by the federal government under congressional mandate in December 2003. However, users of such measures need to exercise care. There are a number of competing sets of indicators, most notably by the NQF and JCAHO. In some cases, the same indicator name is used while the specification of the numerator and denominator may vary. Such indicators are limited to inpatient data due to a paucity of available outpatient data. Finally, indicator tools are a retrospective (versus) prospective tool for examining AMEs.

Retrospective monitoring tools can fill important needs in hospital quality improvement. Hospital boards that are seeking standardized measures for monitoring and benchmarking safety performance have turned to the PSIs. Further, these indicators can be used at the sharp end to generate statistical process control charts that highlight outlier cases where drill down via root cause analysis (RCA) may yield true AMEs. From a systems perspective, we may also turn to another class of tools from probabilistic risk assessment.

---

[1] More on HCUP data can currently be found at www.ahrq.gov/hcup

| Provider-Level PSIs | Area-Level PSIs |
|---|---|
| Accidental puncture and laceration | Accidental puncture and laceration |
| Birth trauma–injury to neonate | Foreign body left in during procedure |
| Complications of anesthesia | Iatrogenic pneumothorax |
| Death in low mortality DRGs | Postoperative wound dehiscence in |
| Decubitis ulcer | abdominopelvic surgical patients |
| Failure to rescue | Selected infections due to medical care |
| Foreign body left in during procedure | Transfusion reaction |
| Iatrogenic pneumothorax | |
| Obstetric trauma – cesarean delivery | |
| Obstetric trauma – vaginal delivery with instrument | |
| Obstetric trauma – vaginal delivery without instrument | |
| Postoperative hemorrhage or hematoma | |
| Postoperative hip fracture | |
| Postoperative physiologic and metabolic derangements | |
| Postoperative pulmonary embolism or deep vein thrombosis | |
| Postoperative respiratory failure | |
| Postoperative sepsis | |
| Postoperative wound dehiscence in abdominopelvic surgical patients | |
| Selected infections due to medical care | |
| Transfusion reaction | |

**Figure 8-3** AHRQ Patient Safety Indicators (PSIs).

## A Tool for Excavating Adverse Medical Events: FMEA

Failure Mode and Effects Analysis (FMEA) is one approach in the family of methods included in probabilistic risk assessment. FMEA has been widely used in high-risk industries such as energy (nuclear), aerospace, and manufacturing for a number of years. More recently, quality improvement analysts in health care have turned to this tool to attempt to understand system failures and identify opportunities to enhance patient safety. In particular, the literature provides excellent examples of FMEA application to medication safety (Cohen *et al.* 1994; Williams and Talley 1994; Fletcher 1997; Bayley *et al.* 2004).

The health care industry has been receptive to this structured approach for organizing information collected on causes and their effects. FMEA can be used at the process conceptualization, design, and/or assessment stages. It can be consistently applied for continuous quality improvement (CQI) in care processes from planning through performance monitoring. CQI teams can easily interpret and respond to outputs from the FMEA. For this reason, FMEA is one of several methods recommended by the Food and Drug Administration to verify new designs; the Process Safety Management Act lists process FMEA as one optional method to evaluate hazards; and JCAHO requires all medical facilities to complete at least one FMEA per year on high-risk processes. Furthermore, FMEA satisfies ISO 9001 or 9002 requirements.

Briefly, FMEA as a structured approach to AME excavation involves:

- Assembling a team of clinical experts involved in a high-risk care process
- Identifying a trained facilitator
- Meeting to discuss a care process in detail
- Conducting analysis and scoring risk items on the care process maps
- Applying the indicated results

High-risk care processes are typically those involving extensive hand-offs from one department to another or where a care process is highly fragmented, involving people from several different departments and/or disciplines performing various or even the same tasks. Results from the FMEA clearly describe and prioritize failures in such a care process and identify root causes. From these, evidence-based safe practices can be implemented as targeted quality improvement interventions.

| Step or Link in Process | Potential Failure Modes | Potential Effect | Severity of Effect | Probability of Occurrence | Ability to Detect | Risk Score $S \times O \times D$ (Criticality) | Cumulative Sum | Rank |
|---|---|---|---|---|---|---|---|---|
| | | | | | | | | |
| | | | | | | | | |

Figure 8–4  Example FMEA Documentation Work Sheet.

| Process Step | Potential Failure | Effects of Failure | Severity | Occurrence | Detection | Risk Score |
|---|---|---|---|---|---|---|
| List the patient's allergies | Forget to ask | Allergic reaction | 8 | 2 | 4 | 64 |

Figure 8–5  FMEA Scoring Example.

There are a number of excellent resources (Stamatis 1995; McDermott *et al.* 1996; Feldman and Roblin 1997; Juran and Blanton 1999) and training programs that provide an in-depth description of how to conduct FMEA. Basically, the CQI team begins by flow charting the intended process—as it was designed. A flow chart of the selected process—as routinely conducted—is then produced. The team then creates a documentation worksheet (see Figure 8–4) that: (1) lists each step and each link between steps in the process (column 1); and (2) identifies discrepancies between the flow charts (column 2). The product of Severity-Occurrence-Detection (SOD) ratings is used as a risk score for that potential failure. Figure 8–5 provides a FMEA scoring example. The risk scores can be summed or averaged to assess the risk at each step in the care process. Entire processes can be rated and compared in this way *(if the rating method is the same)*.

Since expert CQI team members who judge and rate the probability of risks, and the data to support these estimations are often extremely limited, the rating process method can be highly subjective. Therefore, internal consistency is important and caution should be taken in comparing risk scores. When internal rating consistency is preserved, CQI teams can use the same framework to brainstorm and list causes of failures, detection methods, and potential controls. Later, the same framework can be used to document actions taken and rerate potential failures once new controls are in place.

## CONCLUSIONS

CQI teams committed to providing the safest care possible for patients are challenged to prioritize efforts and direct scarce resources to those safe practices that are both evidence-based and supported by data-driven need identification. Beginning with a comprehensive discussion of adverse medical events from a systems perspective, we have reviewed the evidence for safe practices in this chapter. Next, we described the current state of error detection and monitoring. From this, we offered a set of tools for monitoring and subsequent investigation of AMEs. In particular, we suggested that the FMEA tool allows users to compile and organize root causes in order to give greatest priority to the intervention opportunities with the highest probability of risk reduction.

# CHAPTER 9

# The Human Face of Medical Error: Classification and Reduction

*Joseph G. Van Matre, Donna J. Slovensky, and Curtis P. McLaughlin*

Medical errors are attracting much public attention. Two Institute of Medicine studies have demanded provider action about medical errors, clinical quality and patient safety. The first, *To Err is Human* (2000), emphasized the surprisingly large scale of the problem, while the second, *Crossing the Quality Chasm* (2001), focused more on solutions. While the numerical findings in these reports were debated heavily in the professional literature, there is little doubt that there are serious problems of both system-based and human errors in health care. While reports of unacceptable levels of medical errors have been written about occasionally since at least 1951, these reports appear to have had little impact on the medical profession until Dr. Lucien Leape's article on "Error in Medicine" appeared in 1994 in the *Journal of the American Medical Association* (Millenson 2002). By this time, related issues of quality improvement were already receiving wide attention and these two sets of issues converged to form a fertile joint ground.

Often missing from these efforts, however, was reference to the extensive research done on the etiology and treatment of human error, especially catastrophic human error, in a number of fields, including airline and rail safety, nuclear reactor safety, and workplace accidents. Two notable exceptions are provided by Feldman and Roblin (1997) and by Eagle *et al.* (1992) who recommended using a failure analysis process in health care settings.

The medical profession has often avoided explicit recognition of this problem until recently, for a number of reasons, including protecting fellow professionals ("there but for the grace of God go I") and malpractice costs. Moreover, the overemphasis on blaming the individual in health care, something that quality improvement advocates have been fighting, may have subtly led otherwise knowledgeable individuals to play down the topic of human error. However, a closer look at the literature on human error shows that it emphasizes system improvement and plays down blaming the individual. Stewart and Grout (2001) also suggest that academic research concerned with quality improvement may be biased toward statistical methods and away from detailed process design issues, including their cognitive dimensions. Yet even such an advocate of system-based solutions as Deming, admits that human errors are a part, perhaps 15%, of the problem (1986). Reducing them ought to be a part of the analysis and the solution (Becher and Chassin 2001).

This chapter begins with a review of the definitions used in developing a system for classifying medical errors based on the work of Reason (2002) and Weick and Sutcliffe (2001), among others, and suggests a suitable taxonomy for both active and inactive human errors and for system faults. These are supported with examples and then with suggestions about how these categories of error can be matched with arrays of countermeasures for rapid and effective corrective action. We also outline how a cross-sectional analysis of errors can be useful in identifying systematic organizational problems that might be overlooked when focusing on the multiple causes of a single incident or error.

## MEDICAL ERRORS

An error occurs when a process does not proceed the way that it was intended by its designers and managers. The most frequent error occurs when a step is omitted from an established process (Reason 2002). Note that this definition does not relate directly to the outcome of that process.

> As noted below, "errors can be moderated through targeted... management techniques." Errors themselves are not intrinsically bad—indeed, they are often highly adaptive as in trial and error learning or the serendipitous discovery that can arise from error. However, they can have damaging and even fatal consequences, particularly in the "hands on" often uncertain activities associated with delivering health care to vulnerable patients—although these injurious outcomes are probably far fewer than their contextual opportunities would warrant. Unlike some epidemics, there is no

specific countermeasure for error. Rooted as it is in the human condition, fallibility cannot be eliminated—nor is that a sensible goal—but its adverse consequences can be moderated through targeted error management techniques. (p. 40)

For example, the quoted article is on "Combating omission errors through task analysis and good reminders." In the same issue of that journal, Barber (2002) utilizes Reason's human error classification system to analyze medication noncompliance as a medical error.

Organizations should include near misses and nonadverse events in their studies of errors. Weick and Sutcliffe (2001), for example, identify one of the characteristics of a reliable organization as a focus on failures, not just successes, including highlighting and investigating near misses and nonadverse errors. They suggest a number of characteristics of successful, high reliability organizations, observing that:

- While successful at avoiding disasters, they are still focused on errors in their earliest manifestations
- They try to understand processes in depth. They do not focus on simplification.
- They emphasize knowledge of operations and learning on the front line.
- They build in resilience to overcome the errors that do occur.
- They listen to and respect experience and expertise at the operational level.

They also build on Reason's work (2002), listing four attributes of a "mindful" culture, one which seeks out weaknesses in the system:

- A reporting culture, in which no adverse events are hidden, in fact, they are seen as opportunities to learn
- A just culture in which one does not shoot the messenger and there is no scapegoating.
- A flexible culture in which information flows freely and rank respect local expertise.
- A learning culture in which new understanding is sought after and prized.

These and other sets of observations (Gibson and Prasad 2003; Walshe and Shortell 2004) are very consistent with the CQI philosophy including Deming's "profound knowledge" and with many of the issues raised in Chapter 6 on teams, and operate beside the traditional professional social controls documented in Charles Bosk's *Forgive and Remember: Managing Medical Failure* (1979). They also bring to mind the work of Thomas Kuhn (1962) on scientific revolutions in which he noted that paradigm shifts in science occur when newcomers pay attention to discrepancies (often minor ones) between established theories and empirical observations and generate new hypotheses about system behavior that take these into account.

The cost of medical error in the United States is reported to be great, but estimates of both cost and error rates vary widely. A 1964 article based on data from Yale-New Haven medical center reported that 1.3% of patients died due to complications from some procedure intended for the patient's benefit. However, iatrogenic negative results do not equate to medical error. All procedures carry some risk of negative outcomes. Then, in 1991, Dr. Leape coauthored a study that focused more on medical errors and reported that 4% of patients in the study suffered an injury that prolonged their hospital stay or resulted in measurable disability. Since then, the rate of research and publications concerning medical errors has increased markedly (Millensen 2002).

## WHY A CLASSIFICATION SYSTEM?

The mix of activities (products if you will) in health care organizations is so varied that classification systems become extremely important components of any comparative analysis of health care quality issues. It is no accident that the field of quality improvement in health moved very slowly until the widespread adoption of the Diagnosis-Related Groups (DRG) system for quality purposes. It would also be useful to have and promulgate a common classification system for human errors in health care that could be applied in parallel across institutions and product lines. A classification system is also necessary if we are to encourage knowledge management efforts among institutions concerning medical error.

The existence of a classification system for errors is an important precursor of a systematic method for developing error responses. For example, the JCAHO *Sentinel Events Letter* is very good about citing "risk reduction" steps for each error studied. However, the next step would be to categorize these errors that are human errors and then associate them with corresponding preventive steps using a comprehensive classification structure, so that those responding to other errors could readily transfer such steps to their situations.

## Suggested Starting Points

One widely-cited classification system was developed by James Reason (1990) that he called the Generic Error Modeling System (GEMS). A professor of psychology, he asserts that, despite the wide range of experiences involving human error, a "surprising limited number of forms...errors appear in very similar guises across a wide range of mental activities. Thus it is possible to identify comparable error forms in action, speech, perception, recall, recognition, judgment, problem solving, decision making, concept formation and the like." He defines human error as "a generic term to encompass all those occasions in which a planned sequence of mental or physical activities fails to achieve its intended outcome, and when these failures cannot be attributed to the intervention of some chance agency" (Reason 1990, p. 7). This definition contains three major points. First, there must be *intention* in the action sequence for an error to occur; errors cannot occur absent intention (of the actor or the organization). Secondly, the failure may occur because of *errors in the plan* or in *execution of the plan.* In fact, this dichotomy was more common after and, to some degree, remains a popular classification (Norman 1988). The GEMS approach, however, separates the planning error into two parts: rule-based mistakes and knowledge-based mistakes. Finally, a tragic outcome *need not involve error* because a chance event may occur (e.g., a pulmonary embolism can occur despite all the steps normally necessary to avoid it.)

## GEM's Basic Error Types

This framework extends the popular dichotomy of slips (failure in execution) and mistakes (planning errors) and argues for four basic error types:

- Skill-based slips (and lapses)
- Rule-based mistakes

- Knowledge-based mistakes
- Violations of rules or norms

Splitting the rule-based performance from the skill-based performance was a useful contribution of Reason's work. These categories parallel those of Bosk (1979) who outlined technical errors, judgmental errors, and normative errors while analyzing the training and socialization of surgeons.

*Skill-based performance* is governed by stored patterns of preprogrammed instructions. For example, most clinical caregivers are taught to take blood pressure readings using a procedure that involves a specific sequence of steps. After countless repetitions, the steps become part of the knowledge base and little or no conscious thought is required when the caregivers fits and inflates the cuff and observes the pressure readings. Nevertheless, the individual does have to pay attention and perform certain "checks" to monitor the process, for example, assuring that the cuff is properly secured. A *lapse* occurs when the caregiver fails to check to see whether the cuff is secure. A *slip* occurs when the caregiver writes down an illegible number after reading the gauge correctly. These errors may occur due to being distracted, tired, or otherwise not giving full attention to the process.

*Rule-based performance* is applied to familiar problems in which solutions are governed by stored rules of the "if-then" type. These rules are based on previous experiences and are called into play when a trigger event or situation occurs. For example, when a patient goes into cardiac arrest, the medical team responds to a "code blue" alarm with the cardiopulmonary resuscitation protocol. Errors occur when a new situation is perceived as the same as or similar to a previous situation and the response model for the prototypical situation is wrongly applied.

*Knowledge-based performance* applies to novel problems when actions must be planned in "real time" using attentional control in conjunction with working memory. In other words, this situation calls for "hard thinking." The individual must assess the situation, draw relevant information from memory, and formulate a response. Knowledge-based performance often requires incremental decision making as additional information becomes available. Planning errors can occur, for example, when the relevant probabilities are mis-assessed, perhaps because of experience biases in decision making. Health care examples illustrating these categories of medical errors are shown in Table 9–1.

**Table 9–1**  Health Care Examples Using the GEMS Framework

| Error Type | Example |
| --- | --- |
| Skill-based Slip | A physician orders Inderal intravenously for a patient, but writes the order for the typical oral dosage. |
| Skill-based Lapse | A physician forgets to prescribe beta blockers following myocardial infarction, although he is aware of the strong research evidence that this helps prevent re-infarction and normally prescribes it in such cases. |
| Rule-based Mistake | A patient presents with a high white blood cell count and lower right quadrant pain. The physician's schema defaults to the most frequently observed outcome (acute appendicitis), confirmatory tests are not ordered, and the diagnosis proves incorrect. |
| Knowledge-based Mistake | Confirmation bias: A physician presumes a diagnosis of cancer based on an initial blood chemistry value, and dismisses subsequent counter-evidence from a biopsy. |

## REPRESENTING THE SUGGESTED APPROACH

Given the four types of error shown by the GEMS model and the earlier categories of action-inaction, intention (good or bad), and planning versus execution, we suggest the classification system identified in Figure 9–1. Our criteria in developing it were that it be practically useful, cover a wide range of health care situations, and not support the biases that often occur, namely: blaming the victim, scapegoating the staff, or faulting the system. In complex situations all might be partially involved, although we know that the first two are all too likely.

### Action Versus Inaction

The first question asks whether the error involves action or inaction. The nature of the analysis differs between these two categories. If no action took place, there is no physical evidence and little opportunity to determine whether or not a step in a procedure was omitted. The process to be reviewed is primarily cognitive. The issue of intention is internal to the

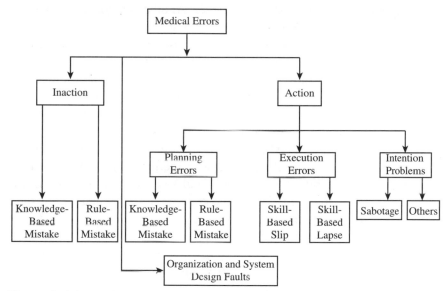

**Figure 9–1**  Potential Classification of Human Medical Errors.

cognition of the decision maker and is difficult to separate out from one's rules and knowledge states. Therefore, we have limited the intention issue to analysis of those cases where there was an action, since many health care situations have multiple actors who might have had differing intentional states that may need to be sorted out.

On the other hand, inaction events are likely to be highly significant in identifying system errors. The much-reported, much-reviewed, much-litigated 1994 death of a patient at the Dana-Farber Cancer Institute, who received four times the intended daily dose of chemotherapy and soon died, could have been dismissed as a single human slip of dosage entry. Yet there were many subsequent system questions raised as to why it went unnoticed over the subsequent three months—why the error was not caught by physicians, nurses, and pharmacists, and why no post mortem was held, etc. These inactions were all revealing of system problems later identified by accrediting and licensing bodies (Bohmer and Winslow 1999; Crane 2001).

Furthermore, attention to inaction may lead to refinement of what is or is not a medical error. One example is Barber's argument that patient noncompliance is a medical error (2002). Another example to consider would be the diabetic patient, obviously in some distress, who presents herself one Saturday afternoon at the local hospital emergency room. She reports having tested her glucose level and found it unusually high. Once her findings are confirmed, the duty nurse calls her physician for an order but is unable to reach him. The patient waits and worsens for several hours until the physician finally responds. Then she is treated and released. In most cases this inaction would not be reported as a medical error.

The patient might well complain to the hospital administration, but this could be treated as a case of patient dissatisfaction rather than a medical error. Unless the quality assurance staff is alerted to the importance of inaction, they are unlikely to address the systematic issues generating such delay and unnecessary distress.

### Planning and Execution Errors and Violations

Step two is to determine whether the error involved planning, execution or motivation. If the issue is primarily related to planning or execution skills, the GEMS categories outline above can be applied.

### *Planning*

Most reported medical errors are in execution, the wrong drug dosage administered or the wrong side operated on, but many of these have their genesis in the planning stage. If one operates on the wrong side of the brain, it is obvious that the physician did not read the chart or X-ray correctly and the numerous other signals were transmitted or ignored before the wrong action was taken. This may be the result of a knowledge error, such as the wrong side of an X-ray being displayed on the light box, or rule-based failure, such as not asking the patient which side they believe will be affected. In all likelihood there was more than one mistake as well as failure of the systems intended to avert such mistakes (Steinauier 2001). A more clearly rule-based mistake occurred when a man was brought to the emergency room in intense abdominal pain. Without ordering a CT scan, the surgeon assumed a kidney stone. None was found and eighteen hours later the patient died of a ruptured abdominal aortic aneurism (Gawande 1999).

*Execution*

No matter how good the planning, however, the individual carrying it out may err. An inexperienced surgical resident doing a thyroidectomy made a horizontal cut across the patient's neck instead of the correct vertical incision (Gawande 1999). This was contrary to his instructions. This would have been a skill-based slip had he not internalized the instructions, and a skill-based lapse if he had learned, but failed to implement the rule.

*Violation*

Other categories refer to motivational problems behind individual *violations* of the plan, stem from organizational factors, or combine both. An example of a personal motivational problem would be an aide who skips steps in a care process because he wants to sneak away early for a date. Barber notes the importance of motivational problems in his analysis of prescription medicine compliance as a medical error problem, using Reason's term, "violations."

> Violations include taking short cuts that bend the rules to make life easier, such as taking several medicines together which should be taken at different times, or taking a non-steroidal anti-inflammatory drug on an empty stomach. (Barber 2002, p 83)

Presumably the patient has been informed of the right procedure and internalized the appropriate rules to follow, but decides to do something else for personal reasons.

Reason suggests three types of violations:

- "Routine violations"—the cutting of corners that Barber cites.
- "Optimizing violations"—individuals pursue personal ends at the expense of the process, like the aide on the telephone, or the case of a Kansas City pharmacist who pleaded guilty to diluting chemotherapy and perhaps thousands of other medications for profit.
- "Necessary or situational violations"—the individual sees no other way out of a bind (Reason 1995).

**Organization and Process Design System Faults**

The literature on continuous quality improvement, especially root cause analysis as it is applied to sentinel events in health care, already provides a highly developed structure for analysis of organizational issues and the design of processes. These are the blunt end of medical error, the much less visible sources, since they do not necessarily involve individual failure to implement a process or procedure properly. They are implicated in many adverse situations, since they produce appropriate or inappropriate information and training, motivate proper teamwork and personal vigilance, and stimulate appropriate or inappropriate intentions. Therefore, this classification has been included in Figure 9–1 to serve as a linkage to the existing literature of quality and process improvement.

## MATCHING COUNTERMEASURES TO ERROR TYPES

The test of the effectiveness of such a classification scheme is whether or not it can categorize experience sufficiently to lead toward the selection of appropriate responses to human error. The schema offered here should be useful because it points toward specific types of remedies.

The easiest types of medical errors to deal with are those which are skill-based, followed by rule-based mistakes, then knowledge-based mistakes, and, finally, intentional problems.

*Skill-based errors* occur when an individual fails to make an attentional check during the process of executing a schema or procedure. These omissions occur most often because an individual is fatigued, pre-occupied, or distracted. Obvious countermeasures involve:

- Attention getters—Reason argues that one should respond with task analysis followed up by effective reminder systems and provides ten criteria for a "good" reminder (Reason 2002).
- Error detection—Stewart and Grout (2001) review the industrial literature on methods of error detection and limitation. Monitoring systems offer many opportunities for error detection in health care.
- In-line inspection—Many health care professionals like working in groups because their "buddy" can serve to inspect ongoing work and help avoid or respond early to errors (Stewart and Grout 2001).

- Error limitation—This is more difficult to achieve in health care than in other settings, but computer-based transactions and records can be programmed to respond when process limits are exceeded and the system is presumed to be out of control (Stewart and Grout 2001).
- Checklists—These can be used to assure that attentional checks are performed. These are often a natural byproduct of the development of practice guidelines.
- Resource input standards—Donabedian (1980) observed that one of the aspects of quality health care was adequate resource inputs. These include establishing reasonable staffing levels as well limits on the number of consecutive hours worked. Such rules already exist in the airline industry, a rich source of ideas for potential error avoidance for the health care industry.
- Substitute a rule-based solution—If there is concern about operating on the wrong knee, write "NO" on the incorrect limb and "YES" on the correct one (Steinauer 2001).

*Rule-based mistakes* involve the inappropriate use of an "if-then rule." Several possible rules may appear appropriate. Then the choice of a rule depends on how completely the competing rules match the situation and the strength of the rule—how many times it has been applied successfully to such situations in the past. Reason suggests that the number of contingencies that their "if-then" rules cover distinguishes experts from trained novices (Reason 1990). However, one must be careful to avoid application of a "strong, but wrong" rule. For example, Reason (1995) reports a case of a patient who died of radiation burns. He was receiving his ninth treatment of 200 rads following removal of a tumor from his shoulder. The machine had two modes of delivery, with the second using 25,000 rads and a metal plate to transform the beam into therapeutic X-rays. A technician had edited the software program to correct a typo, but introduced a new error which caused the machine to correctly remove the plate, but left the setting at 25,000 rads. The radiotherapist activated the machine but received the unfamiliar and cryptic message "Malfunction 54" on her computer screen. She assumed that the treatment had not happened, which is what similar messages had meant in the past, and she set up the machine to "fire" again and repeated the process a third time when the message reappeared—with tragic results.

Countermeasures include:

- Enhancing the search process to include more alternative responses.
- Sharing what has not worked well (past errors) with others.
- Decision support systems to make the preceding two alternatives more feasible.
- Using simulators and simulations to build a larger rule repertoire. Had the radiotherapist encountered that message in a simulated environment, an observer could have pointed out the consequences of her strong assumption.

Simulation can provide excellent learning opportunities with realistic resource utilization and without putting patients at risk (Slovensky and Morin 1997). The radiotherapist would have learned the need to search out the meaning of warnings rather than go on past experience.

*Knowledge-based mistakes* occur during problem-solving situations when one's repertoire of "if-then" rules proves inadequate. There may be a lack of information, the information may be out-of-date, or one's judgmental decision-making heuristics may be biased. Equating ease of recall of an event with its likelihood of occurrence is an example (Tversky and Kahneman 1974). So is weighting local, personal data more heavily than distant, impersonal data. For example, a community may have had an instance when a 20 to 30 year old female had breast cancer. This single episode, pertinent and tragic, is told and retold, causing young women to seek mammograms even though national studies show them to have a very poor benefit–cost ratio. Similarly, a physician may not prescribe a new and effective medication, because one of her first patients to use the drug reported dissatisfaction due to a side effect (Russo 1999).

Countermeasures include:

- Decision-maker education including continuing education and academic detailing.
- Increasing awareness of how biases on the availability and locality of information affect decision making.
- Decision support systems to increase availability of information that meet the criteria of evidenced-based medicine.
- Peer-review of knowledge-based schema used in frequently-seen cases.
- Collaborative discussion of diagnoses and treatments involving rarely-seen cases.

## Motivation Problems

The categories of motivational problems are so numerous and varied that we can only scratch the surface. The best way to think of them in all but the most egregious cases is that they are the epsilon factor in safety and quality. After the indolent, the malicious, and the impaired have been removed (Weick and Sutcliffe 2001), the inability to fix the causation with the four GEMS categories probably means that there are further organizational problems to be considered (Reason 2000). These include:

- Overspecialization of tasks (West 2000).
- Problems of coordination, communication and cooperation (West 2000). These should also show up in process analyses associated with execution performance.
- Diffusion of responsibility (West 2000), which must be addressed by establishing process ownership at the appropriate level of aggregation (McLaughlin and Kaluzny 1999).
- Goal displacement (West 2000; Carthey *et al.* 2001) in which funding, profitability, or performance measures dominate quality and safety measures and damage professional morale.
- Unfair blaming of individuals (Carthey *et al.* 2001) for systems problems and/or denying the existence of systematic error.
- Conflicts between management and staff, leading to a variety of responses, including sabotage (Reason 1995).
- Norms and cultures supporting risk-taking and rule-bending (Reason 1995).

## Organization and Process Design System Faults

Organizational functioning and improved process design are the focus of much of the quality and safety literature. Where they are not the direct cause of medical error, each might certainly be a "latent" factor behind medical error (Reason 1995, 2000; Berwick 2001). Understaffing can easily be a management contribution to the fatigue and inattention that leads to an implementation error by an otherwise reliable staff nurse or, if continued, to motivational problems leading to violations. Some researchers refer to these organizational issues as the "blunt end" of safe operations (Cook and Woods 1994; Ketring and White 2002).

Rather than bore the reader with a laundry list of organization and process design factors, we refer the reader to the numerous existing checklists, for example:

- All of the other items in the "special cause" variations array and those in the "common cause" section in JCAHO "framework for root cause analysis and action" (JCAHO 2002).
- Reason *et al.* (2001) suggest a survey for institutional-level functioning in avoiding medical errors. It involves a 20-item checklist for assessing institutional resilience (CAIR). They also suggest comparing the scoring across internal professional groupings to look for problem areas.
- Another useful set of organizational scales is provided by Weick and Sutcliffe (2001). Their work is also interesting because it emphasizes the importance of organizational resilience, the ability to contain and recover from the errors that will happen despite the best laid plans and designs.

## ADOPTING THE AVIATION INDUSTRY APPROACH

In addition to the specifics, one can adopt an overall approach modeled on the aviation industry approach, conducting in-depth analyses of both actual errors and "near misses." The aviation industry's approach was identified as a useful model by most of the authors cited in this chapter. The Maccabi Healthcare Services, a non-profit HMO in Israel, has been applying the aviation industry investigative approach for more than five years. They report the following features of their successful system as it has evolved:

- An interdisciplinary team with doctors, psychologists, and individuals with aviation experience.
- A support system for supporting the reporting caregivers, including lack of blame and immunity with emphasis on reporting near misses as well as adverse events.
- A hot-line for reporting rapidly ahead of any retrospective reviews.
- A carefully constructed event debriefing methodology.

- Wide dissemination of reports and recommendations throughout its dispersed ambulatory care system. (Wilf-Miron *et al.* 2003).

## MULTI-CAUSATION AND CROSS-SECTIONAL FOCUS

Organizations do not suddenly start making mistakes. They tend to slide imperceptibly into a set of conditions that produce medical error. People start changing the way they do things for convenience or to adapt to perceived management goals. New digital equipment that is supposed to eliminate the human element is not failsafe. New personnel replace those previously trained to respond to a situation. Pressures build that lead to inattention and reduce morale. Supplies and medications are substituted that were not included in formal procedures and so on. Often it is the concatenation of these drifts that lead to major errors. Any error classification system must adapt to this multi-causal reality.

Table 9–2 presents a format for adapting this human classification system to multi-causality and to the fact that multiple events may be reported with a reasonable time period within the same institution. Why not take a cross-sectional look at the number of times that a type of causation occurs? A cross-sectional analysis of commonalities across adverse events may provide a more representative snapshot of systems problems than in-depth focus on a single event (Meurier 2000).

Those familiar with the cause-and-effect diagram and root cause-and-effect tools of continuous process improvement will observe that the first three columns could be derived from such an analysis of the cognitive or procedural processes behind any given medical error situation. Perhaps more importantly the cross-sectional approach encourages the organization to look at the latent conditions behind the errors, the attitudinal and information processing differences among professionals, the patterns of communications within and across teams, and environmental factors such as management pressure to speed up procedures and improve OR utilization or harried nursing staff lacking time to check patient identities and prescriptions (Steinauer 2001; Meurier 2000). It may also lead to greater breadth of tactics applied to such errors rather than relying on one size-fits-all or perfunctory responses such as "nurse counseled" (Bohmer and Winslow 1999).

**Table 9–2** Applying the Classification System

| Type of causation | Indicate # present | Detailed descriptions for each | Recommended responses to each |
|---|---|---|---|
| Inaction—knowledge-based | | | |
| Inaction-rule—based | | | |
| Planning—knowledge-based | | | |
| Planning—rule-based | | | |
| Execution—skill-based slip | | | |
| Execution—skill-based lapse | | | |
| Violations | | | |
| Organization and process design system faults | | | |

## CONCLUSION

Given the complexity of health care situations and how they produce medical errors, it is important to have a conceptual schema for their classification and analysis. We have outlined one schema, drawing heavily on the work of J.T. Reason. It is offered because it is practical, and draws on the extensive work done on the psychology of human error and human factors in health and other fields, as well as organizational antecedents of errors. It is applicable to a wide array of situations and leads to the use of some, if not all, the techniques of continuous quality improvement, but overcomes some of the biases exhibited by both those who espouse such techniques and those who avoid them.

The next step is a continuing dialogue to improve our ability to identify and further codify both individual and organizational responses associated with each category of error, keeping in mind that any system must be capable of handling the multiple individual and systemic causations behind medical errors and enhance access to relevant arrays of responses and tactics.

CHAPTER 10

# Information Management and Technology for CQI

*Curtis P. McLaughlin and David C. Kibbe*

This chapter is designed to help health care leaders visualize the role of information technology in their performance improvement strategy, regardless of the size of the organization or its mission. It presents a framework for the management of informational resources along the continuum from data collection to information and knowledge management to decision making. It also describes how recent advances in information technology, including the Internet, make it possible to support and enhance health care CQI efforts, given the right leadership, technological expertise, and financial investment.

## HISTORICAL UNDERINVESTMENT IN HEALTH CARE INFORMATION TECHNOLOGY

The US health care industry is highly fragmented. Therefore, the decision process for information technology (IT) adoption is complex and its implementation is beyond the financial and technical resources of many small providers (Marchibroda 2004). The major area for growth and change will be the emerging markets of small physician practices, outpatient care settings, and patient homes. During the 1980s and 1990s, large IT suppliers assumed that their traditional markets in hospitals and large health care systems would expand and provide a market for existing or slightly modified products. However, they achieved only limited success and the health care sector fell further behind other service sectors in IT investment. Moreover, attempts to transfer existing approaches to the physician markets have not caught on. Despite word processors, handheld devices,

Internet access, and increasingly robust broadband communication networks, the great majority of physician orders to hospitals, nursing homes, pharmacies, and other care settings require paper, pen or pencil, and information transmission via FAX machines or courier. In 2004, for example, 90% of US health care transactions were transmitted by telephone, FAX, or mail, and only 5% of physicians were entering prescriptions electronically (Marchibroda 2004).

While the financial and insurance sectors were investing 11.1% and 8.1% of revenues, respectively, in IT, healthcare was investing a mere 2.2% of revenue (Marchibroda 2004). The director of the US Agency for Healthcare Research and Quality, Carolyn Clancy, MD, comments that the current IT approach of most hospitals is "brain dead" with disconnects and unnecessary delays and gaps, while physician practices operate like "Marcus Welby" (Masquera 2004).

The implementation of information technology is not an easy process. The requirements of the Health Insurance Portability and Accountability Act of 1996 (HIPAA) and the decentralized nature of these markets represent major barriers to successful transformation. It is no surprise that Christensen and associates (2000) saw the health care industry as one in need of "disruptive innovation" in order to establish a modern, information-savvy, market system of delivery.

Yet even in the context of this underinvestment in information technology, the resources devoted to quality and performance in health care are significant. In 1998, for example, The Joint Commission on Accreditation of Healthcare Organizations (JCAHO) listed over 125 vendors of outcomes and performance measurement information systems as meeting accreditation requirements for the Joint Commission's ORYX initiative. The overall market is even greater. The medical profession, barred by antitrust laws, medical practice acts, and, some would say, a stubborn resistance to modern corporate organizational forms, has largely retained its characteristics of small, independent units, owned and operated by the physician or small clinician group. Among the membership of the American Academy of Family Physicians (AAFP) over 70% of its 56,000 plus active practicing members work in settings with four or fewer providers. The same appears true of other primary care physician groups. Of the nation's 650,000 physicians in active practice, over half are owners/partners in small or medium-sized practices with fewer than ten full-time employees including the physicians. We estimate that there are roughly 100,000 separate medical practices in the United States. By comparison, there are approximately

5,500 nonfederal hospitals, 65,000 US banking branch offices, and 25,000 McDonalds restaurants.

Past accusations that physicians in their cottage industry are technophobic, resisting information technology, are not currently relevant (Wagner 2004). Nowadays, even very small medical offices and outpatient clinics own and operate multiple health information devices and systems. In a recent survey conducted by AAFP, 85% of the responding physicians maintained Internet connections in their practices, a similar number used onsite practice management software to send bills electronically to insurers, and 80% indicated they were contemplating purchasing an electronic health record (EHR) system.

Today's medical practice commonly has a system for practice management (including billing and accounting functions); office productivity suites for letters and other clinical documents; personal digital assistants (often with medical reference sources in memory or linked by wireless systems); and an array of paging, copying and faxing equipment. These devices are increasingly connected to local area networks (LANs) and to internal servers, and it is becoming typical to have Internet connections to a local hospital, or to a corporate data center. Systems for maintaining electronic health records are less common, but are increasing in use. However, it is clear that employer- and payer-supported groups, such as The Leapfrog Group, will eventually force mandated computerized physician order entry (CPOE) for prescriptions which will demand re-evaluation of existing infrastructure and a lot of shopping and buying (U.S. Congress, Senate 2003). Even institutional support may not be sufficient, if physician productivity and net income is not enhanced at the same time (Kolata 2004a).

Current equipment configurations contain many "gauge breaks" because of hardware, software, and network incompatibility (Kibbe and Peters 2003). In general, office administrative and practice management systems do not transfer information directly to other systems, such as those of insurance companies or health plans, except through gauge breaks, known as clearinghouses. EHR software often does not interchange messages with hospitals or reference laboratories, except through expensive interfaces that have been programmed for that purpose. Many medical office computer systems do not enable physicians to submit prescriptions electronically to pharmacies or to pharmacy benefits management companies, whose computer systems contain detailed information regarding health plan formularies.

Much of the hardware, software and networking currently used in small and medium-sized medical practices is old and outdated with respect to the privacy, security, and electronic data interchange (EDI) provisions of HIPAA. Practices will probably have to upgrade or completely replace their current systems to meet the new federal requirements for the protection of patients' health information, the security of the data stored and transferred, and the format and content standards required for electronic exchanges between medical practices and payers and health plans, including Medicare and Medicaid. However, currently available EHR systems developed for large organizations have been costing $10,000 to $15,000 a year per physician. These costs are likely to decline rapidly, but vendors and users have to come up with workable systems that are better scaled to this type of practice and require physician payments of a few hundred dollars per month per practitioner.

"Literally hundreds of products are identified as EMRs" (electronic medical records), many with some Internet capability (Rehm and Kraft 2001). On the surface the current situation looks much like a market with no dominant product form as characterized by Abernathy and Utterback (1978) who used the automotive industry to formulate their model. Their model also fits other situations such as personal computers and consumer electronics. Society, however, cannot wait around for a dominant form of health care information product to emerge. This is not a discrete product. It is a complex system affecting both the quality of care and its availability and there is no clear decision-making process as there is with an automobile or a personal computer. Furthermore, it is a service and Abernathy and Utterback's two-stage model of first product and then process change is very difficult to apply. A review of the history of hospital information systems shows the risks of waiting for any such shakeout (Kibbe and McLaughlin 2004).

The current concern with medical error and patient safety has created a new sense of urgency about information technology for EHRs and data exchange within and among health care providers. The reports of the Institute of Medicine (2000, 2001), pressure from payers, and successful implementation at a few very large institutions (Wagner 2004) mean that there is now demand for change. Information complexity in health care is likely to take a quantum leap as genomic information takes our symptom-based models of disease and replaces them with causative models expanding definitions of diseases and offering new approaches to treatment. The availability of health information (albeit of varying quality) through Internet sources is leading to more patient demands for responsiveness and autonomy from their providers (McLaughlin and Fitzgerald 2001). At the same time, the reality is that the anticipated roll-up of primary care physicians into large practices has not been successful nor have consumers accepted the attempts of health maintenance organizations and insurers to control utilization externally. Internal efficiencies and positive investment returns must be the end objective (Chinn 2002).

## INFORMATION FOR ORGANIZATIONAL IMPROVEMENTS

Both quality and cost can be improved markedly by better information technology. However, it would be a mistake to think that CQI at the organizational level requires expensive, sophisticated equipment and software programs. Easy-to-use general-purpose personal computer applications are available for many of the needs of quality improvement teams and quality managers.

This chapter emphasizes underlying concepts useful for studying health care processes and understanding causes of variation. Information systems do not in and of themselves solve many quality problems. More sophisticated information technology, which brings greater access to more data, more information and more advanced decision aids, does not guarantee better decisions or better decision makers. In fact, modern information systems may sometimes *detract* from a health care organization's overall ability to improve performance. Today's frantic and increasingly impersonal electronic world, replete with fax machines, voice transcription, and e-mail, has as much potential to create confusion in an organization's processes and disorientation or even alienation among an organization's members, as it has potential to improve productivity, enhance quality, or bring clarity to complex decisions. The approach to information management and technology's role in quality improvement efforts, therefore, calls for a balance between skills, methods, and technologies, together with a healthy skepticism about what can be accomplished in the short run through the application of existing systems from software vendors.

### Information Management Under QA and CQI

CQI challenges many of the assumptions held by both traditional quality assurance (QA) and health care information services (IS) bureaucracies regarding health care information and its uses. There are important differences between QA and CQI regarding the kind and scope of data to be collected, who collects it, and where it is used to make improvements in quality. Because of these differences, the shift from QA to CQI calls for an entirely new approach to the management of health care quality-related data and information.

In the traditional hospital clinical QA program, data flow is a convergent path from patient charts located on the hospital wards, through staff reviewers from the QA department, to centralized peer review committees. Reviewers screen cases for adverse occurrences, tally events, and report summary information. Underlying data may not be displayed nor widely disseminated. In fact, clinicians usually receive feedback from this process only when their performance is unacceptable. Finally, any action to address problems or make improvements must originate from the central peer review committees.

Information management systems in hospitals have historically been driven by the requirements of administrative and financial functions, such as billing, purchasing, payroll, and accounting, not by the needs of quality improvement. Typically, a central IS department staffed by systems analysts and managers maintains computers and data systems to service administrative functions. IS-supported hospital data management systems are not linked to quality-related data collection efforts except to supply quality analysts with patient identification information, diagnostic codes, and length of stay data. In effect, administrative data management and clinical quality improvement have remained separate domains, with distinct information needs and uses. The common thread linking administrative data management and traditional quality assurance activities is that they both exhibit a convergent flow of data whose endpoint is upper management.

## CQI Uses Mostly Decentralized Management of Data, Information, and Knowledge

Compared to QA, CQI involves more cross-disciplinary teams composed of managers *and* front line employees participating in the collection and analysis of process- and outcomes-related data, as well as in the decisions about what data should be collected and what actions should be taken to bring about improvements. The scope of the information that could be relevant to such teams is very broad. It routinely includes both clinical and administrative data captured from multiple sources inside and outside the organization. For example, a CQI team charged with improving the emergency room evaluation of patients with chest pain would gather information directly from patients and other customers; from the current medical literature; from suppliers of medical and diagnostic equipment; from data systems containing financial, scheduling, and demographic information; by direct observation (such as waiting times); and from patient charts, among other sources. Furthermore, CQI team members commonly analyze the data and take action at the local level and share data with other teams. This combination of activities performed by improvement teams can be termed *decentralized data management.*

Dispersed and decentralized data traffic of this sort lends itself to personal computing and other network technologies; e.g., groupware and email. In fact, health care organizations implementing CQI have found that quality improvement teams spontaneously reach for desktop-type software to aid them in handling their data management needs. Decentralization also requires wide dissemination of skills in the management of data, information, and knowledge to adequately support organization-wide CQI. When these skills are merely an afterthought, as they often are, problems quickly arise that can place the entire CQI initiative in jeopardy. CQI in complex organizations is a data- and information-intensive enterprise, and it is dynamic. If successful, CQI increases the demands within the organization for access to data, information, and knowledge for a whole new set of "customers" with a whole new set of questions they'd like answered. The leadership must be ready to guide the organization to a new level of expertise with information management and technology.

## The Data-to-Decision Cycle

The Data-to-Decision Cycle provides a framework that recognizes that both centralized and decentralized data management need to be present in complex organizations like hospitals and provider networks. However, the Data-to-Decision Cycle offers all organizational members a framework for understanding how information management and technology is capable of promoting improved organizational performance.

The Data-to-Decision Cycle is illustrated in Figure 10–1. The cycle describes how data are transformed to information, how information becomes knowledge, and how knowledge supports decisions and actions for improved performance. The cycle suggests that in the ideal setting data

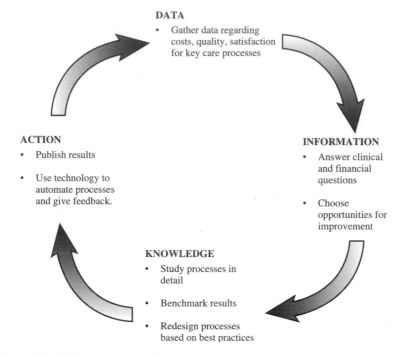

**Figure 10–1** The Data-to-Action Cycle.

collection efforts occur alongside the routine delivery of health care, and that performance improvement decisions should determine the data to be collected, thus improving the feedback between data and decisions.

Data, information, and knowledge are terms commonly used as synonyms. However, information management for CQI requires that they be defined more precisely, and the distinctions between them clarified.

*Data are facts.* Data elements by themselves have no meaning: they are simply isolated facts. For example, in Figure 10–2 we see that in the month of April there were 14 medication errors reported from nursing unit 12BG. Management at the data level is concerned with the problems relating to the accuracy of the facts, their accessibility, their formatting or organization, and their storage. Data that are accurate and structured properly can be retrieved easily and combined with other data elements in a relational database for purposes of analysis. Conversely, data of poor quality, or stored in nonstandard formats, may be next to impossible to find, and therefore useless for performance improvement work.

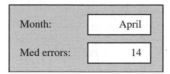

**Figure 10–2** Data on April Medication Errors for Unit 12BG

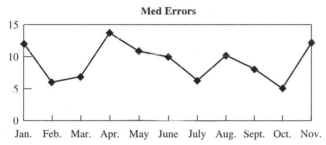

**Figure 10–3** Information on Medication Errors for the Year

*Information is data that has become meaningful.* Data assembled to answer someone's question becomes information. At the information level, management deals with proper framing of questions, identifying sources of data necessary to answer the questions, selecting and combining views of data to provide answers, and the communication of these to people who want them to aid decisions. In Figure 10–3, enough data have been collected, assembled, and displayed to provide information about the behavior of the medication delivery processes on unit 12BG, and to answer the question "what was the average monthly number of medication errors?" One very practical example of a common problem in information management involves the identification of *denominators* when rates or percentages are needed. A denominator requires that the question "how large is the whole population from which the numerator was selected?" be answered.

*Knowledge implies prediction.* Management involves utilizing information to predict and, insofar as possible, control the future performance of processes of care. When our information is robust and plentiful enough to permit predictions about performance, individuals and organizations possess knowledge that can be used to intervene, as required. In Figure 10–4, statistical process control methods have been applied to the information about medication errors on unit 12BG to ask: "Is the behavior of the

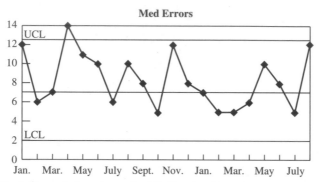

**Figure 10–4** Knowledge about the Medication Error Process

process predictable? Should we intervene? What kind of intervention is required?" Statistical process control techniques can provide knowledge about the causes of variation in a process. Other methods of interpreting and synthesizing information may provide knowledge about the appropriateness of specific treatments for individual patients or populations, or identify patients at risk.

*Decisions lead to action or inaction.* Feedback about the likely results of our actions that is based on knowledge of processes and systems is the best possible motivation for improvement. Some organizations threaten and punish individuals who are "noncompliant"; however, it is preferable to seek improvement based on knowledge and collaboration based on shared goals and on an appeal to evidence. In Figure 10–5, a quality improvement team has used data, information, and knowledge of the medication delivery process to make specific decisions about how to improve the processes. The subsequent data collection efforts shown here illustrate that the desired results; i.e., consistently fewer medication errors, have been achieved.

Over the years a number of other frameworks have been developed for describing the taxonomy of health care information systems, including those that divide systems into layers differentiated by financial or clinical orientation, and more technical schemata that are based on models in which there are conceptual, logical, and physical categories (Tan 1995). These can be useful models and the reader is encouraged to learn more about them. However, for quality improvement the Data-to-Decision Cycle has the advantage of focusing squarely on the ultimate goal of improved decisions in patient care, while providing a conceptual model to

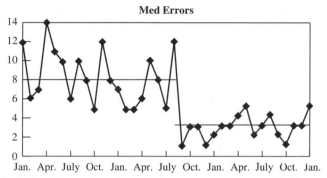

**Figure 10–5** Decisions Have Been Taken To Improve the Medication Delivery Process

guide further discussion and learning about CQI data, information, and knowledge management tasks. This framework also leads us in a systematic discussion of the technological components that can be of assistance to CQI. Finally, the Data-to-Decision Cycle points directly to the issues of data management and data quality as a place to begin any discussion of information systems related to quality improvement. It also leads us toward issues of standards, interfaces and community networks that expand quality improvement efforts beyond institutional walls.

## DATA QUALITY CONCEPTS, ISSUES, AND TECHNOLOGIES

### The Dimensions of Data Quality

Regardless of the information system(s) used, data quality is of paramount importance to quality improvement efforts where management decisions are to be based on data, not opinions or hunches. Health care data, however, often are not of very good quality. And if the underlying data are unreliable, how good are the decisions based on that data likely to be?

Electronic medical records, decision support systems, survey reporting systems, executive information systems, cost accounting systems, and quality management–performance systems all utilize data elements that come from somewhere to be stored in electronic databases. For example, the data most hospitals collect for profiling and administrative analysis comes from the 1992 version of the Universal Billing claims form (UB-92) produced when patients are discharged from the hospital. The UB-92 form provides demographic data about the patient (birth date, sex, race, discharge status), codes for several diagnoses and procedures, and total charges aggregated by type of service such as pharmacy, laboratory, and radiology. The claims data contains no clinical results, nor does it include any measures of the patient's satisfaction or functional status before or after treatment.

How good is the quality of claims data? Not very. Investigators have consistently found serious quality problems in large federal and insurance claims databases, including error rates and rates of discrepancy between similar databases of between 10% and 30% (Fisher *et al.* 1992; Whittle *et al.* 1991; Roos *et al.* 1991). In a study of almost 13,000 patients hospitalized for cardiac catheterization, the authors found that "claims data failed to identify more than one-half of patients with prognostically important conditions." The authors concluded that "insurance claims data lack important diagnostic and prognostic information when compared with concurrently collected clinical data in the study of ischemic heart disease" (Jollis *et al.* 1993).

### Data Modeling for Electronic Data Collection in Databases

Databases store data in a controlled, orderly fashion. The first step in any database design is to decide what data elements will be included, how they are related to one another, what values are permissible, and how the data will be represented or viewed according to certain rules. A data model interprets the real world. It seeks to describe or capture the real world in a structure that will support specific goals for storage, access, and analysis. The basic unit of this structure is termed the data *view,* composed of *entity, attribute,* and *value* (e,a,v). For example, the entity *employee* could contain the attributes *name, address,* and *date of birth.* Each of these attributes has many possible values, for example *Tom Jones, 123 Broad Street,* and *5/10/1950.* It is important to recognize that any data collection involves choices about how the entities, attributes, and values are set up, and these choices may greatly affect what happens (or can't happen) with the data later on. For example, we may choose to create a single attribute called *telephone number* for each employee–entity, or we might choose to create two attributes, one called *home telephone* and the other *mobile.* Similarly, we could choose to collect the date information in the format *dd/mm/yy* instead of *dd/mm/yyyy.* Finally, data have *representations* that have to do with how values are exported and displayed during analysis or reporting. For example, the choice as to how to represent null values is an important one in the design of data collection systems. Will an empty data field represent the *absence* of a value, because for example a reply was not applicable, or will it represent that a datum is *missing?* A general schema for data modeling is shown in Figure 10–6.

As presented in Table 10–1, the ideal data view should be relevant (capture only the data needed by the application), possess clarity of definition (avoid confusion between entities), be comprehensive (include all the attributes necessary to describe the entity), attain appropriate granularity (get the right level of detail), and be precise about the domain (allow for all the right possible values). The data values should be accurate (not misspelled or incorrect), complete (not missing components), current (up-to-date), and consistent (the same in different places). And the data representations should be portable (able to be exported from the database), precise as to format, able to express null values, and efficient in use of storage space. See Table 10–1 on page 256.

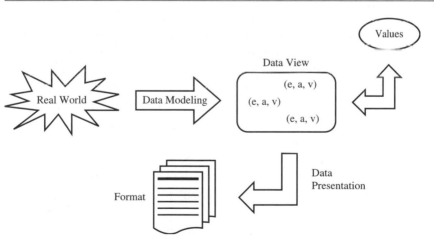

**Figure 10–6** Data Modeling Results in Views, Values, and Representations

**Table 10–1** Data View, Value, and Representation

| Data Model Component | Example | Ideal Characteristics |
|---|---|---|
| Data View | Triplet: entity, attribute, value (e,a,v), as in (employee, first name, John) | Relevant, clearly defined, comprehensive, appropriate level of detail (granularity), allow for all possible values |
| Data Value | The telephone number 919-929-5993, the date May 10, 1950 | Accurate, complete, current, consistent |
| Data Representation | Date formats, expression of null value, e.g. none vs. not known vs. zero | Exportable from one database to another, precise as to format, efficient use of memory |

## Medical Vocabularies and Standardized Data Definitions

There is no "universal language" to describe medical care. Two equally competent nurses or physicians might describe the same patient and his/her degree of severity of symptoms in very different terms. The ambiguity and vague terminology inherent in standard coding systems makes it possible for physicians, practices, and departments whose clinical or financial performance is being examined, to question whether the comparisons made are fair, or to assert that "apples are being compared to oranges." Leaders of these efforts need to understand that until a comprehensive dictionary of valid terms to be used in information systems to support CQI is produced, these problems will persist at the data quality level and are not solvable via more complex or expensive information technology. While efforts can and should be made to code patients correctly and consistently across the organization, for example by encouraging computerized physician order entry and having physicians participate more directly in the structured data process, the lack of uniform descriptors for the patients' experiences in care processes will likely plague CQI efforts in health care for a long time to come.

Medical vocabularies have been developed, of course, but they serve specific and limited purposes. The International Classification of Diseases (ICD) was developed by the World Health Organization primarily to collect health statistics, not to support detailed clinical descriptions. The

ICD9-CM (1977) added Clinical Manifestations extensions to the basic ICD, but the ICD9-CM still cannot express the detailed granularity needed for today's complex diagnoses. For example, the same ICD9-CM code "600" would appear as the primary diagnosis for two men undergoing the same procedure to remove prostatic tissue, even if one of the men had twice as much tissue removed as the other and suffered significant bleeding during the operation while the other did not. Because the ICD9-CM was intended only to classify diseases for aggregate statistical purposes, it cannot describe important aspects of the patient's history or physical exam.

The American Medical Association's Current Procedural Terminology, Fourth Edition (CPT-4), has become the standard coding system for billable physician and hospital outpatient procedures. Like the ICD coding system, the CPT system has no descriptors of patient attributes. Furthermore, there is no compatibility or interpreting between the ICD and CPT coding systems. They remain distinct coding systems for claims and billing purposes only.

The Systematized Nomenclature of Medicine (SNOMEDIII) was developed by the College of American Pathologists to include clinical concepts lacking in ICD9-CM, and to encode concepts of the history and physical exam, as well as laboratory studies, diagnoses, and procedures. The SNOMED system has not gained widespread use, however, in part because there are multiple ways one can link numerical codes to represent essentially the same entity. For example, the entity "acute appendicitis" can be represented as any of the following:

- D5-46210—acute appendicitis, not otherwise specified
- D5-46100— appendicitis, not otherwise specified, G-A231—acute
- M-41000—acute inflammation, not otherwise specified
  G-C006—in T-59200—appendix, not otherwise specified

  Key: D = diagnosis axis, G = general axis, M = morphology axis, T = topology axis (Horn *et al.* 1994)[i]

Medical Subject Headings (MeSH) were developed by the National Library of Medicine to index biomedical literature. MeSH serves well the needs for indexing articles from the literature, but was not designed to describe procedures and patient attributes such as history and physical findings. Meanwhile, a host of other institutions have developed proprietary vocabularies to serve the needs of their specific information management systems.

Given the diversity of proprietary coding systems, the National Library of Medicine has inaugurated a project to map the terms in the widely used vocabularies ICD9-CM, CPT-4, SNOMED, and MeSH. The project, known as the Unified Medical Language System, has created a *metathesaurus* that helps health professionals and researchers retrieve and integrate electronic biomedical information from a variety of sources. It can be used to overcome variations in the way similar concepts are expressed in different sources. This makes it easier for users to link information from patient record systems, bibliographic databases, factual databases, expert systems, etc. It is a very valuable resource for solving the most difficult problem in exchanging healthcare information: the multiplicity of coding systems in use. One on-line use of the UMLS is the Medical World Search site (www.mwsearch.com). When you search the Web for a medical concept, the Medical World Search uses the UMLS to include synonyms in the query. However, The UMLS is not itself a standard coding system; it is a cross-referenced collection of standards and other data and knowledge sources.

## Still Needed—New Vocabularies to Capture the Patient's Experience

So far, we have been considering vocabularies that originated with the medical profession or as a result of researchers' needs to describe the patient's condition. Paul Ellwood, MD, who coined the term "outcomes management" described this field as "a technology of patient experience," and he placed great emphasis on the need for a "patient-understood" language of outcomes (1988). None of the vocabularies mentioned so far meet this definition, but there have been recent attempts to construct data sets and measurement tools that are more patient experience oriented. A prime example is the SF-36, or Health Status Questionnaire, Short Form 36, used to measure patient perception of physical and mental well-being, which was first developed by Dr. John E. Ware, Jr., as part of the Medical Outcomes Study in the late 1980s (Tarlov *et al.* 1989). The SF-36 is administered by the Medical Outcomes Trust. Other health status survey instruments, such as the Outcomes Assessment and Information Set (OASIS) used by Medicare for outcomes study for long term care patients, are gaining popularity among health care quality improvement professionals in a wide variety of settings and institutions, precisely because they get closer to the patient's experience.

## Applying CQI to the Improvement of Data Quality

Data-generating processes in health care organizations can be studied and improved using basic CQI techniques. It is beyond the scope of this chapter to go into detail regarding data quality improvement methods and examples of their application, but the basic approach is one that considers the customer's data quality requirements, studies the current data generating processes for causes of variation in specific quality or performance attributes, acts to change processes in a systematic fashion, and then holds the gains while ascertaining and anticipating new customer requirements. Data-intensive processes can be described in terms of the Data Life Cycle (Redman 1992) a version of which is illustrated in Figure 10–7. Typically, the Data Life Cycle includes stages during which data are created, collected, stored, and accessed. In most situations, data may also be manipulated, cleansed, or used in a variety of ways and returned to storage. Occasionally, data are retired through archiving or actual de-

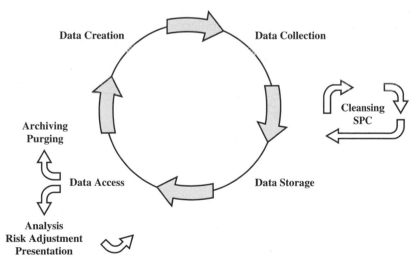

**Figure 10–7** The Data Life Cycle

struction of the data. Once these data-generating processes are described and their performance measured, then statistical process control (SPC) methods can be used to manage them and improve their performance.

### Data Quality Improvement Through Error Checking and Validation

Increasingly information systems are able to assist efforts to improve data quality by checking for data entry errors and performing range validation. In most cases, this "artificial intelligence" is really a set of simple rules that are coded into the application making it impossible or very difficult for the end-user or data enterer to send bad data to the software application. As automated data entry in health care increases, this feature of information systems becomes more valuable as a means of decreasing costly errors that can lead to re-work or unreliable information.

Figure 10–8 illustrates error checking and range validation in progress in a Web-based case management information system designed for a pediatric IPA. Javascript code written into the HTML form viewed on the Web browser software Internet Explorer™ automatically checks to see that the dates entered are consistent with rules in the program. In this case, the data enterer has mistakenly entered the admission date as 9/31/1948 instead of 9/31/98. The rules in this application are that date of birth must *precede* the date of admission, and since this rule was violated, the program returns the error message seen here telling the data enterer to check for data inconsistencies. Note that this online error checking is occurring on the client's computer, that is, on the data enterer's computer, and not in the database computer itself. No communication need take place between the client software and the remote database server for this error checking to occur, saving both time and network traffic.

### INFORMATION MANAGEMENT ISSUES, CONCEPTS, AND TECHNOLOGIES

Information management involves the skills, methods, and technological tools required to answer questions from available sources of data, and, in addition, to communicate information in a timely manner to those in need of answers. CQI in health care has grown increasingly dependent on communication networks or channels that enable health care professionals in distributed locations to share information, simultaneously access in-

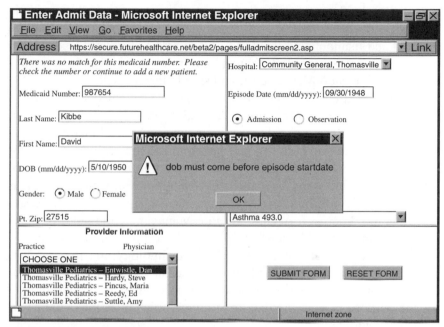

**Figure 10–8** Error Checking Done by Javascript Code in an HTML Document. When the data enterer hit the "submit form" button, the application noted that the patient's date of birth (DOB) was *after* the admit date, and prompts the data enterer to check for errors in the date fields. Here, the admit data should have been 1998, not 1948.

formation stored in electronic databases and merge the data into a working file. Health care professionals involved in CQI need to possess a thorough grounding in information management in order to be good customers of their IS department colleagues and to have reasonable expectations about getting their needs for information met.

### Relational Database Technology: Foundation of the Data-To-Information Conversion

Those interested in health care CQI recognize that many of their work environments are "data rich but information poor." By this, they mean they are in the uncomfortable position of being aware that data that (actually or potentially) hold answers to their questions are stored electronically somewhere in the enterprise, but significant barriers exist to getting the data out and manipulating them in order to arrive at desired analyses. In some cases, this is a purely technical barrier, in others it can be a combination of technical difficulty, cost, and simple lack of will.

Fortunately, almost all new information management systems used in health care organizations employ relational database technology, including those used in general ledger systems, laboratory and pharmacy systems, cost accounting systems, and performance measurement systems. Relational database technology is at the heart of information system applications that are built on databases from popular vendors such as Oracle, Sybase, Informix, and SQL Server, as well as the popular desktop programs Microsoft Access and File Manager. While not a panacea for all the problems of transforming data into information, the almost universal adoption of relational database technology and the standard query language (SQL) has made it much easier for analysts to manipulate data for reports, and to move data from one database into another for the purpose of merging data to study complex questions about performance and outcomes.

The basics of relational database technology are straightforward. All relational databases organize data in tables that store data belonging to specific entities. A table for the entity "patient" would have places to store the attributes first name, last name, social security number, etc. A table for "lab tests" would likely store the test name, the data obtained, and the result. Because each table is independent of the others, new data (e.g., new patients, new tests) can be added almost indefinitely, and new tables can be added as the need arises for new entities to be included. This arrangement is both flexible and expandable, therefore cost effective.

Of course, what we usually want to get out of the database involves knowing how the data in the tables are related. For example, we want to know the test result for a particular patient, or all the test results for a particular patient for a specified date range. Relationships between entities can be one-to-one, as in the relationship "case number:patient last name," or one-to-many as in "case number:laboratory tests." These relationships are mediated or controlled by *keys* that permit all lab tests for a particular patient to be assembled and reported to a computer screen or printer, as illustrated in Figure 10–9. The key number in this case is the social security number. Standard query language (SQL) provides for standard definition of various commands to perform relational

| Patients | | | | Lab Tests | | |
|---|---|---|---|---|---|---|
| **ID** | **Last Name** | **Date of Birth** | | **SSN** | **Test** | **Date of Test** |
| 105-58-1866 | Jones | 4/20/78 | | 346-06-9595 | CBC | 3/16/94 |
| 472-10-3959 | Smith | 7/17/84 | | 833-68-1345 | HGB | 3/8/94 |
| 889-75-1865 | Williams | 3/14/67 | | 346-06-9595 | HGB | 3/7/94 |
| 833-68-1345 | Friedlander | 8/28/44 | | 833-68-1345 | HGB | 3/2/94 |
| 614-41-0798 | Statler | 5/6/40 | | 105-58-1866 | LYTES | 3/1/94 |
| 356-02-0128 | Eddings | 7/3/53 | | 346-06-9595 | LYTES | 2/27/94 |
| 601-20-8124 | Blondel | 1/23/53 | | 105-58-1866 | HGB | 2/27/94 |
| 339-42-9100 | Elfish | 6/17/81 | | 105-58-1866 | CBC | 2/22/94 |
| 346-06-9595 | Adelberg | 6/10/54 | | 105-58-1866 | HGB | 2/21/94 |
| 010-22-4893 | Calvander | 7/11/55 | | 833 68-1345 | CBC | 2/20/94 |
| 662-35-1832 | Delbert | 7/26/60 | | 105-58-1866 | HGB | 2/18/94 |
| 087-11-6498 | Gump | 10/19/88 | | 346-06-9595 | LYTES | 2/17/94 |

< Key Values Are Unique >

**Figure 10–9** Relational Databases Permit One-to-Many Relationships To Be Mediated by Keys

---

operations, and is used by all commercial vendors to provide connectivity between systems.

## Interface Standards are Key to Communications between Medical Information Systems

SQL is an example of an "interface standard" that permits communication between information systems. Standards in general are essential to provide computer "interoperability," which is the ability to access information and manage it independent of the types of computing devices storing the underlying data. Prior to the establishment of interface standards, organizations were burdened with many point-to-point applications existing on mainframe computers. During the 1970s and 1980s, interfaces required an enormous amount of time to build, test, and install, and they typically required a separate interface to be built for each application. Interface standards ameliorate this maintenance nightmare. Standards are also required because data is distributed throughout numerous databases, controlled by different groups and with different rules for access. Some interface standards govern what should be encoded and transmitted, while others cover what information content should be provided to create an adequate record. There must also be standards to assure the security and confidentiality of data that identifies patients.

The Internet uses a set of standards for data communication known as Internet protocol/transfer control protocol (IP/TCP), which have been essential to the creation of a world-wide network. Users can access the same documents regardless of whether their computers are running on Windows, Unix, or Apple operating systems. Hypertext markup language (HTML), the language in which all World Wide Web documents are written, is another standard in use in the information highway.

There are a number of messaging standards specific to health care with which health care CQI professional should be familiar.

- **HL7**—Short for Health Level 7, this system grew out of hospital information system vendors' efforts to design an open standard for transmitting clinical data. HL7 is named for the seventh, the data presentation level and highest layer of the Open Systems Interconnection (OSI) model of the International Standards Organization (ISO). The six lower levels of the OSI, the network, hardware and software, are used to transmit the data through the network. HL7 includes standards for formatting of admission–discharge–transfer (ADT), financial order entry, clinical laboratory tests, X-ray reports, diagnostic studies, and several other areas. The current version of HL7 is known as Version 3 released in 2004.
- **ASTM International**—The oldest of the standards organization, formerly the American Society for Testing and Materials, has been involved in developing health care data interchange standards for many years. Relevant ASTM International efforts include standards for connecting laboratory instruments to computers, standards for ADT transactions, bar codes, and medical records. The ASTM E31 Committee on Healthcare Informatics also has a number of accepted and proposed standards dealing with privacy, interchange, and the structure and content of medical records. Table 10–2 lists a number of examples of the types of standards being addressed by the ASTM E31 committee and its subcommittees. It gives the reader just a hint of the magnitude of the tasks of developing and getting approval for these voluntary standards. The draft standard for the Continuing Care Record (CCR) from its E31.28 Workgroup was planned for

2003 release, but as more individuals developed an interest and more concerns were expressed it has been evolving and is now expected to become official in 2005. HL-7 Version 3.0 planned for 2000 was released in 2004.

The standards also set criteria for an acceptable electronic signature. The electronic signature must assure the identity of the signer (authentication), the unaltered transmission and receipt of the message (message integrity), and must prevent a signer from successfully denying the signature (non-repudiation). The standards explicitly require that a digital signature is the only technology that satisfies these criteria. Digital signatures employ digital certificates to bind user identity to a cryptographic element called a public key pair. The technology generally assumes that a trusted third party creates the certificates and in so doing confirms the identity of a key holder. The collection of certificates created by these trusted third parties is known as a public key infrastructure (PKI).

Standards and guidelines for the electronic maintenance and transmission of health care information will be a "moving target" in the coming months and years, influenced both by public and political opinion and by the rapidly advancing technologies in electronic security areas. The general trend, however, is clearly towards broader use of public communications systems like the Internet, World Wide Web, local area networks (LANs) and e-mail to link providers with consumers and both with ever larger stores of health care data, information, and knowledge.

- **DICOM v3.0**—The American College of Radiology and the National Electronic Manufacturers' Association began developing standards for exchanging radiological images in 1982. A revised version of the standard was published in 1988. In both versions, data transfer was defined for point-to-point connections; i.e., a networked environment was not considered. The third version of the standard was renamed DICOM which stands for Digital Imaging and Communications in Medicine.
- **ANSI ASC X.12**—ANSI stands for the American National Standards Institute, which has accredited an independent organization, X.12, to develop a number of messaging standards for health care provider information, benefits and eligibility information, and insurance claims forms information.

**Table 10–2** Examples of Standards Dealt With by ASTM International E31 Committee on Health Informatics and Its Subcommittees

Vocabulary Standards
   Terminology for medical records
   Terminology for health informatics
Record Content and Structure
   Data specification and formatting of Electronic Health Record (EHR)
   Structure and content of EHR
   Coding for EHR
   Rating scales in EHR
   Representation of personal names
   Representation of personal characteristics
   Representation of locations
   Descriptors for registration, admission, discharge and transfer information
     in EHR systems
   Representation of encoded data
   Descriptors of clinical information systems and how to model them
   Specification of Continuity of Care Record
   Relationships between patient and suppliers of records content
Security and Privacy
   Attributes of a Universal Healthcare Identifier
   Principles relating to confidentiality, privacy and data security
   Procedures of user identification, authentication and authorization
     with related training guidelines
   Other standards relating to security, signatures, certificates
Transcription and Medical Records
   Contracting and quality assurance for medical transcription
   Procedures to manage confidentiality and security during transcription
     and transfer
   Specification and use of speech recognition and dictation technology
   Interface management between digital and voice systems

## A Remaining Information Management Standards Challenge— A Patient Universal Identifier

One of the most imposing challenges to information management in health care is how to develop and gain acceptance for some standard for universally identifying patients and their data. Because patients receive care across primary, secondary, and tertiary care settings, and because numbers that identify patient records in these settings are generally assigned by detached computer databases, patients often end up with many different identification numbers.

Researchers, policy makers, and quality improvement professionals have long recognized that patients' episodes of care commonly span multiple providers, institutional settings, and occur over time. As more health care delivery activity has moved out from the hospital and into the ambulatory care setting, accounting for the activities and experiences of patients has become even more difficult. An episode of congestive heart failure, for example, could include visits to a primary care physician's office, diagnostic studies in an outpatient radiology center, a hospitalization for acute care, and follow-up with a visit to a cardiologist's office. Any attempt to study the processes of care throughout this sequence requires gathering data from each site, which is made very difficult, if not impossible, if each site's computer system identifies patients with its own unique identifier. Some indexing system that maps all those different numbers to each other, and provides a single unique identifier by which all parties could be assured that they were working with the data of the right patient, is a requirement for community-wide or system-wide quality improvements.

Attempts to create "master patient indexes" that would map these various identification numbers to a single universal number have been frustrated by a variety of sources, including social fears that such a system will allow unwanted intrusion into patient privacy. The Healthcare Insurance Portability and Accountability Act (HIPAA) of 1996 mandated Congress to establish a methodology for instituting a national unique patient identifier system. Public debate and political pressure from concerned voter groups have delayed action indefinitely (Moynihan and McLure 2000).


## INFORMATION TECHNOLOGY FOR INTER-ORGANIZATIONAL QUALITY EFFORTS AND POLICIES

### Planning for the Future in the Light of Past History:

The 35-year history of continuous attempts to develop and deploy hospital information systems as well as the current efforts to develop an electronic health record for outpatient settings suggests a lifecycle for health

IT adoption. This must play out before any electronic technology is generally adopted in the highly decentralized US health care system. This six-stage lifecycle, which we have called the ABCs of change (Kibbe and McLaughlin 2004), involves *acceptance* of the need for change, alignment of the actors to fulfill that need, *breadboard* development of the desired, integrated system, a *blueprint* for the system to be commercialized, *configuration* methods for adapting the system to individual provider and patient needs, and *capital* sources for the desired change. It is outlined one level further in Figure 10–10. However, as that figure indicates, this is not a linear process but an iterative one as questions addressed in subsequent stages uncover the need to revise and expand the work done in earlier stages.

This section of this chapter reviews how that six-stage model is relevant to current efforts to bring electronic health records to small, primary-care practices if we are to avoid the earlier pitfalls and delays.

One of the earliest hospital information systems (HIS) was officially implemented at El Camino Hospital in Mountain View, CA in 1971. It had received considerable government development support in the late 1960s. The positive impacts of a workable system were clear to policy makers even then. Lockheed, a substantial local employer, approached the hospital and asked the hospital to be the test bed for the time-shared system that this defense contractor was developing. The hospital board was not convinced of the merits of the system, but agreed, provided it did not add to costs at the hospital. Therefore, the hospital did not provide data entry labor and the hospital's community-based physicians were required to input their own data. There were serious human factor problems due to the programmers' lack of health care experience, so, while the system was not thrown out, it limped along with both champions and detractors. This commercial system has continued to develop slowly, has gone through several mergers and acquisitions, and has evolved into one of the leading vendor platforms available today. In 2003 El Camino was cited as one of the country's top-100 "Most Wired" hospitals. Yet by any metric, the industry impact has been long delayed in meeting a need identified 35 years ago. This very slow pace of adoption is not limited to the United States (Walley and Davies 2002).

What were the barriers to success visible in that experience? It was vendor-driven and was not responsive to a felt need of health care providers. The interested parties were the vendor and the government. There was no linkage between such a huge, risky investment and the competitive

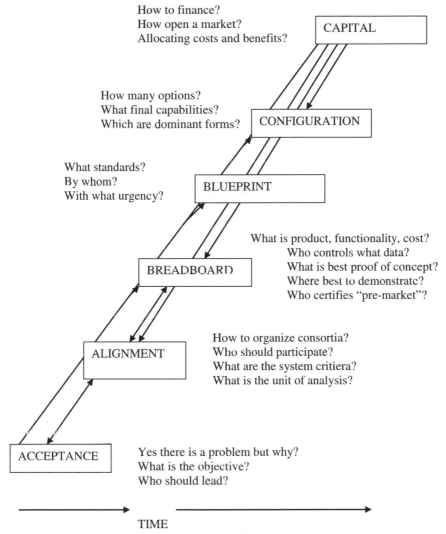

**Figure 10–10** Conceptualization of the Health Care IT System Development Process

strategy of the institution. The vendors were not gaining much from clinician insights in using the system and little information was being developed to justify commercialization. One of the major issues then as now is "Who should bear what share of the cost?" In this case neither doctors, nor patients, nor the hospital wanted to (McLaughlin 1968). In any decentralized system, there must be someone looking out for that issue when the implementation crosses corporate borders.

## Stage 1—Agreement

Many observers as noted in earlier chapters cite information technology as the key to improved quality of care and patient safety, and consumer-managed cost control. Now, for the first time, there is a sense of urgency, first among outsiders, but increasingly among those working in clinical practices. There appears to be the necessary *agreement* among actors to have achieved the first of the six stages outlined in Figure 10–10. Many actors are calling for action now, especially for CPOE, because handwriting and transcription errors are a major source of clinical error. This is almost sure to come in hospitals, but a key issue will be whether the response in the office practice will be yet another stand-alone system, or the long-awaited leap forward to an integrated personal electronic health record (Schuring and Spil 2002).

What is needed in the office-based medical practice is a virtual replacement for both the medical record and the administrative paperwork currently required to practice medicine. Administrative data and paperwork in a practice are essentially byproducts of the workflow and decision process or the clinical notes and documentation. Unless the automation of this process simplifies that flow and reduces the paperwork burden of the practice, it is unlikely to be accepted by overburdened practitioners and clerical staff. If a new system could accomplish that at reasonable cost, practitioners will be anxious to come on board.

With widespread acceptance that there is a problem, at least in patient safety, what is missing is sufficient concerted effort on the right objectives on the right scale. The objectives of patient safety, cost control, appropriate incentives, consumer choice, and smoother workflow need to be incorporated into such an effort, even though they are often conflicting. Therefore, the other five stages of this life cycle have to be implemented effectively. At the crucial primary care level, American Academy of Family Physicians (AAFP) has set up a new division, its Center for Health Information Technology, to make this transition feasible. Its efforts have followed the model in Figure 10–10 and involve a number of interesting projects to move this lifecycle agenda forward.

## Stage 2—Alignment

By focusing on the office practice as the logical target for change in health care information technology, we may have reached a major milestone in achieving the alignment necessary to improve the health care system. Practitioners, vendors, service providers, regulators, and payers have all begun to take the necessary steps toward a common achievement. To this end the AAFP has put together a consortium of interested parties to come up with a practical system that is scaled to this type of practice at an appropriate cost.

One issue that the aligned system must address is the ownership of the electronic health record. We have already mentioned some type of community clearinghouse. Another alternative, recommended by HMO pioneer, Paul Ellwood, MD, of the Jackson Hole Group, is that the patient should "own" the record (2003). A surprising number of individuals receive care from multiple providers, change their health plans, or move to new locations. If the locus of control were with patients, they could take an active role in maintaining and updating their records. However, no one knows what proportion of the population would be motivated to carry out that assignment effectively or could afford computer access of sufficient sophistication to manage it.

The aligned participants need to be in agreement on what functions the system should to perform. We suggest that such a system must integrate:

- Claims processing transactions and exchanges between medical offices, hospitals and health plans
- Order entry for diagnostic and therapeutic tests and ancillary procedures
- Laboratory, radiology, and pathology results reporting
- Automated prescriptions, including automated transmission, and standardized links to formulary and patient safety information
- Standardized electronic health records and continuity of care records (CCRs)
- Automatic access to eligibility determination and master patient identifiers
- Standardized communication links to paging, Internet, and specialized data bases with appropriate mobility features

- Patient scheduling and other office management functions, including letter generation, follow-ups, health maintenance reminders, accounting, purchasing, and inventory control.

We would also like to see real-time claims adjudication, but our own sense of urgency makes us unwilling to wait for payers to replace their legacy claims systems and establish the network capabilities that are required.

## Priniciples to Guide Development

AAFP's coalition partners have all had to agree to four principles:

- Affordability—Recognizing the limited capital available to small medical practices, partnering firms will discount their prices and work with AAFP to increase the volume of their sales of hardware and software.
- Compatibility—a plug-and-play feature of the hardware and software that does not require customized and/or expensive interfaces within the EHR system, or with key resources for electronic prescribing, laboratory results reporting, and hospital information systems.
- Interoperability—that data, such as the Continuity of Care Record, can flow among physicians, other providers and patients without specialized equipment, software or clearinghouses.
- Data Stewardship—a transparent system that meets prescribed ethical and legal standards for collection, storage, management, and use according to the highest standards of medical ethics.

Certainly, these will not be the only principles that will guide the aligned parties, but they represent a bedrock base from which to work.

## Achieving Critical Mass

On November 12, 2003 in Washington, DC, the AAFP and a consortium of vendors announced Partners for Patients, a joint effort to work in accordance with those principles with GE Medical Systems Information

Technologies, Siemens, Hewlett-Packard, Medplexus, A4, NextGen, PMSI, and Welch-Allyn. This group of vendors is not intended to exclude competition, but just the opposite, to convince the public, the providers and the vendors that this is a market that is worth exploiting. Since then more than 50 organizations have adopted these principles and joined in the development of suitable, but competing systems for the office practice. In addition to their commitment to work with AAFP on standards based on these principles, the companies have agreed to significant reductions in the prices of their products and services to AAFP members.

In July 2004, fourteen prominent medical organizations representing 500,000 primary care and specialist physicians announced the creation of the Physicians Electronic Health Record Coalition (PEHRC) to speak with unified voice about the development and implementation of "affordable, standards-based electronic health records and other information technology to improve quality, enhance patient safety, and increase efficiency." Its press release identified PEHRC's guiding principles with the acronym, QUALITY.

Quality
Usability
Affordability
Long-term commitment
Interoperability
Trust—data stewardship, financial stability, integrity
Yield—work must provide tangible benefits for physicians.
   (AAFP 2004)


**Stage 3—Breadboard**

The first task after alignment is to produce and test a workable office system that meets these principles in the field. With so many promises and so many disappointments in health care information systems, most actors are content to wait and see. As the Institute of Medicine observed:

> There is no accepted blueprint for redesigning the health care sector, although there is widespread recognition that fundamental changes are needed in health care and the financial and legal environment that shapes it. The sheer size and complexity

of the health care sector, with tens of thousands of health care providers and a myriad of public and private insurance and delivery arrangements, makes wholesale change difficult. For many important issues, we have little experience with alternatives to the status quo. For these reasons, the committee sees the launching of a carefully crafted set of demonstrations as a way to initiate a "building block" approach to health system change. (IOM 2002b, Executive Summary, p. 3)

One of the five areas for demonstrations recommended by the IOM committee was health care IT with the objective of the "paperless" health care system. These demonstrations are underway and AAFP is participating with CRMI, the California medical review organization, in project DOC-IT (Doctors Office Quality Information Technology). This program is designed to promote the adoption of the EHR, electronic prescribing, electronic laboratory results management, and electronic care reminders and registries. The focus here is on measuring quality of care and documenting quality improvement, but the same systems can accomplish a broad array of objectives. This demonstration is to involve at least 1,000 physicians in hundreds of offices. Work on the measurement and validation part of this program will go forward while the appropriate systems of hardware and software are being specified, so that both the measures and the systems can be implemented to show the waiting profession what can be done effectively and efficiently.

Hospital inpatient information systems have advanced much more than those for office practices, but we can learn from them as well. One advanced system is the Veterans Administration's excellent VistA EHR system, some of which can be adapted for the office setting. However, it is designed for large institutions with extensive computing resources available and only limited dispersal among communities.

AAFP and the Health Information Management Systems Society (HIMSS) are leading a small-scale collaborative pilot project in 18 family medicine practices, each paired with a sponsoring organization in their community. Each office will implement the Medplexus XML- and Java-based EHR system with application hosting and management, software, training donated by Medplexus, Siemens Medical Solutions and Hewlett-Packard. The pilot project's main objective is to provide proof-of-concept for the applications service provider mode of delivery of scalable electronic health records systems. The barriers and keys to success will also be studied extensively.

## Stage 4—Blueprint

Once the concept is proven, it will be time to implement standards for interchange of information to meet the principles of compatibility and interoperability. ASTM's Committee 31 has taken on responsibility for issuing standards in electronic health. It has already worked on a standard for the internal EHR. But that may be one of the easier tasks. A current effort is the Continuity of Care Record document standard for a core set of health information on each patient- problem list, medications, allergies, etc. This would be a referral document or "face sheet" or mini-medical history that could be imported or exported from a number of vendors' software products or via secure e-mail attachment, or carried by the patient on a smart card or USB memory stick. AAFP is co-sponsoring this development with ASTM, Massachusetts Medical Society, HIMSS, American Academy of Pediatrics, and others. This is just one of the standards that will have to be developed to assure compatibility and interoperability of the entire system within the practice and among authorized users.

Once the demonstrations have been evaluated, system specifications can be developed and finalized. Then hardware and software vendors can scale and optimize their systems for efficiency and effectiveness. These new systems can then be tested and the results disseminated.

## Stage 5—Configuration

It is too early to say how this fifth stage will play out in a competitive marketplace. Some entity will have to be an honest broker in evaluating outcomes from the prior stages and recommending how practices can effectively and economically retool to meet the demands of the Internet age. Certainly, having evaluative information come out of existing demonstration projects will be a key input to this stage of the process. Developing this information has been a key component of each AAFP-directed project. Meanwhile, the US Agency for Healthcare Research and Quality (AHRQ) has identified this need and is offering up to $10 million in grants for research to "assess the value derived from the adoption, diffusion, and utilization of health information technology to improve patient safety and quality of care." The RFP also calls for attention to the financial and organizational impacts of these systems (Department of Health and Human Services 2003).

## Stage 6—Capital

The cost of this conversion will not be cheap. There is the cost of new practice systems, supplier and payer hardware and software, storage systems and network development. Vendors would certainly expect to recoup their research and development costs and payers their conversion costs. 2003 data indicates that the health care industry spent only 3.9% of gross revenues, despite its prior lagging position, compared to 5.3% in the already automated financial services sector, and 6.6% in the government sector (Wagner 2004). This is expected to rise, but there is still the question of how to pay for it.

Given the financially strapped position of the industry right now, there has to be either a subsidy for improvement, a source of capital, and/or excellent cost justifications for the program. This has to go beyond positive anecdotal evidence such as that supplied by CareGroup on its CPOE system at Beth Israel Deaconess Medical Center in Boston (Wagner 2004).

Yet we know that primary care physician income has been dropping year-by-year and most practitioners are averse to cost-increasing decisions. Several alternatives have been suggested:

- Payer incentives
- Mandating costs
- Government grants or loans

For example, Empire Blue Cross-Blue Shield in New York City has offered hospitals a 4% bonus for meeting the two Leapfrog Group standards of CPOE and board-certified or qualified critical care physicians in their ICUs. Many other organizations are experimenting with pay for outcomes performance which should also enhance the value of e-health efforts (Glaser and Phillips 2003).

Efforts by payers and accrediting agencies can mandate investments just as effectively as direct government efforts. The CPOE requirement, as it becomes effective, will mandate practice and hospital investments at a new level through the pressures of the marketplace.

The role of governments as sources of capital is well established for health care. Tax-exempt health care bonding authorities exist in many states. However, it would take a major change of attitude and mission to support financing equipment for physician practices.

We expect to see some aspects of all of these, but would also like to see some more novel arrangements. An example would be a contribution to the upkeep of the network by vendors who would experience reduced costs thereby, such as regional laboratories that now spend large amounts faxing results reports to the practices.

While the federal government seems to be an active participant in the process at the research and development and demonstration stages,

> New federal activism is required to assure not only interoperability of clinical data systems, but also that providers who lack capital and technical resources can make the digital conversion. (Goldsmith *et al.* 2003, p. 45)

Another area of need for federal support is to "remove barriers to hospital's propagation of their EHR systems to physician's office practices by amending fraud-and-abuse statutes to provide a legislative safe harbor for carefully-defined cooperative IT activities between hospitals and physicians" (Goldsmith *et al.* 2003, p. 53).

## FUTURE DIRECTIONS AND TRENDS FOR INFORMATION TECHNOLOGY IN CQI

The fundamental importance of data—collection, storage, protection, analysis, and use—has emerged as a key characteristic of the changing health care delivery system in the United States. No matter what the health care setting or population, the dual imperatives of controlling costs and improving quality can be achieved only through managing with data, that is, through careful evaluation of how the processes of care are linked to the outcomes of health care delivery, and through the application of information systems that help us to achieve the best possible outcomes. This means that outcomes data collection, the assurance of health care data quality, and the methodologies for accessing health data and information when needed have become almost overnight highly desirable capabilities—indeed, core competencies— for professionals involved in producing health care services whether the issues are organizational or national or in between. This is underscored by the Center for Medicare and Medicaid Services' new requirement that the reimbursement of the purchase of expensive new drugs, services and devices include the on-going gathering and analysis of data on patient use and outcomes financed by the vendor (Kolata 2004b). It is also evident in two of the cases in this book: Case 7 that involves the State of North Carolina's attempt to assure the use of evidence-based practices in its public mental health system and Case 2 about efforts organizations certifying medical specialists to require process improvement activities as a condition of recertification.

# PART IV

# Application

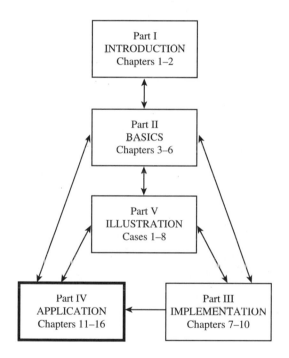

Part I
INTRODUCTION
Chapters 1–2

Part II
BASICS
Chapters 3–6

Part V
ILLUSTRATION
Cases 1–8

Part IV
APPLICATION
Chapters 11–16

Part III
IMPLEMENTATION
Chapters 7–10

# Integrating Approaches to Health Professional Development With Approaches to Improving Patient Care

*Julie J. Mohr and Paul Batalden*

*All health professionals should be educated to deliver patient-centered care as members of an interdisciplinary team, em phasizing evidence based practice, quality improvement approaches, and informatics.*
*–A vision for health professions education,*
*articulated by the Institute of Medicine, 2003*

The purpose of this chapter is to provide a brief background on current reform efforts in health professions education and to explore health professional development from the perspective of three quality improvement strategies—organization-centered, issue-centered, and clinical microsystem-centered.

## BACKGROUND

In 2001, the Institute of Medicine (IOM) published a report, "Crossing the Quality Chasm: A New Health System for the 21st Century." This report was a culmination of the work of the Committee on the Quality of Health Care in America, which was formed in 1998 (Institute of Medicine 2001). Among the many points the Committee made, it acknowledged that

most health professionals have had limited education in extracting information directly from their own practice experience and using it to redesign
their everyday care systems.

The Committee recommended that strategies be developed for

> (1) restructuring clinical education to be consistent with the prin-
> ciples of the 21st century health system throughout the contin-
> uum of undergraduate, graduate and continuing education for
> medical, nursing, and other professional training programs and
> (2) assessing the implications of these changes for provider cre-
> dentialing programs, funding, and sponsorship of education pro-
> grams for health professionals (Institute of Medicine 2001).

The Committee also recommended that an interdisciplinary summit be
held to develop next steps for the reform of health professions education
to enhance patient care quality and safety. This summit was convened in
June 2002.

The calls for educational reform and the work of the interdisciplinary
summit were based on several points:

- Health professionals (e.g., physicians, nurses, health administrators) are not adequately prepared—in either academic or continuing
  education venues—to address shifts occurring in the US patient
  population such as changes in diversity, aging of the population, increasing incidence of chronic illnesses, and improved access to
  health information.
- Once in practice, health professionals are expected to work as part of
  interdisciplinary teams, yet they have not been trained as part of an
  interdisciplinary team and they often lack team-based skills.
- There is a rapidly expanding evidence base for making health care
  decisions, but there is a lack of consistency in training about how to
  search and evaluate the evidence base and to apply it to practice.
- There is a mismatch between what is known about quality and safety
  of care and coursework that is available to health professional students about how to assess quality and safety-of-care information and
  design and test solutions.
- There is lack of a basic foundation of training on informatics
  (Institute of Medicine 2003).

The Committee concluded by recommending a set of "core competencies" that all health professionals should acquire during training, regardless of their discipline. These competencies include (1) providing patient-centered care; (2) working in interdisciplinary teams; (3) employing evidence-based practice; (4) applying quality improvement; and (5) using informatics.

Many organizations that govern medical education—from medical schools through the specialty boards—are focused on identifying these core competencies and what they mean for professional education in their field. For instance, the Accreditation Council for Graduate Medical Education (ACGME) in increasing its focus on educational outcome assessment in residency programs identified and endorsed six general competencies that residents must demonstrate—patient care, medical knowledge, practice-based learning and improvement, professionalism, interpersonal skills and communication, and systems-based practice (Accreditation Council for Graduate Medical Education 1999). Specialty boards (e.g., the American Board of Pediatrics, American Board of Internal Medicine, and the American Board of Medical Specialties) have followed suit, recognizing the need for physicians to demonstrate core competencies as part of initial specialty certification and for maintenance of that certification.

The concept of acquiring, demonstrating, and maintaining these core competencies presents new challenges to health professions education. Although most residency programs focus on providing physicians with substantial training in patient care and medical knowledge, only a few expose residents to systems-based practice and practice-based learning and improvement (Eliastam and Mizrahi 1996; Weingart 1996; Weingart 1998; Mohr *et al.* 2003b; Ogrinc *et al.* 2004). Developing these two competencies challenges residency programs to find innovative ways to integrate quality improvement and systems thinking into training and evaluation.

## THE PROCESS OF PROFESSIONAL PREPARATION AND DEVELOPMENT

Health professionals have long been proud of their personal commitment to lifelong learning and to their role as leaders in the design and delivery of health care.

The exact process varies for each professional discipline, but at a high level the processes resemble one another and can be illustrated with the case of medicine. The process can be described by the categories of formal educational preparation:

- *basic health professional preparation* leading to an MD degree,
- *graduate health professional preparation* leading to specialty certification,
- *postgraduate health professional preparation* for continuing medical education and maintenance of certification.

Each step of the process has a defined content of learning. That definition of content has been based on some expert assessment of what is now known, what is appropriate for the learner at this stage of his/her preparation, and what the profession in general has established as knowledge needed for competency as a professional at that stage of development. State, national, and professional exams have been designed to assess the candidate's knowledge and skills at that level.

While everyone seeking professional training goes through the same formal education process, each person also progresses through an individually unique process of skill and knowledge development. The Dreyfus Model, developed by brothers Stuart Dreyfus and Hubert Dreyfus, suggests seven stages, five of which—novice, advanced beginner, competent, proficient, and expert—seem relevant to medical practice (see Figure 11–1). The model was developed based on work commissioned by the US Air Force to describe the development of the knowledge and skill of a pilot. They later identified a similar process of development in the chess player, the adult learning a second language, the adult learning to drive an automobile, and many others (Dreyfus and Dreyfus 1986). For example, when applied to medicine, in the *novice stage,* the freshman medical student begins to learn the process of taking a history and memorizes the elements, chief complaint, and history of the present illness, review of systems, and family and social history. In the *advanced beginner stage,* the junior medical student begins to see aspects of common situations, such as those facing hospitalized patients (admission, rounds, discharge) that cannot be defined objectively apart from concrete situations and can only be learned through experience. Maxims emerge from that experience to guide the learner. In the *competent stage,* the resident physician learns to plan the approach to each patient's situation. Risks are involved, but supervisory practices are put in place to protect the patient. Because the resident has planned the care, the consequences of the plan are knowable to

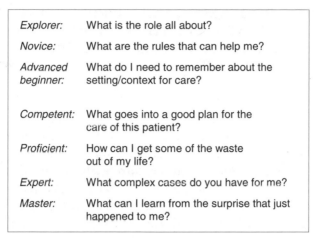

| | |
|---|---|
| *Explorer:* | What is the role all about? |
| *Novice:* | What are the rules that can help me? |
| *Advanced beginner:* | What do I need to remember about the setting/context for care? |
| *Competent:* | What goes into a good plan for the care of this patient? |
| *Proficient:* | How can I get some of the waste out of my life? |
| *Expert:* | What complex cases do you have for me? |
| *Master:* | What can I learn from the surprise that just happened to me? |

**Figure 11–1** The Modified Dreyfus Model of Skill Acquisition
*Expertise in Nursing Practice: Caring, Clinical Judgment, and Ethics*, P. Benner et al., 1995. Springer Publishing Company, Inc., New York 10036. Used by permission.

the resident and offer the resident an opportunity to learn. In the *proficient stage,* the specialist physician early in practice struggles with developing routines that can streamline the approach to the patient. Managing the multiple distracting stimuli in a thoughtful way is intellectually and emotionally absorbing. In the *expert stage,* the mid-career physician has learned to recognize patterns of discrete clues and to move quickly, using what he or she might call "intuition" to do the work. The physician is attuned to distortions in patterns or to slow down when things "don't fit" an expected pattern (Batalden *et al.* 2002).

Initial professional formation occurs within disciplinary channels, even though health professionals of varying disciplines usually work together. Further, health professional education does not occur in isolation. It occurs within the context of a setting: the organization in which formative professional development occurs. In combining the existing process of preparation of the health professional with the newly-defined core competencies of health professionals, we must consider how the formative processes of health professional development and the context of the setting—that is, the organization and delivery of patient care—can interact and adapt to deployment strategies for the continual improvement of health and health care.

## ORGANIZING, DELIVERING, AND IMPROVING PATIENT CARE: ORGANIZATION-CENTERED STRATEGIES, ISSUE-CENTERED STRATEGIES, AND MICROSYSTEM-CENTERED STRATEGIES

Traditionally, there has been an organization-centered and an issue-centered deployment strategy for continual improvement of quality and value of healthcare. Both have specific implications for health professional development—and each has strengths as well as important vulnerabilities (Batalden 1998). With the current efforts for health professions education reform providing the context for this discussion, this chapter explores these strategies. We also add a third strategy to the mix by considering the role of the clinical microsystem and outlining the contribution that it can make in training health professionals for quality improvement.

### Organization-Centered Strategies

Organization-centered improvement in health care has been alive in the United States for several decades, ever since the American College of Surgeons began accrediting hospitals (Brennan and Berwick 1996). This focus on the macro-organization as the unit of attention began when health care organizations, particularly hospitals, began to explore the lessons of continual improvement that were being learned concurrently in other sectors. In 1980, new visibility for organization-wide efforts to improve quality came from the public television documentary, "If Japan can, why can't we?" (Dobyns and Crawford-Mason 1991) Early visibility in the US for "Company-wide Quality" (Mizuno 1988) or "Total Quality" came in manufacturing settings, most prominently in the automotive sector. By the middle of the 1980s, efforts were underway in health care in the Alliant Hospital System in Kentucky and the Hospital Corporation of America in Nashville, Tennessee (McEachern and Neuhauser 1989; Walton 1990). Many more in health care became interested as the Joint Commission on the Accreditation of Healthcare Organizations and subsequently the National Committee on Quality Assurance incorporated this thinking into the accreditation processes. Important characteristics of the organization-centered strategy include a focus on the context for work, knowledge of work as a system/process, attention to patients–payers–communities as beneficiaries/customers, the leader's role in promoting learning, and organizational networks. These features are described below.

*Focus on the context for work:* Efforts were made to clarify what it meant to engage "quality" as a business or organizational strategy, including work on organizational policy statements of mission, values, and vision to create visibility for the objectives of continual improvement of services and products. These efforts were aimed at fostering a work environment that recognized and celebrated the value of learning at work. Deming wrote a set of guidelines for Western management, widely known as "Deming's Fourteen Points," that were extensively studied as descriptive of a workplace that was to be encouraged (Deming 1986). Health care versions of these points were made, and they facilitated study by health professionals and their organizations.

*Knowledge of work as system/process:* Building on and complementing the work of many general systems thinkers (Bertalanffy 1968; Churchman 1971; Brockman 1977; Ackoff 1981; Checkland 1981; Forrester 1990; Mitroff and Linstone 1993), Deming offered a view of the work of organizations as a system (Deming 1986). Adaptations of this model were made and used in health care (Batalden and Stoltz 1993; Batalden and Mohr 1997). With the focus on health care as a system and process came adaptations of process and system change strategies in the form of "projects" where, in many cases, the people leading the change had never been active in those roles. This newfound opportunity gave them additional pride in their work. "Tribes" grew up around particular improvement methods and approaches. The language of one approach was sometimes difficult for others to understand—it was easier to classify the label than to understand its relationship to the underlying phenomenon. Sometimes the proprietary interests of authoring individuals and organizations got in the way of dissemination and critical methods analysis. Some evaluation efforts were aimed at assessing what happened when people were engaged in "doing quality improvement" rather than seeing "improving the quality of what you do" as a key aspect of work. Despite these limits, these new methods and skills for understanding and changing health care in usual practice settings gained new visibility.

*Attention to patients, payers, communities as "beneficiaries" or "customers:"* The focus on the design and delivery of patient care required better understanding of personal preferences, values, and aims of the person receiving that care. Many methods for creating the new knowledge and understanding were offshoots from the "customer" focus in sectors other than health care (Batalden and Nelson 1990; The Joint Commission on Accreditation of Healthcare Organizations 1992; Nelson and Batalden 1993). It was no longer a matter of "patient relations" or "patient satisfaction," as it became clear that we needed more insight into our efforts to design care. Coping with the reality of multiple—and sometimes apparently conflicting—customer requirements placed health care alongside many other sectors with similar struggles.

*Leader's role in promoting learning:* To bring these changes about, leaders had to move beyond "command and control" understandings of their own work (Taylor and Taylor 1994). Work done by Argyris and Schön (Argyris 1991; Argyris and Schön 1996) expanded our understanding of what it meant to learn in the work setting. The work of Peter Senge and his colleagues at the Massachusetts Institute of Technology provided great visibility to the idea of a "learning organization", identifying five disciplines as fundamental to the creation of such organizations (Senge 1990; Senge *et al.* 1994)

*Organizational networks:* The desire to create opportunities to share learning underway in similar organizations led to the creation of multiple networks of organizations. (Institute for Healthcare Improvement's Quality Management Network [QMN], Group Practice Improvement Network [GPIN], The Healthcare Forum's Quality Improvement Networks [QINs], and HCA's Healthcare Quality Technology Network [HQTN] all had active, regular meetings and cross-network learning.) These networks provided settings in which organizations and their leaders came together to share and accelerate their own efforts at organization-wide improvement.

Such organization-centered efforts led to positive changes in how we organize and deliver healthcare, but at the same time other changes occurred in health care organizations that were toxic to the organization. Organizational definitions changed weekly with the flurry of new partnerships, mergers, acquisitions, divestitures, joint ventures, etc., which added confusion and complexity at the level of the caregiving personnel as new procedures for connecting their services emerged continuously. Old patterns of working wherever you wanted as a graduated medical specialist were supplanted by the need to go where there was work as layoffs, cutbacks, and hiring freezes targeted oversupplied medical specialties. As documented in the Dartmouth Atlas of Health Care, there were huge variations in care-giving and health resource capacity: beds, MDs, nurses, care-giving practices per thousand population (Wennberg *et al.* 1996).

These variations prompted many to ask why they were bearing the additional costs and morbidity experienced in their geographic region.

Furthermore, as comparable clinical outcomes were being documented, purchasers accelerated their pressures for cost reductions. With minimal agreement about measures of quality, assumptions that "all care is about the same, only the costs are different" led purchasers to engage in demand or target pricing strategies: the purchaser tells the health plan how much less they will pay for their health care premiums the next year. These pressures further contributed to the "disconnect" between the senior leaders and the front line caregivers who were being asked to work harder to achieve these external demands. This would have been of little consequence if real changes in the value and quality of care were not desired. However, real changes were sought by recipients of care and by those paying for care. They perceived that provider "unresponsiveness" was a matter of will and they sought political, regulatory, or "contractual" relief. At the same time and outside of health care, we witnessed changes in the way manufacturing and service enterprises were led. Expectations about customer-driven design, process and system analysis, and improvement were built into the public's assumption structure. While the leaders in other sectors were often able to make these changes, it has been difficult for many leaders in health care to consider these as relevant and deserving of the same priority. Though we have learned the names and terms, we have had difficulty learning and incorporating these basic insights offered by W. Edward Deming and others (Batalden and Stoltz 1993; Deming 1993). Some in health care see this requirement for new knowledge and its application (McLaughlin and Kaluzny 1999). Market pressures and regulatory pressures have helped increase the recognition of the terms and the pace of such change.

Few macro-organizations engaged in both organization-wide improvement of patient care and health professional education combined the two initiatives. Each initiative seemed to have its own "home" within the organization. Strategic initiatives for improvement of care were much more common than strategic initiatives for professional education and development, and few common initiatives linked the improvement of patient care with professional development. Line leaders were more comfortable asking for accountability around patient care improvement than around professional development.

In summary, organization-centered strategies for the improvement of health care gave new emphasis and new energies to many features of organization life that were helpful to improving quality. However, the fundamental realities that organizations of all kinds were becoming less stable, organization-wide efforts of all kinds were becoming less dependable, and "quality" was becoming only another theme for the harried top leaders left the unmistakable impression that complete dependency on organization-centered strategies for the improvement of health care quality left these efforts vulnerable. In addition, health care delivery is highly fragmented in ownership and control. In most hospitals, physicians are not employees and in some communities can move their business among institutions at will. The reality is that at the macro-organization level there is a limited ability to directly improve quality and value of care. Organizations don't provide the care, individual professionals do. It is the same phenomenon with professional education and development—macro-organizations don't "educate physicians and nurses"—people do. Further, most individual health care professionals working in complex organizations do not provide care as individuals; they work together as part of interdependent systems.

## Issue-Centered Strategies

Improving health care by finding topics or conditions that could be improved, conducting tests of change, and disseminating those efforts is as old as the application of empiricism to health care. What seemed new was the public identification of gaps between what was known and what was usually done coupled with strategies to accelerate closing those gaps. In his 1994 keynote address to the annual National Forum of the Institute for Healthcare Improvement, Donald Berwick, MD, challenged the group by naming specific conditions and clinical situations where the scientific evidence suggested one path for practice and the increasingly available data about our common practices suggested that another path was in use, indicating a real performance gap. Later, these observations were prominently featured in a widely-circulated medical journal (Berwick 1994).

These observations arose from increasingly available comparative practice data made public by purchasers, private data companies, and public sources, including states. These data invited comparisons across provider settings and revealed wildly varying care processes and outcomes. Variation in care across small areas had been known for years (Wennberg and Gittlesohn 1973). What was new was the extent of the variation and its significance for both clinical outcomes and costs (Wennberg et al. 1996).

Under the auspices of the Institute for Healthcare Improvement, a series of issue-specific efforts began in May 1995. This model brought together a panel of knowledgeable subject matter experts and a panel of people who had been able to make change in their practices. Together they developed a set of "change concepts" worth trying. Other teams of subject matter practitioners were invited to join a cooperative effort to rapidly test these concepts in their home settings and to compare experiences through closely networked communications and return meetings. Their collective experiences were then made public in publications and a national "congress" for the larger interested public. The gains were impressive. Stretch goals of change: more than a 40% change in practice was achieved by more than 25% of participants, and more than a 20% change in practice in 78% of the first 147 organizational participants (Kilo 1997). The rush of issue-centered activity sharpened the focus for improvement. Many changes were made and networking increased among similarly motivated clinicians and other health care leaders. At the same time, it became clear that all this highly visible activity masked real unevenness in execution—sometimes within the same organization. The idea that improvement could occur without explicit attention to the context for work grew. The popularity of "naming the issues" caught on and the impatience to "name" the next issue seemed to take precedence over deployment of systematic change. The longevity for an "issue" seemed to be getting shorter. Improving patient care, issue by issue, became the same as creating a "quick-fix skunkworks": delegating the responsibility for improvement to that group and assuming that they would accomplish all that was needed. Privately, some wondered about the sustainability of the larger numbers, faster issues, and activity vortex, that seemed to obscure unresolved deployment challenges and threatened to exhaust dedicated (but finite) professional resources. Some also wondered about the cost of this "late education" and wondered why the acquisition of this knowledge and these skills could not become a part of the regular preparation of health professionals.

It did not occur to many to actively couple the professional learning and development with issue-centered improvement. Students were busy learning the "tried and true" ways, which—somewhat paradoxically—were the focus of change and of the "improvement hot houses" within organizations. Graduate level learners could only be helpful players in these efforts if their faculty were actively engaged in these efforts. Yet faculty were rarely recruited to join improvement teams. As a result, it seemed appropriate to keep professional education and issue-centered improvement separate.

With the vulnerability of organization-centered strategies and the questions about the sustainability and overall impact of issue-centered programming, the future for the improvement of health care seemed less than certain. Further, the two strategies were not seeking explicit linkages to professional development. Fortunately, another option began to emerge.

### Microsystem—Centered Strategies

Systems of care exist at multiple levels—the individual patient involved in a self-care system; the physician–clinician–patient dyad; the clinical microsystem that recognizes the multiple people, activities, technology, and information involved in providing patient care; the larger macro-organization that provides an institutional home for multiple microsystems; and finally the external environment surrounding the macro-organizations. These multiple systems can be depicted as the series of concentric circles shown in Figure 11–2.

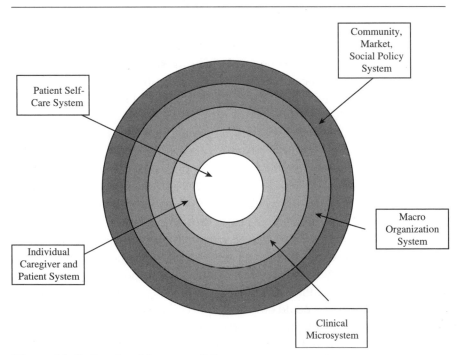

**Figure 11–2**  Levels of Systems of Care.

The focus on the clinical microsystem provides a conceptual and practical framework for thinking about the organization and delivery of care. A clinical microsystem is a group of clinicians and staff working together with a shared clinical purpose to provide care for a population of patients (Batalden *et al.* 1997; Nelson *et al.* 1998; Mohr 2000). The clinical purpose and its setting define the essential components of the microsystem. These include the clinicians and support staff, information and technology, the specific care processes, and the behaviors that are required to provide care to its patients. Microsystems evolve over time, responding to the needs of their patients, providers, and external pressures. They often co-exist with other microsystems within a larger (macro) organization. This initial focus on the clinical microsystem suggested that the aim of good patient care could be the sole focus for the daily work of the microsystem. Eventually, it became clearer that at least for academic clinical microsystems—those existing within academic health centers—the dual mission to provide excellent patient care and excellent professional development–learning was their reality.

The emerging nursing shortages and mounting physician frustration and dissatisfaction signaled that the need to focus on both patient and providers at the level of the clinical microsystem might not be limited to academic medical centers. Most patients get health care from health professionals who work in very complex organizations. Patients interact with multiple microsystems as they navigate through the health care system. The handoffs between microsystems, even for the most savvy consumers of health care, can be difficult and confusing. Similarly, health care professionals rotate through multiple microsystems as they receive their initial clinical training. They often receive little orientation to the way an individual microsystem works; indeed, they are often members of that microsystem only for a few weeks before rotating to a different microsystem. As students and trainees, they are "rewarded" for finding ways to work around the system to accomplish patient care activities. As they are immersed in the daily work of caring for patients as part of a microsystem, students, trainees, and the fully trained health care professional can see the system issues that impede high quality care, yet they lack the tools and resources needed to make changes in that work environment. Not surprisingly, they become frustrated with their own ability to respond to the macro-organization and societal pressures to remove cost while maintaining or improving the quality of care. After graduation, these students assume practitioner roles and in them they experience their continued professional formation and development. Unless the work settings are explicitly aimed at good patient care *and* good professional development, the results will reflect the shortages and frustrations currently being experienced widely in US health care.

In the late 1990s, under the aegis of the Institute of Medicine (IOM) and with funding by the Robert Wood Johnson Foundation, Mohr and Donaldson investigated high-performing clinical microsystems (Donaldson and Mohr 2000; Mohr 2000). Their research was based on a national search for the highest-quality clinical microsystems. Forty-three clinical units were identified using theoretical sampling and their leaders were interviewed using a semi-structured interview protocol. The results of the interviews were analyzed to determine the characteristics that seemed to be most responsible for enabling these microsystems to be effective. The results suggested that eight dimensions, shown in Figure 11–3, were associated with high quality of care.

Recognizing both the role of the microsystem in training health professionals and in providing patient care offers several advantages. Training within the clinical microsystem allows for cross-profession development. Traditionally, health professionals have been prepared within her or his disciplinary, professional "silo." However, once practicing in a professional setting, they work together in processes that require them to reach common understandings about the design of change and improvement of care. Moreover, models of professional development that offer a theory of knowledge and skill acquisition that crosses disciplines have the added attraction of offering special opportunities for those faculty who under-

---

1. Constancy of purpose
2. Investment in improvement
3. Alignment of role and training for efficiency and staff satisfaction
4. Interdependence of the care team to meet patient needs
5. Integration of information and technology into work flows
6. Ongoing measurement of outcomes
7. Supportive from the larger organization
8. Connection to the community to enhance care delivery and extend influence

**Figure 11–3** Eight Dimensions of Effective Microsystems

stand the new information and skills and who can integrate them into their own way of teaching the current subject matter.

Such an integrated model of front line work offers health professional faculty the opportunity to demonstrate what the continual improvement of care and systems-based practice means in the daily work of the faculty and other learners. Learners acquire the knowledge and skill as part of their experiential learning

This model emphasizes the context within which students and trainees learn and are assessed and provides insight into how to link the development of learner competencies to the specific environment. Improvement efforts—educational as well as clinical—may be more effective when designed and implemented at the microsystem level and supported by the larger organization. Clearly, there is a role for the organization-centered strategy as well as the issue-centered strategy. By explicitly including students and trainees in designing and testing interventions, we can enhance our efforts to achieve the mission of teaching and assessing specific core competencies within the academic clinical microsystem.

An example of this idea at work can be seen on 1East at Dartmouth Hitchcock Medical Center—a busy in-patient general medicine clinical microsystem that determined it wanted to do better with pneumonia immunization in the adult patients it cares for and earlier treatment of adult patients with community-acquired pneumonia. A resident learner in the Dartmouth Hitchcock Leadership Preventive Medicine program began to work along with the faculty and nursing leadership. New practices for discharge and admission were co-developed by the resident, medical faculty and nursing leadership with the result of higher levels of immunization and more prompt administration of antibiotics on admission.

Linking health professional development and improved patient care with the macro-organization policy and practice, issue-centered innovation and change, and enhanced front line operations in the clinical microsystems where patients and providers regularly meet offers many challenges. Faculty need to be encouraged and recognized for leading in these ways. Infrastructure—such as information and human resource policy and practices—that has served good and improved patient care needs to serve both professional development and patient care. Educational requirements that have celebrated frequent rotations in and out of front line systems of care need to be re-examined for their effect on the total system of patient care and professional development. Learning about professional work depends on role models who are able to integrate providing and improving care. Accreditation practices must explore both learning and patient care. Fortunately, such changes invite a more satisfying professional life and are likely to be attractive to many, though many existing systems and operational habits are likely to need re-examination and probably modification.

## CONCLUSION

Health care improvement that is undertaken with any one of the strategies as the major driver can expect to experience the strengths and weaknesses we have already seen. Improvement that is part of the fundamental processes of health professional development and able to attract the synergy of an integrated approach-organization—centered, issue-centered, and microsystem-centered—has the possibility of creating a potentially more robust strategy. Such an effort offers the health care sector a potentially transforming and more durable model for the continual improvement of health care.

# CHAPTER 12

# Quality Improvement in Primary Care: The Role of Organization, Collaboratives, and Managed Care

*Leif I. Solberg, Thomas E. Kottke, and Milo L. Brekke*

*"Occupational organization . . . constitutes a dimension quite as distinct and fully as important as its knowledge."*
—Elliot Friedson: *Profession of Medicine,* p. xi, 1970a

In recent years, both the care delivery system and concerns about its quality have undergone many important changes. While managed care plans still finance the care of most Americans, their ability to regulate care patterns has been reduced by a counterbalancing power shift to purchasers, consumers, and large provider organizations. As cost pressures have again cycled higher, purchasers are paying more attention to costs and are shifting more of this burden to consumers, who are simultaneously refusing to accept many of the previous restrictions on their care choices. At the same time, a series of reports from the Institute of Medicine (IOM) have heightened everyone's concerns about the quality of American medical care, expressed most clearly in the 2001 *Crossing the Quality Chasm* (IOM 2001). Perhaps the most memorable comment in this report was "Between the health care we have and the care we could have lies not just a gap, but a chasm." That report was preceded by the IOM report highlighting the frequency of medical errors and followed by the RAND Corporation study of 439 quality indicators showing that, on average, only 55% of the time was the desirable care provided to adults in 12 metropolitan areas of the United States (IOM 2000; McGlynn *et al.* 2003). Nearly all of these indicators measured care that is provided in large part in primary care, so that setting in particular must rise to the challenges raised by these data.

The net result of all of these changes has been to focus attention and pressure on clinicians, especially those in primary care. They are feeling both stressed and unappreciated as they have to run faster to keep up, while being constantly told that what they do is not good enough. At the same time, it is becoming clearer that if we are to address the cost and quality conundrums we face, clinicians must not only be involved, they must take the lead in making change happen.

This chapter reports on what is happening in the effort to improve quality in the primary care setting, and the role and approach of what we shall call quality improvement (QI). If there is any overriding lesson from the past 20 years of CQI/QI experience, it is that Eliot Freidson's observation in 1970 and our observation in 1993 hold true today: As individuals, clinicians are rarely able to make significant changes but they will usually accept and support office systems that simultaneously improve their work life and patient care (Freidson 1970a,b; Kottke *et al.* 1993). After all, the care gaps identified in the Chasm Report and other studies are primarily gaps in the consistency and comprehensiveness of care, and closing these gaps requires systemization previously lacking from medical care. Thus, a critical question is how to motivate primary care delivery organizations of all sizes to want to implement systems, and how can we best facilitate such implementation? There is clearly an important role for care delivery leadership and infrastructure, but there is also a need for help from purchasers, managed care plans, and improvement collaboratives. This chapter first addresses these factors and then provides a specific example of a randomized controlled trial of an intervention to address the improvement of preventive services through an improvement collaborative sponsored by two managed care organizations.

## INTERNAL FACTORS: THE CARE DELIVERY ORGANIZATION AND QI

Care delivery organizations, especially those organized to provide ambulatory care are currently part of a slowly evolving revolution in the structure and function of care: one from largely solo doctor practices to medical groups, some of which are now huge multispecialty organizations integrated to provide every type of medical service. Some of this revolution has been hastened by the need to create negotiating power with managed care plans, but it was being fostered in any case by technological changes, cost pressures, physician attitude changes, and heightened consumer and purchaser expectations.

Since so many policymakers and researchers seem to lack a good understanding of care delivery organizational structure, we focus on this first. Doctors initially banded together to share after-hours calls, billing systems, and other infrastructure in a common office or clinic site. These sites usually consist of 2 to 10 doctors, typically of the same specialty, with 3 to 5 being the most efficient unit size. Later, and particularly in regions with high penetration and pressure from managed care plans, these single-site groups merged or were bought out by large care systems, hospitals, or care plans hoping to create a captive referral network. While some of these larger aggregations continue to contain largely a single primary care specialty, many become multispecialty as well as multisite. We refer to these larger organizations as medical groups, while recognizing that some medical groups continue to practice at a single site or to have much smaller satellite sites, particularly in rural areas.

Another factor of tremendous importance for QI is the lack of integration within these medical groups. Formed largely for economic or cross-coverage reasons, early medical groups tended to maintain separate medical practices, with each physician retaining individual autonomy in care decision making. However, this meant that unless an individual physician was unusually interested in organizing care patterns, there was little consistency, comprehensiveness, or outreach involved in patient care. Each patient and each visit was unique and any care actions had to be recalled or created anew. Over time, this individualization of practice (which we characterize as the "motel syndrome" to illustrate the shared solo-ness) tends to disappear as it becomes clearer that both efficiency and effectiveness can be improved by systems that cross individual clinician boundaries. Nevertheless, this integration has continued to vary enormously among different medical groups, and sometimes even at different sites within an individual group.

Of course, this increasingly complex organization also requires leadership, so medical groups found a need for a medical director, a chief administrator, committees, and boards of directors. As they become larger, multisite groups also usually create medical and administrative leaders for individual sites.

As pressures to improve quality increase, medical groups usually find that it is necessary to develop greater integration and to create an infrastructure that can develop and maintain common systems to support consistent care. This infrastructure necessarily seems to include a specific QI approach, personnel, a coordinator, and a physician leader who can connect the QI efforts to organizational priorities, plans, and resources.

## The Complexity of the Task

In order to better understand and identify the factors important to QI in medical groups, we identified the most experienced and insightful physicians and coordinators for QI in our region among the medical groups with the most success in improving quality. Over one year, we led them through a series of interviews and formal group process rating exercises aimed at identifying and ranking the factors and strategies that they considered most important for QI. We published this synthesis of their opinions as well as a related literature review that highlighted the need for greater recognition among QI advocates and researchers of the importance of organizational factors and systems (Solberg 2000; Solberg *et al.* 2000a).

There were several important lessons from these experienced leaders of change in medical groups. One was that they needed to keep in mind a great many factors as they attempted to improve quality, which we pragmatically divided into five categories:

1. Characteristics of the guideline or quality improvement topic
2. Medical group characteristics
3. Organizational capability for change
4. Infrastructure for implementation
5. External environment.

Both by their ratings of individual items within these categories and by their ratings of each one's overall relative importance, these subjects chose organizational capability for change and infrastructure for implementation as the most important. Table 12–1 displays the 21 factors that received the highest rating out of the 87 that they had identified as of value in their work. Most of these 21 are directly or indirectly related to systems and organizational change.

**Table 12–1** Factors Ranked in Order of Rated Importance to Ability to Improve Quality

| Rank | Factor |
|------|--------|
| 1 | **Presence of Organized Systems** in the clinic |
| 2 | **Commitment to Change** by leadership |
| 3 | **Voluntary Leadership** by enthusiastic volunteers |
| 3 | **Internal Clinician Champions** for the guideline |
| 3 | **Priorities** for quality vs. finance by the group |
| 6 | **Resources Available** for guideline implementation |
| 6 | **CQI Understanding and Skills** in the organization |
| 6 | **Collaborative Psychological Working Environment** |
| 6 | **Clinician Cohesiveness** to shared mission/policies |
| 6 | **Relative Advantage** of the new care process |
| 6 | **Importance** of the guideline topic to clinicians |
| 12 | **Standardized Org. Process** for making change |
| 12 | **Change Management Infrastructure** well-developed |
| 12 | **Internal Clinician Interest** in making the changes |
| 12 | **Internal Turmoil** present from internal changes |
| 12 | **Leadership Support** for steps to fulfill their vision |
| 17 | **Management Authorization** of resources for guidelines |
| 17 | **Strategic Plan Inclusion** of implementation in annual goals |
| 17 | **Resource Agreement Process** at all organizational levels |
| 17 | **Active Leadership Involvement** personally in the change |
| 17 | **Organizational Culture** supportive of planned change |

These "insightful implementers," as we called them, also identified and rated QI change strategies in terms of their effectiveness when used appropriately. They also concluded that one needed to use many strategies, rather than the single strategy approaches usually studied in research. The strategies receiving the top 10 ratings out of a possible 25 were:

1. Using system supports like reminders, registries, and task delegation
2. Focusing on changes that would make physician work easier
3. Reducing or removing barriers
4. Measuring for improvement periodically
5. Providing information or training
6. Delegating authority to the implementation planners
7. Providing comparative feedback of relevant measurements
8. Pretesting change through pilots and rapid cycling

9. Tailoring implementation to each practice setting
10. Focusing on changes that make it better for patients


**Need for Simplicity**

It is not enough to understand the factors affecting the ability to improve quality and the most effective strategies for change. Medical group leaders must also understand and adopt an efficient and effective approach to QI, one that is feasible and understandable for internal change agents. When CQI was first imported into medical care in the late 1980s (mostly in hospitals) (Berwick 1989; Laffel and Blumenthal 1989), it usually used a formal process with many separate steps. These steps began with extensive data collection efforts to understand the process needing improvement and progressed through developing an entirely new and detailed process, which was then implemented en mass after a year or more of work. While there was usually a theoretical dictum to evaluate the change through more measurement and then cycle back through the steps for further improvement. In practice this usually did not occur because of participant and group fatigue. The culture of medical practice, the focus on administrative rather than clinical problems, insufficient appreciation for the importance of leadership support, and other problems also contributed to a discouragement about this model in the mid-1990s (Bigelow and Arndt 1995; Early and Godfrey 1995; Shortell et al. 1995; Goldberg 1998).

At about the same time, a new model of QI was being developed through leaders connected with the Institute for Healthcare Improvement (IHI). This model is described in detail in The Improvement Guide but it has also been discussed in many articles (Langley et al. 1994, 1996; Berwick 1996; Nolan 1997; Berwick 1998). Instead of many detailed steps, this model asks that QI teams first answer three questions:

1. What are we trying to accomplish?
2. How will we know that a change is an improvement?
3. What changes can we make that will result in improvement?

These QI teams then start making small tests of change, using the PDSA cycle (Plan-Do-Study-Act) as they gradually develop the pieces of a new system. As they do this, a solid understanding and application of systems thinking, measurement, variation, and change management are needed, no matter what change they are trying to accomplish.

An even more recent modification in approach has suggested that the real focus of QI should be on microsystems, "the small, functional, front-line units that provide most health care to most people." Although this term is also used for the units that provide front-line specialized or inpatient care, the concept is particularly important in primary care, especially because it focuses on the strong multidisciplinary teamwork that appears necessary to improve quality in primary care (Grumbach and Bodenheimer 2004). Microsystems are discussed extensively in Chapters 11 and 15.

## EXTERNAL FACTORS: THE CARE DELIVERY ORGANIZATION AND QI MANAGED CARE AND PURCHASERS

The founders of the health maintenance organization (HMO) concept that evolved into managed care health plans believed that HMOs would have "a vested interest in regulating output, performance, and costs in the public interest" through better organization, integration, and coordination of care (Ellwood *et al.* 1971). While that belief hasn't fully lived up to its promise, the latest Miller and Luft (2002) summary of the published evidence suggests that HMO-style plans provide roughly comparable quality of care to other types of plans. While they note that HMO (managed care) enrollees do report worse access and satisfaction with care, they conclude that quality is very heterogeneous, varying widely among providers, plans, geographic areas, and degree of market penetration.

Goldsmith *et al.* (1995) developed a conceptual framework for thinking about the possibility that managed care plans evolve from cost to quality and value through three stages. During Stage I, all of a managed care plan's focus is on the management of costs, primarily through the reduction of inpatient care by various administrative and regulatory mechanisms. There is no need to work with hospitals and physicians to restructure the way that they provide care. McEachern *et al.* (1995) describe the strategies typically used during this stage as making superficial changes in care delivery as compared to the fundamental changes required in later stages. However, as all types of health insurance organizations achieve similar levels of hospital use and costs, and as managed care becomes the dominant form of coverage locally, this strategy no longer works to differentiate among health plans. They must find new ways to compete or engage in destructive price wars.

In Stage II, competition forces a focus on value, combining more sophisticated approaches to cost containment with efforts to change the actual delivery of care. These care delivery changes require clinicians not only to cooperate with their implementation but to provide leadership for the change (McEachern et al. 1995). Since these changes are really process improvements, QI is a potentially valuable tool. Once health plans have successfully made some headway on these challenges in Stage II, Goldsmith et al. suggest that the new strategies identified in Stage III will become necessary, focusing on population-based health status improvement. Although Goldsmith et al. did not include QI as a method in this stage, we believe that it is equally important here. (1995)

But how will these stages impact on primary care? Managed care plans can certainly undertake some population-based strategies without involving primary care organizations or clinicians at all. They can provide financial incentives, information and behavior change support, specific self-help tools, and other resources directly to members. They can also provide disease management services (and are increasingly doing so) through contracts with companies that are largely divorced from any primary care clinicians or organizations. While some plans believe that they have achieved significant cost savings along with some quality improvements by carving out disease management, (Gold and Kongstvedt 2003) the general consensus of objective observers is that there is little good evidence on either side of the question (Bodenheimer 1999; Selby et al. 2003). However, most primary care clinicians appear to dislike this arrangement and feel threatened by it (Bodenheimer 1999).

Whether in Stage II or III, it seems likely that most QI for managed care plan members will still require clinician-led QI efforts, and the ability of managed care plans to influence that is limited. The most promising strategies at this time appear to be some type of pay-for-performance approach for clinicians and a tiered system that costs more for members who choose care from providers who have lower quality and/or higher costs (Endsley et al. 2004; Epstein et al. 2004; Rosenthal et al. 2004). These approaches are usually combined with some type of public accountability measures of selected quality indicators (Epstein 2000; Marshall et al. 2000). Casalino et al. (2003) in their study of 1040 large primary care organizations, found that external incentives and information technology were the two factors most closely associated with care management systems.

Purchasers, both private and governmental, clearly have a role in providing needed external motivational support for QI. Health plans are clearly very sensitive to the needs and desires of their large customers and they are loath to do anything that hurts their ability to contract with any source of many members. As health care costs have increased at double-digit rates over the past few years, these purchasers have become alarmed about the effect on their own bottom lines. That has been reinforced in the past by a commonly-held view, at least among private purchasers, that all of their suppliers should not be asking for more pay to guarantee the quality of their product—that is simply an expectation by the purchaser.

Despite those barriers, large purchasers have been surprisingly receptive to new large demonstration projects that test the ability of performance payments to stimulate improved quality and costs (Endsley *et al.* 2004). The two projects receiving considerable attention are:

1. *Rewarding Results*—funded by the Robert Wood Johnson Foundation (RWJ) and the California Health Care Foundation with grants to Blue Cross of MI, Blue Cross of CA, IHA (a coalition of CA health plans), Excellus Health Plan, and Massachusetts Health Quality Partners
2. *Bridges to Excellence*—funded by RWJ and the Center for Medicare and Medicaid Services in cooperation with many large employers and health plans and physician groups in Boston, Cincinnati, and Louisville with incentives of up to 10% of annual income for providers who meet quality targets.

## QUALITY IMPROVEMENT COLLABORATIVES

Assuming that managed care and/or purchasers establish external incentives that motivate the leaders of primary care medical groups to work hard on QI, it seems likely that some way must be found to facilitate these efforts. At the very least, most groups will need knowledge and skills in QI and in the content of systematic ways to increase the consistency and comprehensiveness of care. One of the most promising ways to provide this appears to be through participation in local, regional, or national quality improvement collaboratives (QICs).

The most well known of such QICs is that run by IHI, the so-called Breakthrough Series (Kilo 1998). This grew out of an IHI reappraisal of the lack of demonstrable impact of its previous focus on courses and an annual national forum on quality. At the same time, Davis *et al.* confirmed the ineffectiveness of most standard approaches to continuing medical education (Davis *et al.* 1995). In the Breakthrough Series model, IHI hosts collaboratives of 20 to 40 organizations that work together on a particular quality topic for 9 to 12 months through three two-day "learning sessions" and a final presentation at a national congress, with work at home in between. These series have been popular, but they are very expensive for participants and tend to attract mainly large care delivery organizations.

A wide variety of other QICs have developed, mostly on a regional basis or within a large organization like the VA, but also in other countries. One of the oldest and most successful has been the Institute for Clinical Systems Improvement (ICSI) in Minnesota, now cosponsored by all the managed care plans in the area and jointly run with medical group and hospital members now consisting of 70% of the state's physicians (Reinertsen 1995; Mosser and Reinertsen 1996; Farley *et al.* 2003). Founded well before the Breakthrough Series in 1993, ICSI began as a way to develop local buy-in for evidence-based guidelines (available at www.icsi.org) and soon moved on to emphasize implementation and improvement of broad quality topics beyond any particular guideline. Each year for the last decade, Brekke has conducted in-depth interviews with a range of ICSI participant medical group leaders to help keep the organization aware of its member needs. Over the years, he has observed a tendency for medical groups to evolve in their understanding and work on quality through four stages as they participate in the ICSI collaborative:

1. Implementation of specific guidelines, one at a time
2. Implementation of combinations of guidelines that use similar systems (e.g., all preventive services) or relate in common to a specific condition
3. Developing or remodeling the group's general systems and infrastructure for improvement of care
4. Redesigning the entire approach the group takes to providing health care

This natural history of changes in their perspective and understanding of what they are doing gives evidence of evolution in

1. recognition that QI is a systems issue;
2. awareness of the complexity and interrelatedness of factors in systematic improvement;
3. belief that improvements are likely to be more efficiently accomplished through an holistic perspective, approach, and action than by an accumulation of piecemeal efforts, even when intended to be well coordinated;
4. confidence that sustainable improvements require significant resources and must be aligned with, recognized as, and budgeted among the medical group's goals as an organization.

There are numerous anecdotes and case studies suggesting that these QICs generate enthusiasm and possibly some improvement among participants but, as yet, little clear evidence of their effects. Even Ovretveit *et al.*, representing a group of researchers conducting evaluations of QICs, agreed with this, stating "there is little evidence that they are more cost effective than other methods, and little knowledge about how they could be made more effective." (Ovretveit *et al.* 2002) Mittman's review concluded that "the widespread acceptance and reliance on this approach are based not on solid evidence but on shared beliefs and anecdotal affirmations." (Mittman 2004) Nevertheless, these evaluators seem to share the view that such evidence is needed because it seems likely that QICs are an important methodological way to address QI.

## IMPROVE: A TEST OF A MANAGED CARE-SPONSORED QIC FOR IMPROVING PRIMARY CARE PREVENTIVE SERVICES DELIVERY

In the late 1990s, we conducted a randomized controlled effectiveness trial of a CQI and QIC intervention in primary care clinics that was sponsored by two large managed care plans with funding by the Agency for Healthcare Research and Quality (AHRQ). At the time, there was only one published trial of CQI (Goldberg *et al.* 1998), so this trial provided us with an extraordinary opportunity to increase our understanding of the potential of this strategy. Although this trial focused on the delivery of clinical preventive services, the concepts, methods, and lessons should apply to any effort to facilitate QI actions by medical groups.

## IMPROVE: Background

The primary stimulus for this trial was the need to improve preventive services in primary care. There was a fairly extensive literature on the need for a systems approach to this problem; a need to build office systems that change the care environment to make it more likely that needed preventive services will be provided during any office visit. The system components are outlined in Table 12–2 (Solberg *et al.* 1997b). Such systems had been largely missing or disorganized in primary care settings, so preventive services were dependent on the memory and actions of individual clinicians who were often too busy addressing the immediate needs and wants of their patients (Kottke *et al.* 1993).

The trial focused on the improvement of rates of providing eight diverse preventive services that had strong evidentiary and clinician support: mammography, clinical breast exam, pap smears, influenza and pneumococcal immunizations, blood pressure, smoking, and cholesterol.

## IMPROVE: Trial Design

This trial was called IMPROVE (Improving Prevention through Organization, Vision, and Empowerment). It was all the more unusual because it was actually sponsored by a collaboration of two HMOs who otherwise compete in the same regional market (Magnan *et al.* 1998). Forty-four primary care clinics contracting with one or both of these HMOs agreed to participate in response to a joint recruitment letter from the medical directors of the two plans, and were randomized into 22 intervention and 22 control clinics. These were fairly typical clinics for the area, representing 33 of the 71 medical groups contracting with these plans. They averaged 7 to 8 adult primary care physicians and 45% prepaid patients (although only 20% were from the two sponsoring plans).

The intervention involved training two people from each intervention clinic at group learning sessions in how to lead and facilitate an internal multidisciplinary team through a seven-step CQI process that was fairly

**Table 12–2** The Component Processes of the IMPROVE Prevention System

1. Guidelines: developing, obtaining buy-in, and updating a set of preventive services for defined age/gender/risk groups by and for a specific medical group
2. Screen: obtaining health risk and previous preventive service information at visits in a standard way about all patients of a clinic in order to identify their specific needs
3. Summarize: organizing and updating the information obtained in the screening process so that it is all in one place and easily reviewable by those needing to know the current prevention status of a particular patient
4. Cue/Remind: reminding clinic staff and clinicians about their need to undertake necessary prevention system tasks
5. Follow-Up: communicating to patients the results of preventive services along with appropriate explanations and recommendations
6. Resources: selecting, organizing, making accessible, and maintaining patient education and referral information needed by both patients and clinic personnel.
7. Counsel: assisting patients and their families to make needed behavior changes
8. Track and Recall: reminding patients about their needs for specific preventive services between visits
9. Patient Activation: encouraging patients to take greater responsibility for their own preventive services and behavior changes.
10. Prevention Visits: providing all needed preventive services during a single visit designed and organized for that purpose

typical for the early 1990s (see Table 12–3). The training and improvement process addressed each of the ten philosophical elements and most of the eight structural elements described in Chapter 1 of this book. However, the training was not theoretical but very task-oriented around the QI process, preventive services, and the systems that have been demonstrated to be effective. It was spread out over a six-month period to be *just in time,* followed by bimonthly opportunities for the trainees to meet for networking about their techniques, tools, progress, and problems. In addition, consultants from the project visited or called them periodically over the 22 months of the intervention to reinforce their efforts and to problem-solve with them.

In order to evaluate the trial, surveys were completed by all clinic personnel, by the clinic CQI team members, and by patients visiting the clinics, both before the intervention began and near its end. The charts of the

**Table 12–3** The Process Improvement Model

1. Identify the problem
2. Collect data to understand your current process and customer needs and expectations
3. Analyze the data to understand root causes
4. Develop alternative solutions that address the root causes
5. Generate recommendations to implement the best alternatives and pilot test them
6. Implement the tested new process using systematic preparation steps, including orientation and training
7. Use an iterative cycle through these steps to evaluate the new process and continue to improve it until it is good enough

surveyed patients were also audited to provide another way of assessing clinic behavior. Both quantitative and qualitative data were gathered to document the intervention experience. These data provided us with many lessons about both preventive services and CQI in this setting.

### Findings of the IMPROVE trial

Measurement of the rates of these services before the intervention began was especially valuable in understanding the problems of low rates. Actually, the rates at which visiting patients reported being up-to-date for these services before the clinician encounter were fairly good by national standards (Kottke *et al.* 1997). However, if they needed a service, they only had a 6% to 29% chance of receiving a recommendation for the service during their visit (except for blood pressure measurement, which was performed about 90% of the time whether it was needed or not). Thus, after the visit the up-to-date rate for these services had only increased an average of 6%. Interestingly, the 20% of patients who were there specifically for a complete physical were only a little more likely to be offered needed services. Since patients reported making an average of four visits to the clinic a year, and since patient reports tend to overestimate both the recency of services and recommendations by clinicians, it was unlikely that the current rates would improve without a major change in approach.

In order to better understand the reason for these low rates, we measured the presence of functioning prevention systems in these clinics and confirmed that most of these processes were not present in any organized way (Solberg *et al.* 1998). Where present, they were only in effect as isolated processes for individual services, with *follow-up, guidelines,* and *resources* accounting for 60% of the total existing processes. Since none of the three has much to do directly with the delivery rates of the services we were measuring, it is not surprising that the rates were as low as they were. We also demonstrated that there was great variation not only between clinics but, more importantly, within clinics in the relative rates at which various services were provided (Solberg *et al.* 1997a, b, or c). In other words, a clinic that had the highest rate of the 44 clinics for providing mammography was just as likely to be among the lowest as the highest for other services. This tended to confirm the lack of systems.

Unfortunately, the post-intervention measurements revealed that only a few services increased in intervention clinics more than they did in control clinics (Solberg *et al.* 2000). This was confirmed by both patient report and chart audit. In retrospect, it was surprising that these teams and clinics had stuck with their task as well as they did. Not only was the CQI process we used a slow and time-consuming one, but it had been carried out through a period of enormous turmoil in these clinics and the region. We measured that turmoil and found that during the first year of the intervention, 64% of the clinics had undergone a change in ownership or affiliation, 77% had lived through change in at least one major internal system (e.g., billing, lab, records), and 45% had changed clinic manager, medical director, or both at least once (Magnan *et al.* 1997). Moreover, six teams changed leaders, seven changed facilitators, and eight experienced a change in sponsor during this time.

### IMPROVE: Postlude

At the end of the intervention, we asked the control clinics whether they wanted to receive a comparable but improved version of the intervention. Everything they had heard from the intervention clinics was so positive that 17 of them said they wanted to and were able to undertake it at that time. In addition, the project team used this opportunity to train and involve regular staff members from both HMOs in the new intervention and they identified another 18 medical groups that they would like to have had participate. Eleven of these groups chose to do so; thus, a total of 28 clinics/groups went through the experience with even more enthusiasm than the first group. It is unfortunate that we do not have similar measurements of this experience or its outcomes because both the training and the team efforts seemed to go much more smoothly and quickly than they had the first time.

## Lessons From IMPROVE

IMPROVE has many lessons for those interested in QI in primary care. Some of these come from what went right but, as usual, there is more to learn from what did not go right. We believe that the immediate reason that the rates we measured did not increase significantly is because the systems put in place to accomplish them were incomplete and perhaps misdirected. However, the situation is much more complicated than that, with many factors contributing to the lack of rate change. In fact, it seems to us that a whole chain of factors must be satisfied to obtain the desired improvements. Each of these factors need to be satisfied in order to obtain quality improvement in clinical settings, regardless of whether the means chosen are called QI.

1. *High priority organizational commitment to change*
    In order to achieve the type of fundamental system change that the IOM reports called for, both clinic leadership and the clinicians must see the change as a very important priority and become deeply committed to it. Usually that means that there must be either a financial or personal benefit in the new way of behaving, as well as a belief that the change is possible. Most of this tension for change may need to come from the external world in the form of incentives, comparative performance feedback, professional peer pressure, or regulatory/purchaser requirements, but ultimately it must be seen internally as important for organizational survival. A strategy of generating tension for change from multiple sources may be more effective than focused efforts from a single source.
    Our survey of clinicians demonstrated that, despite belief in the importance of these preventive services, they did not have a sense that much improvement was necessary (Solberg *et al.* 1997a). With the possible exception of tobacco cessation advice, nearly as many respondents disagreed with the need to improve each service as agreed. It seems likely that improving prevention just did not have sufficient organizational priority at a time when a great many issues seemed more

likely to affect survival. Both of the sponsoring HMOs as well as the local business coalition on health had emphasized the need to improve preventive services, but until very recently there was no financial carrot attached to that. Thus, change motivation appeared to be borderline at best.

## 2. *Organizational Ability to Manage Change*

This is a very complex factor that includes a variety of knowledge and skills at both top and middle leadership levels, along with a supportive organizational structure and culture as well as successful experience with previous change efforts. The role of senior organizational leaders is particularly important in assuring the presence of this ability as well as in supporting specific improvement efforts. There are many barriers in typical medical practices that interfere with their ability to undertake these changes. Although we have worked with hundreds of clinics and medical groups over the past 15 years, we have seen very few examples where this organizational ability is in very good shape.

Even so, there must also be what we have come to speak of as a "tolerable level of turmoil," both externally and internally, for a clinic to be ready for successful change. As noted above, that was clearly not the case for most of these clinics. One clinic team had to stop functioning for six months after the clinic was bought by a hospital that eliminated most benefits and made everyone fearful. Other teams told us that they hung on to their IMPROVE team activities as the only thing happening that they could feel good about. In some ways it is remarkable that prevention rates did not deteriorate during this time.

The type of QI process being used may have been key to this ability to manage change. We hoped that we were basically providing a vehicle and the training/support needed for change. However, the QI model we used was probably not up to the task, requiring so much time and effort that most teams lacked the will to evaluate the success of their efforts and learn that more change was needed.

Even with an effective change model, however, leadership of the change by our trainees probably was not optimal. Although they were mostly creative, dedicated, and industrious, for many this was their first experience with this kind of change leadership. Our later change efforts have demonstrated how much faster a team can work with experienced leadership. Finally, we also learned that senior leadership of the group and site must really be determined to support the changes.

3. *Substantive change content*

Clearly the best change management in the world will accomplish little if the changes made are not substantial and based on good reason to believe that they can result in significant improvement. Skeptics of QI have correctly noted that there is often so much emphasis on the process of identifying problems and on original thinking by team members unaware of existing knowledge, that they develop only superficial changes like educational programs or new chart forms that will be as unused as previous ones have been. Goldberg has gone so far as to suggest limiting the scope of a QI team's activities by having them concentrate on tailoring a change with demonstrated efficacy rather than picking or freshly designing one (Goldberg 1998). We have seen this work especially well in the ICSI collaborative, where the most successful example has been that of Advanced Access. Here an expert prescribed, taught, and trouble-shot the new process, while medical group QI teams' main task was to tailor it to their setting and facilitate implementation.

In order to minimize this problem, we emphasized from the beginning that this was a test of the combination of a change process plus proven care process content knowledge. However, to the contrary, most teams failed to implement a reminder process to stimulate the clinicians to make use of the information about prevention needs that was identified for individual patients by screening and using a summary sheet. A bigger problem may have been our reliance on reminders, rather than building the new system around task delegation to nonphysicians. In retrospect, adding prevention topics to a clinician's agenda that was already too busy for a brief visit may not be a successful strategy in real life.

4. *Effective development and implementation of improvements*

Even if there is high motivation, good readiness, and sound content, the teams and their clinic leadership must effectively carry out the development and implementation of system changes. This requirement overlaps with motivation and readiness, but the slow pace of the improvement process in most clinics, the fact that only 60% reported implementation after 18 months, and the lack of evaluation and a second cycle of improvement by that time suggest that whatever changes were made were less than likely to achieve their goals.

We do not blame the teams or clinics for this problem. In fact, their enthusiasm and dedication was a constant inspiration to the intervention group. It may have had as much to do with our CQI model, their inexperience, and the motivation and readiness issues noted above as anything else. An equally important barrier may have been the major paradigm shift required by patients and clinicians to include a clinic agenda (identification and delivery of needed preventive services) in a brief visit already filled with other patient and medical needs.

### 5. *Time—sufficient but not too much*

Even if everything else works well, any change of the magnitude required by this project requires enough time. Other experiences with a medical group collaborative working on the improvement of preventive services suggest that at least two years and perhaps as much as three to five years are needed if the changes require a dramatic paradigm shift for patients and health care professionals. Many of the team leaders and facilitators told us that IMPROVE has been very helpful to them in this larger task of changing the whole approach, and they continued to make use of the lessons learned for addressing all types of challenges facing them.

On the other hand, allowing too much time for specific innovations to evolve probably also impedes adoption. The IHI strategy of rapid cycles and ambitious stretch goals is based on this experience. Implementation of preventive services systems in the IMPROVE project may have been more successful if we had been more aggressive with the participating clinics to keep preventive services on the change agenda and with the teams to shorten their PDSA cycles. The trick is to push for change while understanding that real change takes a lot of time.

## CONCLUSIONS AND RECOMMENDATIONS

Although the IMPROVE trial did not result in significantly increased rates of the targeted preventive services, it did generate a great deal of information about clinics, the change process, and the delivery of preventive services. We believe it also helped the participating clinics to increase their readiness to confront other organizational changes that might be necessary in the near future. In most cases, IMPROVE seems to have helped them begin an important transformation of their managerial and operating styles. In the long run, QI may turn out to be more valuable for assisting in this transformation than in facilitating specific process change.

What this trial says about the ability of QI concepts and techniques to produce measurable changes in the quantity or quality of clinical services (much less patient outcomes) is much less clear. We have identified a number of barriers to change with this trial, any one of which might have prevented the rate changes desired. Not least of these barriers was the type of QI process we provided and the magnitude of change in thinking and action from the traditional approach to care. In addition, it can be argued that QI may not be as good for designing and creating an entirely new system where none previously existed, as it is for making refinements and even major changes in a system that already exists. Successful improvements in any other aspect of medicine or in other industries have typically required many cycles of failure and disappointment before the correct approach is identified.

In order to make future efforts more likely to be successful, we make the following recommendations based on the lessons of IMPROVE and subsequent experience and research:

- Before beginning to facilitate a clinic change process, be sure that adequate incentives are in place, that disincentives for improvement are eliminated, and that the targeted medical groups and their leaders have indeed committed themselves to the desired changes. This is best evidenced by the commitment of adequate budget and personnel to the specific QI endeavor.

- In order to learn whether the groups and clinics are adequately ready to engage in the change, use some type of assessment process. Unfortunately, there is no validated tool currently available for this assessment, but giving the clinics a small task to complete may help distinguish between clinics that have little probability for change from those more likely to accomplish change.

- Be sure that the proposed changes in content are substantial enough to lead to real improvements. Ideally, the selected change concepts should be based on both research and real life demonstration of feasibility and value. Then insure that the change agents in each clinic thoroughly understand these concepts and have access to both detailed examples and expert consultation in the application of those concepts.

- Be equally sure that the improvement process chosen fits with the size and nature of the task and that it is on an ambitious but feasible time line.
- Make extensive use of measurement in repetitive cycles, both in the improvement process and in assessing the value of that process. However, be sure to understand the differences between measurement for improvement and that for research or accountability so that excessive measurements do not get in the way of the goal (Solberg *et al.* 1997c).

# CHAPTER 13

# CQI in Contract Research Organizations[1]

*William A. Sollecito and Kaye H. Fendt*

Clinical contract research organizations (CROs) provide a range of services from consulting to labor-intensive tasks such as data processing. Organizationally, they range somewhere between academia and industry. Successful CROs have drawn the best techniques from both. One common characteristic of most successful CROs is the application of continuous quality improvement (CQI) techniques. The distinguishing characteristics of their CQI include four major areas described below.

1. Customer focus
2. Training and empowerment
3. Leadership
4. Statistical process control/statistical thinking

The objective of this chapter is to examine CQI characteristics demonstrated by CROs. To better understand the application of CQI in the CRO industry, the chapter begins with a brief review of the development of CROs as an organizational form within the larger context of health services.

[1]Portions of this chapter have been adapted from W.A. Sollecito and A.D. Kaluzny, Continuous Quality Improvement in Contract Research Organizations—The Customer Focus, *Quality Management in Health Care,* Volume 7, Number 7, pp. 7–11. Copyright 1999. Aspen Publishers, Inc.

## GROWTH OF CROS

From 1980 to 2000, the clinical contract research industry grew at a remarkable rate for at least two reasons. First, the pharmaceutical (pharma) and biotechnology (biotech) industry in the United States and throughout the world underwent a transition that included strategic use of outsourcing in drug development. Second, contract research organizations responded to this demand through entrepreneurial leadership rooted in the application of sound scientific and business practices. The scientific procedures developed by CROs have focused strongly on techniques to provide customer satisfaction and enhance the strategic value of their role in pharmaceutical development.

This discussion is limited to the use of CROs by the pharmaceutical and biotechnology industries, which have accounted for the majority of CRO growth. In this context a contract research organization can be defined as an organization contracted by a sponsor (client) to perform one or more of the functions and duties related to carrying out clinical trials designed to obtain regulatory approval to market a new pharmaceutical or biotechnology product. The services that CROs perform for their clients range from consulting and advice related to the design of drug development programs to labor-intensive services that are part of the drug development process; these include clinical monitoring of investigatorial sites, data management and statistical analysis, and presentations of regulatory submissions for review by regulatory agencies such as the U.S. Food and Drug Administration (FDA). Figure 13–1 lists the most common clinical services provided by CROs.

### Pharmaceutical Industry Trends

The process of developing a new pharmaceutical product is time consuming and very expensive. During the most rapid growth phase of the CRO industry, it took ten years on average from the time a molecule was discovered until a product was marketed, at a cost of 259 million (in 1990) dollars (DiMasi *et al.* 1991). The expense of this process was offset by the profits to be gained through marketing of successful products; however, only about one in 60,000 compounds discovered resulted in a highly successful marketed product (U.S. Congress OTA 1993). The reasons for this

- **Site Identification and Coordination**
- **Project Planning/Management**
- **Clinical Monitoring/Auditing**
- **Data Management and Biostatistics**
- **Clinical Trials Laboratory Services**
- **Regulatory Affairs**
- **Medical Support**
- **Safety Monitoring**
- **Health Economics/Outcomes Research**
- **Management of Clinical Trial Materials**

**Figure 13–1** Typical Clinical* Services Performed by a CRO.
*Performed during clinical stages of a drug development program (Phase II - IV)

include the complexity and number of stages (phases) a product must pass through (Pocock 1983) in the drug development process. One of the most important limiters of profitability is the relatively short length of patent protection given to pharmaceutical products. For many products developed in the 1980s and 1990s, patents had a lifetime of 17 years from date of issue, although in 1995 this was extended to 20 years from date of first filing. There have been other extensions based on recent legislation in the United States and other major health markets (Schweitzer 1997).

During the 1980s, there was significant variation among pharmaceutical companies in drug development time. Figure 13–2 presents the average time (prior to regulatory submission) of the clinical phase (human testing) of new pharmaceutical products approved during the period 1981 to 1989. For the ten companies listed, each bar represents development time in years for all products developed by the company during that time

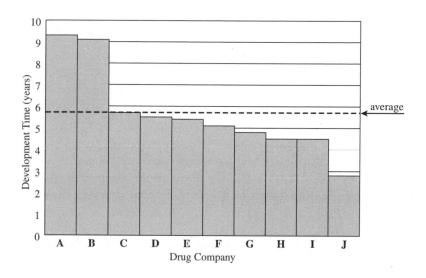

*Development times for foreign companies may be understated where
substantial pre-IND work was carried out overseas.
Sources: FDA, BCF Analysis

**Figure 13–2** IND Filing to NDA Filing Time (All NMEs Approved 1981-89).

frame. The average clinical development time ranged from a maximum of
almost ten years for two companies to less than three years for one company. This wide range in clinical development time indicated significant
variability in the efficiency of drug development. Some companies were
clearly more efficient than others and there was room for improvement in
the process.

As a direct consequence of the lengthy drug development time relative
to short patent protection, there was, and continues to be, intense interest
in accelerating the process in order to improve profitability. This is also a
concern from the medical care and public health perspective, since
a shorter development time for important therapies brings earlier benefits
to patients and communities. Thus, it becomes critical for all concerned to
define efficient processes for drug development and regulatory review and
to continuously improve these processes over time.

**Regulatory Issues**

In reviewing drug development, it is important to emphasize the role of worldwide regulatory agencies in guiding the process. Regulatory agencies, such as the FDA in the United States, have a clear mandate to protect the public's health through laws, regulations, and guidelines that provide oversight of the drug development process. The stages that define this process are well documented (Miller and Millstein 1996) and are carefully adhered to by all pharmaceutical and biotechnology companies, as well as by CROs. One of the key development rules, directly related to the underlying philosophy of CQI, is that process errors should be prevented or detected at their earliest stage. In no case is it acceptable for errors to be detected first during review by the regulatory agency. This is an important basis for CQI in the pharma, biotech, and CRO industries and is visited again later in this chapter.

In summary, drug development is a long and complex process involving clinical trials that may involve several thousand patients and requires adherence to guidelines and laws that are enforced by regulatory agencies. In this setting, efficiency and continuous quality improvement are essential for achieving success.

**Cost Containment**

The introduction of cost containment in medical care by managed care organizations and government agencies also had a significant impact on the pharmaceutical sector. From 1982 to 1996, the percentage of private sector employees receiving health benefits through a managed care plan grew from 8% to 77%, with HMOs having an estimated 59 million members in 1996 (PHRMA 1998).

Virtually every health care organization that reimburses for drugs, whether public or private, utilizes some form of cost containment strategy with regard to pharmaceuticals. These include manufacturer discounts, formularies, generic and therapeutic substitution, and drug utilization review (Schweitzer 1997). In 2004, the debate over Medicare reform again focused on how to cover or at least reduce prescription drug costs. The pharmaceutical sector has a continuing need to improve efficiency and effectiveness in drug development.

## The Biotechnology Challenge

Another important challenge came from within the pharmaceutical sector itself as biotech companies emerged in the 1980s to develop products that would directly compete with pharmaceutical products. Many of the biotech companies made a strategic decision not to become the same as "Big Pharma" companies. They decided that to be truly competitive, they had to develop new procedures and processes with an emphasis on lean organizational structures and efficient R & D processes. This led to alliances with pharmaceutical and financial partners and a development strategy that emphasized outsourcing to CROs rather that building infrastructure. The biotech industry quickly embraced the "Virtual Model" (Byrne *et al.* 1993) as a way of improving the process of drug development, including the use of CROs as virtual partners.

Biotechnology companies have a very high risk R & D process that receives intense scrutiny by financial partners and other investors. As a result, they have focused on the use of high tech innovations and CQI procedures to assure maximum efficiency for themselves and their (virtual) partners, including CROs.

## Outsourcing Trends

The primary impact on the CRO industry of the trends described above was that during the 1980s and 1990s, there was a significant increase in outsourcing by the pharmaceutical and biotechnology industry, which led to the foundation and then substantial growth of CROs worldwide.

What started out as piecemeal consulting evolved into full scale clinical services in the early 1990s and then evolved further to include diverse services such as contract sales and disease management services. In 1992, the top ten CROs in the world had approximately 4,000 employees and revenues of $350,000,000 (excluding investigator grants) (Tassignon 1992). Meteoric growth occurred after 1992; for example, in 1996, the top ten CROs had doubled in size compared to 1992, and worldwide the total number of CROs was approximately 600. Several large companies grew to the stage where they "went public" to raise capital to support further growth. For example, Quintiles Transnational, one of the largest CROs in the world, averaged 50% growth per year from 1994 to 1997 and had revenues of 800 million dollars in 1997. Revenues for the top four CROs were about 1.8 billion dollars (Quintiles Annual Report 1997).

Outsourcing from the pharmaceutical industry has also led to the growth of other contract services, including contract clinical laboratories to provide specialized blood and other tests required during clinical trials. A more recent trend, which broadened the clinical contract services market further, was the growth of site management organizations (SMOs). During the clinical trial stage, actual patient testing is carried out by clinical investigators who cover the entire range from investigators in academic medical centers to private practitioners. These independent contractors work directly for pharmaceutical companies or as subcontractors to CROs. A direct consequence of the independence of these highly valued practitioners is that there is sometimes little control over some of the nonmedical procedures that make up the clinical research process such as data processing. This has resulted in the need to monitor quality because of the importance of the data collected during patient testing. The development of SMOs represents an attempt to form organizations of investigators with the goal of improving efficiency through standardized training and improved administrative procedures. The use of SMOs in drug development is another example of how CQI procedures can be applied and may lead to further growth in the contract research sector.

## HOW CROs WORK

Initially, when CROs worked with clients, the scope of work was fairly narrow and working relationships were often fairly informal. As the use of CROs increased, new suppliers emerged and CROs had to compete in order to sustain critical mass and grow. They had to develop a reputation for high quality, which in turn led to greater acceptance and increased utilization of CROs. This emerging relationship was described as:

> The unwritten deal between the pharmaceutical industry and clinical CROs can be defined as follows: "you, the sponsors, delegate the conduction of the clinical studies to us, CROs, and we guarantee you quality, timeliness, adequate manpower and predictable costs. (Tassignon *et al.* 1992, p. 38)

Early on, CROs had to compete on two levels, among themselves and against the internal clinical development teams at sponsor companies, many of whom initially felt that no CROs could offer the same level of services they could. However, senior management in pharma and biotech companies soon began to advocate outsourcing as a way to replace the fixed costs historically associated with drug development infrastructures by the variable costs of contracting with CROs. In addition, with CROs the expectation was that timelines could be enforced and the highest levels of quality would be guaranteed. CROs had to rise to these challenges: to manage operations efficiently and meet the difficult challenge of delivering products and services that were of the highest quality, on time, at the lowest cost. Tassingnon provides an historical perspective on why CROs emphasized quality above all else:

> Quality first. The history of drug development is unfortunately tainted with stories of fraud and negligence. . . . The CRO industry is, of course, not immune to fraud, but such temptations would mean the death of a CRO. The higher the reputation of the CRO for quality data, the greater the "exportability" of clinical reports to regulatory bodies worldwide. . . procedural sloppiness would cost them the client. Timeliness has traditionally been the nightmare of drug developers. . . CROs can offer an improvement, for several reasons. First of all, they are accountable for the agreed upon milestones in the contract that binds them to their clients. Secondly, CROs work on very innovative drugs. . . Thirdly, the CRO is organized exclusively for the purpose of conducting clinical studies. Speed of execution as well as cost effectiveness are decisive competitive advantages. Whereas the industry tends to promote strategic thinkers to the top, CROs tend to reward "doers," people who get the job done within time and budget constraints. (Tassingon *et al.* 1992, pp. 39–40.)

As the CRO industry matured, pharmaceutical sponsors began to develop standardized ways to manage CROs. These included the formation of contract research management teams and the implementation of formalized proposal, bidding and contract procedures. This fostered the use of CQI because CROs often had to bid against each other in order to "win" the contract and the pharma industry often awarded contracts not on the lowest bid, but rather on the CRO's ability to implement innovative solutions to development problems. Many innovations by CROs were process improvement initiatives. This was particularly true in data management, an area where the pharma industry had been plagued for many years by inefficiency, high costs, and long delays. During the 1980s and 1990s, when the CRO industry was maturing, many breakthroughs occurring in information technology were directly applicable to improving large scale data management in pharmaceutical clinical trials. These included the introduction of microcomputers and improvements in telecommunications such as fax and touch-tone technology for transmitting data. Later this was followed by advanced uses of electronic data capture (EDC) processes that took maximum advantage of the internet as a data transfer medium. As a wide variety of options and approaches became available, there was concern for the need for standards as part of the quality assurance process. During the 1990s and the first decade of the 21st century, CROs and industry worked together with academia and government agencies to develop standards that would best utilize the breakthroughs to increase the efficiency of drug development for all sectors (Fendt 2004).

Once awarded, the contract between a sponsor and a CRO is very specific in defining procedures for interacting and includes such CQI tools as production flow diagrams, Gantt charts, patient enrollment graphs, and performance metrics that allow both the CRO and sponsor to monitor and improve performance.

The project management systems employed by CROs also contributed to the implementation of CQI. Many of the large CROs, such as Quintiles Transnational, structured themselves as matrix organizations with a mission-oriented project management system (Gillings 1997). The Quintiles' project management system uses a value-added approach that emphasizes "the why and how of serving the client" and eliminates waste, i.e., anything that does not add value. The essential components of this approach are a clear understanding that every project has a customer and a sense of serving the customer by the project team (Dotson and Wallman 1994). Another CQI component, illustrated by the Quintiles' project management system, is careful focus on the importance of communication and development of systems that facilitate clear communication between the CRO and sponsor as well as within the CRO project team (Sollecito and Dotson 1995). Effective application of project management techniques is a major reason for the growth and success of CROs in their earliest stages of development.

These techniques have allowed CQI processes to be implemented on a large scale, involving networks of sponsor affiliates, clinical investigation sites, and even other CROs. Many CROs have introduced improvements in project management techniques in the pharmaceutical industry, which led to the evolution of virtual drug development models, sometimes involving multiple sponsors and multiple CROs (Sollecito and Dotson 1994). The use of virtual drug development models is expected to lead to the creation of cooperative virtual organizations with the responsibility of using the resources of all partners (CROs and sponsors) to get the job done (Rudy 1996, p. 42). At each stage in the evolution of the CRO industry, innovation and continuous improvement have been keys to success and further growth.

## CQI CUSTOMER FOCUS

By its very nature, the CRO industry is customer-driven. The customer defines the projects on which CROs work and every project has a specific life cycle. The decision whether or not to award additional work to a CRO is determined largely by performance on the most recently completed project for that customer. Two unique aspects of CRO projects are that, first, the work performed by CROs is scientific in nature requiring a high level of expertise and, second, sponsors make a conscious choice to assign work to CROs that in an earlier time they might have done themselves. Thus, the CRO is asked to meet and exceed standards that are defined not only relative to other CROs' performance, but also relative to the expected internal performance standards of the sponsor.

However, the pharmaceutical sponsor represents only one component of the customer matrix with which CROs deal. As depicted in Table 13–1, this matrix of customers can be divided into two dimensions along the classic definitions of external and internal customers. The primary distinction is that all internal customers supplement, support, or are part of the virtual team that provides services along with the CRO to meet the needs of external customers.

The complexity of implementing CQI procedures in drug development is directly related to the interrelationships of the various customers and suppliers depicted in Table 13–1. This is especially true for CROs, which are frequently at the very center of this complex matrix in terms of coordinating the needs of both internal and external customers.

**Table 13–1** CRO-Drug Development Customer Matrix

External Customers

| Internal Customers/ Supplies | Sponsors | Regulatory Agency(ies) | Physician-Practitioners | Patients |
|---|---|---|---|---|
| Other CROs | | | | |
| Other Divisions (within CROs) | | | | |
| Clinical Trials Laboratories* | | | | |
| Drug Supply and Distribution Facilities | | | | |
| Physician-Investigators | | | | |

*Includes clinical laboratories that provide blood and urine analysis as well as laboratories that provide other specialized evaluations.

## External Customers

### Physician-Practitioners and Patients

Because of their important role in funding all drug development activities, typical pharma or biotech companies may perceive themselves as the ultimate customer for work performed by CROs. However, both sponsors and CROs are actually working to meet the needs of patients and their representative, the physician-practitioner who treats them.

The needs of patients must be kept in mind throughout the drug development process. The ultimate goal in drug development, as in all medical care, is to prevent and treat illness; thus the patient is the ultimate customer. Feedback on the needs of patients and patient satisfaction does not usually come directly from patients themselves, but rather from their caregivers. Thus, in the pharmaceutical industry, great attention is paid to working with physicians to make them aware of new therapies that are available and to seek their feedback on the effectiveness of new therapies in treating patients, i.e., in meeting the ultimate customer's need. Other measures of patient satisfaction come from patient surveys.

CROs are most directly involved in this process through provision of contract sales or post-marketing safety monitoring services. The ultimate responsibility for patient satisfaction rests with the sponsor, but, in a true CQI environment, this is shared by the CRO. One direct measure of quality that is a direct reflection on the drug development process is the number of safety problems that occur in a treated population after a drug is approved and distributed. By its very nature, the drug development process does not allow for all potential safety problems to be identified in advance, due to sample size and other clinical design considerations. When these problems occur, the most serious concern is the negative impact on the health of the population. Other negative impacts include criticism of the sponsors and their agents, including CROs, and criticism of the regulatory agency. However, sponsors, regulators, and CROs share a responsibility for responding quickly to any information about safety problems occurring in the patient population and preventing any reoccurrence of those problems. The most dramatic form of response is the recall of a newly-approved product. Most often the response is less dramatic and, in the spirit of ongoing improvement, involves the issuance of revised guidelines about use of the drug with possible additional warnings to be observed. It is the joint responsibility of the regulatory agency and the sponsor to provide a patient safety monitoring process and act quickly once problems are detected. Hospitals and health advocacy organizations, such as Public Citizen, that monitor and publish guidelines about the use of drugs, are other agents of patient care. Another important component of this patient representative hierarchy is the managed care organizations and the Federal agencies responsible for health care (e.g., Medicare). All have an impact on the assessment and feedback regarding newly approved pharmaceutical products. Their impact is almost entirely on the sponsor and the regulatory agency, but their feedback is a source of information for continuous improvement by all of the drug development customer matrix, including CROs.

*Regulatory Agencies*

One of the most important external customers for CROs and sponsors alike is the regulatory agency. In this discussion, comments are limited to the FDA, although they are applicable to other agencies as well. The FDA defines customer expectations in a pyramid that includes laws, regulations, and guidelines (Miller and Millstein 1996). The purpose of these hierarchical prescriptions is to share information and ensure compliance in the development of new pharmaceutical and biotechnology products. The goal is to make the process of approval as simple as it can be, while still focusing on the most critical mandate—to protect the health and safety of the U.S. population.

The FDA laws, regulations, and guidelines provide a roadmap of expectations from a customer who has complete authority over the approval process. Failure to meet these expectations may lead to costly delays in the approval of new drugs and may also lead to punitive actions (e.g., blacklisting of investigators who are found guilty of fraud). In extreme cases, the FDA has authority to pursue legal remedies.

CROs and others in the drug development process have an obligation to understand and comply with FDA regulations and guidelines. Although in most cases legal responsibility remains with the sponsor, the CRO must be fully aware of FDA requirements. Because of these obligations, CROs include regulatory personnel in their organizations. More importantly, some have adopted procedures that are designed to promote the view that the FDA is a customer rather than a bureaucratic impediment to the drug development process.

An important aspect of interacting with the FDA is compliance with quality assurance (QA) regulations. FDA inspectors have the legal right to periodically audit sponsors and have done so on many occasions as part of their ongoing QA process; they also carry out "for-cause" audits when a problem is encountered during a regulatory review. These same procedures apply to CROs and other participants in the drug development process. Thus, the concept of "conformance-quality" is an important part of the drug development process. As a result, drug developers, including CROs, have instituted mechanisms for demonstrating compliance, such as standard operating procedures (SOPs), which include detailed training records for all employees.

Training processes and records are a critical part of complying with FDA regulations and represent CQI components within most large CROs. Smaller CROs subcontract with professional training organizations to accomplish the same task. Most training focuses on good clinical practice (GCP) guidelines established by regulatory agencies throughout the world to maintain consistency and high quality throughout the drug development process.

Drug developers, CROs, and regulatory agencies make use of benchmarking to develop consistent worldwide standards. Formal initiatives such as the International Conference on Harmonization (ICH) (1996) help to ensure consistency in standards. Informal benchmarking is carried out continually by reviewing public documents that record policies and summarize outcomes of drug reviews within and between regulatory agencies. An example of this was once illustrated by a Japanese sponsor who said: "when the FDA gets a cold, the Japanese regulatory authorities sneeze."

Most CROs and sponsors pay close attention to presentations, publications, and other documentation of FDA opinions or revisions to guidelines. For CROs it is a benchmark, a source of pride, and also good business practice to be able to demonstrate knowledge of and conformance with current FDA guidelines.

An example of how the FDA functions as a customer is the fact that the FDA has undergone CQI processes to improve their performance with "suppliers," i.e., pharmaceutical sponsors and CROs. Part of this process has included charging "user fees" to sponsors as they submit new drug applications (NDAs). These fees have been used to hire staff and provide for other FDA needs in order to facilitate speedier and more efficient review of NDAs (Miller and Millstein 1996). The user fee initiative also enabled the FDA to undertake a careful review of internal processes and led to improved management processes, such as changing to a team-based review process. A customer-focused result was development of "good review practices" and work with sponsors and CROs to develop standards for electronic submission of new drug applications to the agency. These standards include organization of text-based documents, linkage structures for navigation, and content interchange standards for data files. The FDA also participates in quality improvement initiatives through the Product Quality Research Institute (PQRI) (www.pqri.org) and the Data Quality Research Institute (DQRI) (www.dqri.org).

CROs and sponsors interact with the FDA as a customer through an interactive review process. Following predefined rules and guidelines, CROs and sponsors meet with FDA reviewers during the drug development process to review and improve study design, study protocols, and overall strategy prior to submission of NDAs. During and after NDA submission there is a dialogue on the review of findings that sometimes speeds up or clarifies the review process. CROs and sponsors use these interactions to continuously review and improve processes for future submissions, as well as to make changes in current applications. One clear advantage to this process is that it helps to clarify the "unwritten rules" that some FDA reviewers have. Knowledge of these rules facilitates improvement in design of future studies. Sponsors, CROs, and the FDA also interact in public meetings on scientific and regulatory topics. Taken together, these activities serve as customer feedback loops.

Another example of the FDA's customer impact on CROs and sponsors is the cooperative development of technological improvements, such as Computer Assisted New Drug Applications (CANDAs). As new technology became available to facilitate data transfer electronically, the FDA, sponsors, and CROs worked cooperatively to use it to improve the NDA submission and review process. Through formal and informal discussions, meetings, and presentations, CROs and sponsors developed CANDAs that would meet and exceed the expectations of their customer, the FDA. This benefited the FDA, simplifying the review task, and it benefited sponsors, approving products in a more efficient and timely manner.

### Sponsors

The primary customers of CRDs are the pharmaceutical and biotechnology companies that make the decision to develop new drugs and "hire" the CRO. CROs keep in close touch with sponsor demands in several ways. First, CRO–sponsor relationships are defined by carefully crafted contracts that spell out expectations and often include performance metrics that are used to trigger payments and evaluate conformance to expectations. CROs also obtain customer feedback through formal client satisfaction surveys usually conducted after project completion. In most contracting businesses (construction, etc.) and especially in scientific endeavors such as drug development, it is widely assumed that "you are only as good as your last project."

In the same way that regulatory agencies audit both sponsors and CROs, sponsors conduct their own periodic audits of CROs and other subcontractors and suppliers, including investigator sites. These audits take the form of site visits at various times during a project. They are most often conducted prior to awarding a contract. CROs present their overall procedures and experience, including training processes and SOPs, as well as project-specific plans. This audit process is an important reason for having CQI procedures be in place. It is part of the "survival plan" of most CROs since it is a critical means of guaranteeing awards of contracts. Audits and site visits are also conducted periodically by sponsors during the course of a program's execution. The site visits made prior to the award of a contract are conducted by clinical (scientific staff) and members of corporate QA teams and coordinated by specialized contract management groups. Post-award audits are usually conducted by independent corporate QA personnel. Feedback from audits is usually provided in a formal manner and can be used by the CRO to make improvements or changes where needed.

*The Role of Project Management in Ensuring External Customer Satisfaction*

The most important mechanism for assuring customer satisfaction and continuous improvement during the execution of a drug development project is the CRO project management system. Although project teams vary in structure among CROs, the common denominator is that each project team has the responsibility for maintaining close communication with and meeting the needs of the client–sponsor. Project managers are the primary contact with the client, and part of their responsibility is to maintain ongoing communication with clients as well as with team members, other affiliates of the CRO (e.g., on worldwide projects, teams in other parts of the world), suppliers, and other internal customers. Adhering to contract metrics and project timelines is the direct responsibility of the project team. Most important, the overall quality of the project is the shared responsibility of the team, under the direct leadership of the project manager.

In a typical matrix organization (Grove 1983), the project (mission-oriented) team is responsible for interacting with corporate (function-oriented) departments to ensure that customer requirements are met (or exceeded) and that improvements are implemented as necessary. Thus the project management team is critical for guaranteeing not only that improvements are made where necessary on specific projects, but also that the corporate side of the matrix organization maintains the strict CQI focus required to succeed on all projects.

The underlying philosophy of project management in the CRO industry is that every project has multiple customers whose needs have to be identified and the CRO project team becomes an extension of the sponsor's team (the extended team approach). This requires open communication with a sponsor, including sharing of problems and solutions, i.e., maintaining trust. The goal of a project team is to add value to the process regardless of whether the CRO is one component of a larger drug development program or is managing an entire program (Dotson and Wallman 1994). The CQI tools and procedures used by project management teams in the CRO industry include formal communication mechanisms such as defined team structures (see Figure 13–3 as an example), clearly identified communication lines, and regular meetings with internal customers (e.g., project team), suppliers, and external customers (sponsors and FDA) to provide status reports and seek feedback for continuous improvement. They also make use of traditional management tools such as Gantt charts.

## Internal Customers and Suppliers

In addition to working with a range of external customers, CROs are involved with a variety of internal customers and suppliers. Depending on

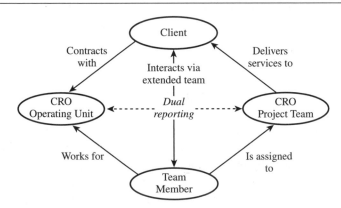

**Figure 13–3** CRO/Client Management Network.

the nature of the contractual relationship with the sponsor, a CRO can be a small part of the supplier chain or play a very large "coordinating center" role. As the role and experience of CROs have grown, CROs, especially the larger worldwide CROs, have been in a central coordination role such as that depicted by the network in Figure 13–4. In a drug development program, the components of the internal customer–supplier network include four major pieces that the CRO often has to manage:

1. Clinical laboratories
2. Other CROs or divisions of the same CRO
3. Drug supply and distribution facilities
4. Investigative sites

### Clinical Laboratories

Safety monitoring is a critical part of every large clinical trial, and with few exceptions clinical trials include "routine" laboratory testing of blood and urine samples, often at multiple time points. The process can also involve specialized testing that goes beyond blood and urine tests, such as MRIs in neurology programs. When CROs play a central coordinating

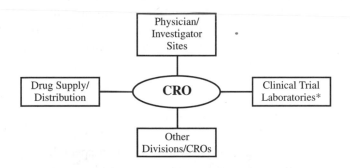

*May include specialty tests.

**Figure 13–4**  Contact Research—Internal Customer/Supplier Network.

role, it becomes their responsibility to coordinate the completion of appropriate lab tests between clinical sites and the transfer of "machine readable" data into the database for statistical analysis. In the early 1980s, it was recognized that lab tests required for clinical trials can be carried out most efficiently in centralized laboratories dedicated to this purpose. As a result, clinical trial labs developed overnight air service to deliver specimens and highly automated procedures to avoid cumbersome reentry of laboratory results. Automation facilitated overnight analysis of safety data and allowed for quick identification of safety problems. This is another example of continuous quality improvement in the drug development process; not only have data transcription errors and problems related to spoiled samples been virtually eliminated, but the use of overnight processing allows for rapid flagging of outliers and other problems.

From the customer–supplier perspective, this process improvement has also changed and simplified relationships between the CRO and laboratory. The automated centralized clinical trial laboratory represents a state-of-the-art supplier that greatly improves the outcomes for all. As an internal supplier, the lab requires that CROs develop specialized procedures to deal with the direct receipt of computerized files and that CROs become familiar with the process of how lab samples are collected and shipped via overnight carriers.

As a further example of continuous improvement, some larger CROs developed their own automated laboratories and made this part of their overall package. Specialized testing laboratories represent a special problem for CROs. Although CROs are ultimately responsible for delivery of all data, specialized studies often require specialized tests that can only be made in large academic centers and do not have high priority compared to tests being carried out for the center's own patients. This represents a timing and coordination problem that often challenges the planning skills of CROs.

*Drug Supply and Distribution*

In every drug development program there is a specialized process for supplying test drugs to be used in the clinical trials. The process involves considerations as to how to "blind" the test product and comparator and how to package the blinded test materials. When CROs are in a coordinating role, it is their responsibility to work with drug suppliers to assure the availability of all clinical trial materials (CTM) and the timely distribution of all materials to investigative sites. In addition, attention must be paid to the needs and requirements of external customers since CTMs are often highly regulated and their distribution must be carefully managed in regard to accountability and quality.

CROs use a variety of methods to achieve this coordination. Some CROs use partners who are responsible for specialized modes of packaging, while some of the larger CROs operate their own packaging facilities.

### Other CROs or Divisions

In worldwide drug development programs, CROs are required to coordinate activities with other CROs or, if the CRO itself is a large worldwide CRO, with other divisions of their own company. The CRO may also be a supplier (to another CRO) or an internal customer (receiving data and services from another CRO). In either case it is critical to establish procedures that are highly compatible with internal customers and suppliers and transparent to the external customer. Coordinating centers such as the CRO depicted in Figure 13–4 have this primary responsibility. This is another situation where efficient project management systems are critical. As teams interact, it is important to treat each other as internal customers, rather than competitors, and work together for the benefit of all. A customer focus by all parties is the key to success. Some components of a project are absolutely critical and cannot easily be shared, so one partner must have the responsibility to develop the process for all.

A simple example of this is the responsibility for coordinating data management in a worldwide program. Small variations in data collection or coding on variables can lead to substantial inefficiencies and quality problems. This is easily avoided by giving one party the responsibility for defining data management procedures for all and then monitoring the process over time through a series of interim data base transfers or reports to verify that the process is being followed. The process can involve not only multiple CROs but also multiple laboratories and drug suppliers, perhaps in different parts of the world. Simple procedures such as standardization of reporting units and attention to time zone differences become very important and remain "simple" only if they are addressed with a CQI focus on "customer delight."

## Investigative Sites

Perhaps the most difficult and most important part of the internal customer–supplier network in clinical trials is the physician-investigator site. All data and decisions in drug development, especially in the later stages, emanate from physicians who are treating patients with the new test therapies. Investigative sites represent "mini-organizations" that have strong scientific and patient care missions but essentially function as businesses that have access to patients and can provide data on patients who receive the experimental treatments being tested. From a production perspective, investigators are suppliers in the initial stage of the drug development process. However, this relationship is complicated by the fact that the physicians and their patients are also representatives of the patient-providers who are the ultimate (external) customers in drug development. Investigators sometimes also play the very important business role of helping to increase awareness about the benefits and risks of new drugs after they are approved, through publications and presentations at professional meetings.

Perhaps the most important complicating factor is that physician investigators are carrying out scientific missions in the drug development process and are subject to all of the uncertainties and complications of the scientific process. As a result, this is the one area in which CQI principles have been applied least effectively in drug development. The industry has seemed to be content to accept that the benefits of investigators' involvement far outweigh the problems and the system has been structured to compensate for their problems rather than eliminate them.

For example, one of the most cost intensive aspects of clinical trials is clinical monitoring. This is essentially a quality assurance process in which experienced clinical personnel, often nurses, review data generated by investigators and make site visits to check data quality (vs. source medical records) and correct case record forms. These processes are focused on correcting errors after the fact, rather than preventing errors before they occur. The CQI principle that error prevention is more cost effective than error correction clearly has not been fully realized in this aspect of drug development. There is, on the other hand, a recognition that time and money are saved by detecting errors early by in-process inspection, since in most drug development programs clinical monitoring of individual cases occurs as soon as possible after a patient visit. Quality improvement initiatives have included more formal training and certification of clinical site investigators and greater emphasis on data standards. Greater use of electronic means of data transmission to obtain patient (case report form) data as soon as possible has facilitated error prevention and early detection and allowed more timely review by clinical monitors. For many years technology such as remote data entry had not been fully utilized to facilitate this process. As these technologies became more accepted by sponsors and regulatory authorities (e.g., through the use of "electronic signatures"), even greater strides toward achieving greater efficiency and higher quality were made.

The adoption of these new technologies to improve quality has rested primarily with clinical investigators, who traditionally have been slow adopters. We can look at the literature on the role of physicians in medical care in general to better understand ways to speed up adoption of new technologies and other quality improvements by clinical investigators. Labovitz and Lowenhaupt (1993) point out that

> Unfortunately physicians—the most critical group of internal customers—are unaccustomed to collaborative efforts and are often unwilling to participate in CQI training. The solution is to use the customer-supplier dialogue to understand physicians' unique needs so that they can be trained effectively and drawn into the CQI process. (1993, p. 39)

Training opportunities for investigators do exist within the drug development process and CROs can play a stronger role. At the beginning of each clinical trial, a series of investigator meetings are held to explain the unique features of the new therapy and the study protocol to investigators and their study coordinators (non-physician study staff who carry out trial-related activities at the site). Very often when CROs are involved in trials, they are given the responsibility of running investigator meetings and it is at such meetings that CQI dialogue and training similar to that described by Labovitz and Lowenhaupt (1993) could be carried out.

Attempts by CROs to implement CQI methods at investigator sites have included: (1) training of study coordinators by CROs and provision of recruiting services to hire study coordinators, and (2) establishment of alliances between large CROs and academic medical centers. For example, in 1997 and 1998, Quintiles announced alliances with several academic medical centers, including the Cleveland Clinic (CenterWatch Weekly 1997a). The purpose of such alliances is to facilitate better interaction and sharing of resources and scientific knowledge between institutions, including training capabilities. Similarly, in 1997, Parexel, a large CRO, which has a separate division devoted to training, announced an alliance with the School of Nursing of the University of North Carolina at Chapel Hill (CenterWatch Weekly 1997b) for the purpose of training study coordinators. These relationships clearly illustrate opportunities for dialogue as part of the CQI process.

Site Management Organizations (SMOs), a new arm of the drug development industry, were developed in the late 1990s and had the potential to promote CQI processes between investigator sites and the CROs and other participants in the drug development supplier-customer chain. These organizations are associations of clinical investigative sites in various forms, some more structured than others. They have multiple purposes, some business and some scientific, but most include improving the consistency of operations and training; all include speeding up (improving the efficiency) of the patient enrollment process. The potential for CROs and SMOs to work together to improve the quality of the entire drug development process is clear.

In summary, CROs have played a unique role in coordinating the various elements of the drug development customer matrix. Because CROs serve a dual role as a party without a vested interest in the success or failure of new pharmaceutical products and as a scientific member of a virtual team to facilitate the introduction of new beneficial therapies, they are able to apply the customer-driven procedures of CQI. Successes in project management of large development programs have sustained the growth of the CRO industry and can provide further opportunities for adding value to the drug development process through the application of CQI.

## TRAINING AND EMPOWERMENT

According to Deming's classic, *Out of the Crisis* (1986), the transformation of an organization into a high quality operation involves two major aspects of employee empowerment: training and employee involvement. In achieving a CQI management style, CROs have invested in both of these areas.

In the startup CRO industry of the 1980s, it was critical to train employees in the basics of drug development first, and then later in more advanced skills necessary for success. The founders of the first CROs had experience; however, many of their early employees were drawn from academia or other areas and formed cohesive teams only through formal and informal (on-the-job) training.

Continuous learning and training, as prescribed by Deming and others, were carried out by the top management of the company and were usually driven by their vision of how CROs could provide uniquely efficient services and in the long run transform the drug development process. As the CRO industry matured, formalized training, in many cases still provided by senior managers, became a standard part of the recruitment and development of new employees. This was especially important for clinical monitoring and data management skills, and eventually led to CROs developing formal training programs and the requirement for certification of their employees by professional organizations.

One critical skill area that emerged as CROs took more direct control of the drug development process was project management. In contrast to pharmaceutical sponsors whose project management process often required that physicians or other "senior staff" be in charge of project teams, CROs tended to assign project managers based on management potential, including an ability to understand and meet customer needs. Like many small businesses, the early CROs required employees to "wear many hats." The key skills for success were a willingness to accept challenges and a desire to excel and succeed. The project management process in these CROs involved employees in all of the major aspects that Deming associated with quality management (1986). Project management team members participated in operating decisions, made suggestions and took a high degree of responsibility for overall performance. Their role often included planning and monitoring performance and always included direct interactions with clients.

## Empowerment and Project Management Processes

The key to empowered project management teams is the close identification with the customer and the customer's product. Project teams in CROs often become extensions of the sponsor's project team, with a high degree of interaction among team members in the sponsor and CRO organizations. For example, statisticians on the sponsor team and CRO team interact directly to decide on analysis plans and carry out the data analysis, and they collaborate on the summary of findings. Project managers coordinate efforts between the two teams and facilitate communication, but they also have responsibility for guaranteeing that timelines are met and budgets adhered to. All members of both the sponsor and CRO teams share the responsibility for quality; all members of both teams are empowered to make the project a success.

An important source of empowerment, which develops over time once trust is earned on both sides, is the ability to share, rather than cover up, problems as they occur. Despite the fact that a CRO may be carrying out the day-to-day activities, upper management at the sponsor company holds its employees along with the CRO responsible for delivering the expected products. Thus a sense of shared responsibility and trust become a critical way of working.

Another important source of team empowerment is a shared sense of ownership of the sponsor's product. The CRO team is not merely providing services that are specified in a contract, rather they develop a sense of pride and desire to exceed customer expectations. This comes directly from the desire to add value, rather than just meet deadlines, and it is even further enhanced when the drug being developed has the potential to improve quality of life or save lives.

Why do sponsors empower project teams in CROs? The answer to this question has two components; both are historical. In the early days of CRO involvement, the work was essentially piece-meal. Later, because CROs consistently delivered high-quality services on time, trust was built and the pharmaceutical industry expanded the depth and breadth of CRO services used. Pharmaceutical sponsors, especially biotechnology companies, were willing to give up control of certain phases of drug development to other partners, including CROs. This is very empowering, not only to the individual teams involved, but also to the CRO industry as a whole.

The second driver for empowered project teams at CROs involved the growth of the industry. As CROs became larger entities, clients no longer identified with founders or principal managers; instead, the linkage and identification with a CRO came through the project manager and project team, who became an extension of the sponsor's internal team. The process by which CROs are chosen has tended to increase this identification. As the industry has expanded, the process for awarding contracts to CROs has become one that requires CROs to prove in great detail that they are qualified to carry out a project. This process includes establishing performance metrics and timelines to be adhered to, as well as establishing scientific credentials and process improvement initiatives. As a result, once a sponsor awards a large contract to a CRO, there is great confidence in the choice made. As a safety net, contracts specify what additional data about the project status the CROs will provide to reassure the sponsor of the soundness of their decision. As CRO teams continue to meet their deadlines and adhere to contract metrics, greater confidence is developed which leads to further empowerment.

Thus the project management process expanded as CROs took on more responsibility for managing or co-managing drug development programs. The empowerment associated with this growth has provided a structure within which CQI became a standard mode of operation.

## CRO Recognition and Experience

As noted by Melum and Sinioris (1992), recognition plays an important role in motivating successful team performance. There are two forms of CRO recognition: first, formal acknowledgement by a sponsor of the important role a CRO has played in a successful drug development program and, second (and most important), the awarding of new contracts to a CRO based on high quality performance. One of the highest forms of recognition comes when the ultimate client, the regulatory agency, recommends a CRO to a sponsor.

Through awarding of new contracts based on high performance, CROs build experience and training of teams. Carrying out additional work for the same client builds further trust. The other major benefit that CROs derive from repeat work is that on-the-job training across a wide range of projects creates a high level of knowledge of the various kinds of drug protocols, clinical trials, and drug development programs that are being used. As CROs develop extensive knowledge of the "art" of drug development, i.e., "what works and what doesn't work," their experience becomes invaluable intellectual capital for continuous quality improvement. It also is an important source of empowerment as project teams become more confident of their ability to predict, prevent, and resolve problems efficiently and, once again, add value as members of a drug development team, not merely as service providers.

This kind of experience has also led pharmaceutical and biotechnology sponsors to adopt more of a "virtual development" model in recent years. Further, there have been formal initiatives to create drug development partnerships and alliances between sponsors and CROs. Such initiatives provide a high level of recognition and empowerment and also foster a high level of education and training as partners become willing to share technology and training resources.


## LEADERSHIP

The importance of leadership as a component of CQI has been noted by many authors and is discussed elsewhere in this text. Melum and Sinioris (1992) speak to the importance of leadership "from the chief executive officer (CEO) and chief operating officer (COO) to vice-presidents, middle managers and frontline supervisors—and leadership throughout the organization."

A definition of leadership applicable in CQI has been proposed by Crosby (1979): "Leading means stating objectives in a way that is precisely understood, ensuring the commitment of individuals to those objectives, defining the methods of measurement and then providing the impetus to get things done." (p. 155) Leadership has been crucial for CROs. Taking a historical view once again may be useful. Many CROs were founded by pharma industry personnel who had inside drug development experience and saw ways to "do it better." Others who founded CROs were academic consultants who could view the process objectively from the outside and who had experience in solving many of the problems confronted by the industry. Both groups had common visions of how to improve the process of drug development. These founders of CROs also had an entrepreneurial approach which allowed them to go beyond the traditional limits that industry had imposed on itself.

One of the greatest barriers to effective leadership is a belief in the infallibility of the leader (Crosby 1979). CROs have avoided this pitfall over the years by the very nature of their business. Every contract has to be won on the basis of a competitive bidding process and, as stated earlier, CROs have had to compete both with other CROs and with the internal drug development teams of sponsor organizations. CROs have had to constantly reevaluate customer demand and find new, more efficient ways to meet them. The need to maintain profitability and protect the welfare of their employees gives CROs a further impetus to focus on CQI. Finally, in order to win additional contracts CROs have to prove that the methods they have developed do work; each new proposal is judged not only on the merits of what is proposed, but also on past successes or failures. Thus, CROs must demonstrate another critical leadership skill—the ability to lead by example. As the CRO industry matured, an expression that was often heard from sponsors during the proposal process was: "Don't just tell me what you can do, show me what you have done!" This justifiable attitude on the part of sponsors led to very detailed site visits and presentations by CROs to demonstrate that they truly could "walk the talk". This also empowered teams to be the best and to apply technologies and new approaches to maximizing efficiency in the drug development process.

Another aspect of leadership that CROs demonstrate is the ability to manage resistance. Melum and Sinioris (1992) cite this in relation to CQI/TQM. They note that resistance is a fact of life for whatever involves change. In the CRO environment, resistance can come from within and from outside of the organization. Although sponsors have consciously chosen CROs to assist them in their drug development efforts, being middle managers and experienced scientists, they tend to be more comfortable with tried and true methods of drug development. CROs have to manage this resistance at the same time they are balancing the need to evoke customer satisfaction. It is through the skills of experienced project managers and senior scientists within the CRO that sponsors can be convinced to "think outside the box" and try new approaches. The ability to train project managers in such skills is critical to CRO success. Sometimes senior managers of the sponsor company, who have more of a "big picture" view, encourage their own development staff to allow CROs to test and evaluate the effectiveness of new approaches.

Also of concern is the need to manage resistance to change within the CRO. This problem becomes more acute as a CRO grows and has to "juggle" many different project needs. It is sometimes possible under stress for CROs—especially the large CROs—to fall into the trap of doing it only their way. This problem has multiple dimensions. For example, the CRO may stop paying attention to customer needs because it is easier to do things in a standardized format that has worked for other sponsors, or the CRO may refuse to look for new ways to improve. This loss of momentum in the application of CQI requires attention and diligence at all levels.

The solution to both problems is leadership, from the top levels and throughout the ranks of CROs. Once again, the project management system provides a powerful vehicle for addressing the problem. The project manager must be a strong leader who promotes the goal of meeting and exceeding client expectations. One important way is to explain clearly and carefully why and how to accomplish these goals. Each team member, in turn, has a leadership role in motivating other team members. In a typical matrix structure, each team member will be drawn from a function-oriented department or section within the CRO. In addition to leading within the team, the team member also has the role of leading and motivating other staff members within his or her own functional department, including managing resistance to any changes being proposed.

### Value Added

One of the key objectives of visionary leadership in a CRO is to add value not only to the sponsor's drug development program, but also to the sponsor organization itself through interactions with the CRO team and the leadership and innovation demonstrated by the CRO. A further important goal is to add value to the CRO from the experience gained on each completed drug development program. This is accomplished by developing long-term relationships with sponsors and sharing knowledge and resources wherever possible. Value is also added within the CRO by identifying organizational leaders from among the ranks of successful project managers and project team members, and by using the knowledge and experience accumulated from each drug development project to build the overall expertise of the CRO. This, in turn, demonstrates a "track record" of successful projects and CQI to potential clients, and opens doors to new challenges and chances to improve further.

In summary, leadership can yield a high level of excellence that is achieved by knowing and doing. This level of excellence raises the quality not only of CROs but of the entire industry as CROs and sponsors work together to develop new standards of excellence in drug development.

### STATISTICAL PROCESS CONTROL–STATISTICAL THINKING

The need to apply statistical process control as part of an ongoing evaluation of system variability and improvement is an important aspect of CQI that has its roots in quality assurance. Much has been written on this topic, especially by Deming (1986), who describes the careful use of statistical analysis in CQI. While statistical thinking should be emphasized, it is important to avoid the use of statistics to instill fear or to create artificial reward systems. In Chapter 1, statistical thinking is discussed as part of CQI implementation; it includes:

- How to look at variation as a generator of errors and costs;
- How to speak with data and manage with facts;
- How to take the guesswork out of decision making; and
- How to reduce variation and unnecessary complexity through the use of the seven (or more) standard tools of data analysis and display.

Statistical thinking requires the understanding and effective use of statistical measurement and analysis. The CRO industry is a data-driven industry requiring the collection and analysis of large amounts of data. Statistical process measures have been developed and used in a variety of ways in the CRO industry. Some are "performance metrics" that help sponsors gauge compliance with contract specifications. CROs also benefit from using these as measures of quality improvement (see Figure 13–5). A common example of this is the use of patient enrollment graphs that plot the number of patients expected to be enrolled in a study during a given time period against actual members enrolled (see Figure 13–6). Taken by itself, this not a CQI tool, but a measure of supplier (investigative site) performance. However, it can be very effective as a CQI tool when combined with other quality metrics, such as the proportion of patients enrolled who are later identified as protocol violators or the proportion of dropouts or other non-evaluable patients. Such statistical tools have been used by CROs to measure and improve on their own internal performance—while at the same time meeting the customer's need to have performance metrics written into contracts.

A good example of statistical analysis of process measurement and improvement is data management.

## Data Management; Process Measurement

Nowhere has CQI had a greater impact on drug development and the work of CROs than in the data management arena. This is a direct result of technological advances, in both hardware and software, such as the availability and use of electronic data capture (EDC) processes. It also reflects the recognition by those in the drug development industry and at the federal level (Institute of Medicine 1999) of the gains in

### Quantitative Evaluation

- Number of Patients Enrolled in Study
  - Expected vs. Actual (by time point)
- Number of Pages of Data Processed
  - Received
  - Edited
  - Entered
- Number of Patients Completed
  - Completed Trial
  - All Data Clarifications Resolved
  - Locked in Database

### Qualitative Evaluation

- Number of Patients Excluded Due to Protocol Violations
- Number of Dropouts/Lost to Follow-up
- Number of Clinically Evaluable Patients
- Number of Tags/DCFs Generated
- Data Management Error Rate

**Figure 13–5** Examples of CRO Performance Metrics.

efficiency that follow from the implementation of quality assurance and improvement processes and the way in which data management technologies can facilitate these processes. For many years, despite technological breakthroughs, data management in pharmaceutical clinical trials remained limited by manual activities. Even as the process became more automated, it still relied on labor-intensive procedures starting with paper data collection forms or case report forms completed by investigators and culminating in an electronic data base which is compatible for statistical analysis procedures (Figure 13–7). Despite the

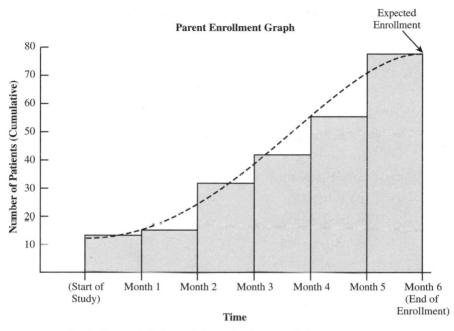

Note: Bars indicate cumulative total of actual patients enrolled.

**Figure 13–6** Patient Enrollment Graph.

large investments made in the clinical trial process, data management has traditionally been the weak link in the chain, and because new drug applications relied so heavily on manually processed data, it was a critical path to success.

In the early 1980s, data management operations in many large pharmaceutical organizations were "black boxes." The process was not well understood and represented a bottleneck in the clinical trial execution. This presented an opportunity for newly developing CROs to improve the process, and in fact this was one of the key contributions of Quintiles, which started as a statistics and data management company. It was also a classical example of how to apply CQI processes.

The first step was to describe the process in a traditional production flow chart including the components in Figure 13–7. This figure represents the process as it was carried out prior to the use of electronic data collection steps and the process still used by many organizations.

## Components of Data Management

- CRF Design
- Data Collection
- Clinical Monitoring
- Document Logging/Tracking
- Data Editing
- Data Coding
- Query Resolution
- Data Entry
- Database Audit
- Data Archiving

**Figure 13–7** Components of Data Management.

---

Because of the number of manual procedures that were performed, various quality control and quality assurance steps had to be built into the data lifecycle to assure the quality of the database. Data management error rates are a good indicator of the quality of the entire system, including clinical monitoring effectiveness, data collection, data editing, and data entry, and are more amenable to quantification and review.

As technology and sophistication improved some of the process improvements that were introduced and became part of standard procedures in most clinical trial operations are:

- Electronic data capture
- Implementation of data (element) standards
- Electronic range and consistency checks
- Automated data clarification forms (DCFs) to document queries
- Double entry of all manual data
- 100% source verification of key safety information
- Automated transfer of laboratory data files
- Audits of final databases

*Electronic Data Capture–Implementation of Data Standards*

Three of these processes warrant further discussion as examples of the impact of CQI and because they are also applicable to other areas of health care. The first is the use of electronic data capture (EDC) and the many improvements that followed from the adoption of this technology. The basic components of the management of clinical data are described in Figure 13–7. EDC not only represents a more automated and efficient way to carry out these steps, but also represents a new way of approaching quality improvement in clinical research.

EDC emerged in the 1970s and has developed steadily ever since into a suite of processes and tools to enhance the acquisition, management, quality control/quality assurance, and archiving of clinical trial research data. Adequate return-on-investment has been proven for the automation of data management processes from the keying through the summarization and archival processes. Newer electronic data capture tools now make it possible to electronically process clinical trials research information from data acquisition through final database lock and archival.

With the issuance of specific data management regulatory guidelines (FDA, 21CFR 11) in March 1997 and the FDA Guidance for Computers in Clinical Trials in April 1999, it became feasible for CROs and the pharmaceutical industry to begin incorporating EDC into their regulated data collection procedures; thus enabling implementation of automation from the beginning to the end of the clinical trials information management process. Areas where this has had the greatest impact include:

- Adverse event tracking and reporting
- Data capture, transfer and validation
- Drug inventory tracking
- Laboratory data management
- Medical coding
- Patient randomization
- Patient recruiting and screening
- Statistical analysis and reporting

The value of this technology as a quality improvement tool continues to be better understood. For example, an investigator site survey conducted by Center Watch in 2002 to 2003, in which over two-thirds of North American sites and eighty-three percent of sites that responded outside of North America felt that the use of EDC is a major strategic initiative that will improve data quality and safety. This response is directly associated with a trend toward increasing use of EDC during this same time period. For example, as reported by Center Watch, PPD, one of the world's largest CROs, indicated that EDC is being used on 15% of its clinical trials worldwide; two large sponsors, Procter and Gamble and Serono, reported EDC usage to be as high as 50% worldwide on Phase II/III trials (Center Watch 2004).

The use of EDC was also coupled with an increase in the development and use of consistent data standards. Standards have been implemented for software development, data management, and data transfer formats. With standard data elements, efficiency of the drug development documentation and review process is improved. This improved both the CRF (case report form) design and development time and improved quality and consistency across trials. With standard data elements the cost of trial design, conduct, submission, and review can be reduced and improved in overall quality (Kush 1999). The development of standards has been achieved through a collaborative effort of CROs, sponsors, and regulators. Two examples of standards that are now in common use are Good Clinical Data Management Practices (GCDMPs) and those of The Clinical Data Interchange Standards Consortium.

GCDMPs (www.scdm.org) provide guidance and establish standards on accepted practices for the many areas of clinical data management (CDM) not covered by existing regulations and guidance documents. This document is consistent with regulatory practices in related areas of clinical research and applies the concepts contained in those regulations and associated guidance documents to clinical data management. The GCDMP recommends guidelines and provides practical suggestions and proven means for meeting these guidelines. The GCDMP addresses the CDM areas of responsibility in ten sections. Each section provides minimum standards as well as best practices. Each section also contains recommended standard operating procedures (Society for Clinical Data Management 2003).

The Clinical Data Interchange Standards Consortium (CDISC) (www.cdisc.org) is an open, multidisciplinary, nonprofit organization committed to the development of industry standards to support the electronic acquisition, exchange, submission, and archiving of clinical trials data and metadata for medical and biopharmaceutical product development. CDISC has developed platform-independent data exchange standards for use in clinical research to improve data quality and accelerate product development in the drug development industry (Fendt 2004).

The adoption of EDC and the implementation of standards have led to many improvements in quality and efficiency among CROs and other drug development organizations. Technology, such as EDC, will continue to improve and will receive even greater attention in the future. Most important will be the need for CQI processes that assure the quality of drug development data. This is especially critical because pressures to adopt new technology may be driven by the need to shorten clinical development time, which, if not managed properly, can have an adverse effect on the ability to prevent and detect data errors. As with the earliest automated manufacturing processes that first led to the development of CQI procedures, new approaches will be required to evaluate these new automated data management systems and find ways to continue to make improvements in quality.

### Data Processing Error Measurement

Another example of a CQI application is the use of data audits to verify the error rate in a database. This is a classical example of how industrial production methods for batch error checking have been applied in clinical trials data management. These procedures are applicable whether data are collected using EDC or more traditional methods. They are also easily applied in other health care settings.

The overall objective of this audit process is to assure the sponsor that the error rate in a data processing operation is below a predetermined acceptable level. For example, an acceptable industry standard in drug development is 25 errors per 10,000 fields checked. Some CROs are so confident of their data management quality that they cite error rates in marketing materials and write them into contracts. Error rate measurement is a process improvement that uses scientific sampling approaches, now standard in industry, to avoid 100% verification of all data, a policy that would be very inefficient and often introduces new (unmeasurable) errors.

Figure 13–8 describes this process. Briefly, the key to the system is that it is carried out after all data management steps, including all query

## ❖ Process

- **Proofreading of Original CRF vs. System Printout**
- **Document Findings By Source of Error**
- **Error Correction**

## ❖ Sampling Approach

- **Statistical Sampling Techniques**
- **Simple Random Sample/Ratio Sample of Patients/Fields**
  - **Stratification by Investigator**
  - **Audit 100% of Data for Sampled Patients**
  - **Audit 100% of Patients for Key Safety Measures**

## ❖ Summary of Results

- **Formal Report/Control Chart**
- **Primary Goal – Systematic Errors/System Problems**
- **Secondary Goal – Documentation of Random Errors**
- **Target: Error Rate <25 Errors/10,000 Fields**

**Figure 13–8**

---

resolutions, have been completed, and just prior to formally locking the database. A sampling methodology, either a ratio sample or a true random sample, is used to select patient cases to be audited. In multicenter clinical trials, the sample is stratified to ensure representation of all investigators, because they are an important possible source of variation. Once the sample is selected (usually representing no more than 10% of the cases), a 100% audit is carried out for all data items in the sampled CRFs. All errors found are documented, investigated, and corrected. An important goal of this process is to identify systematic errors, for example, those due to an electronic/programming problem in the system or to inadequate training. In addition to this sample, critical information such as listings of adverse reactions, a key safety indicator, may be audited on a 100% basis.

All findings of the audit are documented and summarized in a format similar to that used for standard control charts, to allow for ongoing process improvement internally and externally. In cases where error rates are higher than expected, additional sampling or other investigations of the process are carried out.

As new technologies become more widely available and especially as more electronic methods are used to simplify "the black box" of clinical data management, it becomes critical to use existing process improvement technologies and to develop new techniques to continually assess quality and make further improvements in the process.

## CONCLUSIONS

The CRO industry is relatively young, but it has achieved rapid growth and success. Much of its success in the pharmaceutical sector can be traced in part to the implementation of CQI processes. CROs have exhibited each of the three CQI strategies described by Linder (1991). Because of the regulatory nature of pharmaceutical development, CROs have had to conform to requirements. They have used CQI to gain a competitive advantage, not only in competing with other CROs, but also in competition with internal drug development teams in sponsor organizations. They have also used CQI as a process improvement tool and, together with their sponsors, have developed many new techniques and approaches to drug development. Wherever possible, technology has been used to seek solutions to bottlenecks and to accelerate the approval process for new products. Quality improvement has been critical in order to meet the requirements of the ultimate customers—regulatory agencies, which are responsible for approving new drugs; physician-practitioners who must have confidence in the safety and efficacy of new drugs being dispensed; and finally and most importantly, patients, whose well-being depends on the quality of the new drugs they are taking.

In carrying out these processes, CROs have made very effective use of complex project management systems and have applied virtual approaches to emphasize cooperation and partnership with sponsors. Their approach can be described as co-configuration, a concept described in

Chapter 1 as a futuristic approach to the application of CQI. This approach is one example of how the CRO industry has been ahead of many of the other components of health and medical care. It also helps to explain why so much success has been achieved so quickly.

The challenge of the future for this industry is whether it can maintain the customer focus and the level of empowerment and the leadership that it has built into its organizations. CQI processes are hard to develop and maintain. When CROs were small and growing, CQI was necessary for survival; now that many CROs have achieved financial and business success, the key question is whether they will be able to sustain the CQI philosophies and processes that have brought them to where they are today.

# CHAPTER 14

# Continuous Quality Improvement in Public Health Organizations

*Glen P. Mays and Paul K. Halverson*

Although a strong public health infrastructure is essential for preparing for and responding to health threats on a population-wide basis, studies from the past two decades have found evidence of substantial gaps and wide variation in the performance of essential public health services at state and local levels. Concerns about such gaps have grown exponentially in the wake of recent acts of terrorism and bioterrorism, newly emerging diseases such as West Nile Virus and SARS, and rapidly advancing preventable health threats such as obesity. The federal government has begun spending $1 billion annually to strengthen the capacity of the nation's public health organizations to respond to public health emergencies. In this environment, public health organizations face more pressure than ever before—and also have more opportunities and resources—to improve the quality and efficiency of their operations.

This chapter examines key issues in implementing continuous quality improvement (CQI) processes within public health organizations. It first identifies the defining features and critical dimensions of quality improvement efforts implemented within public health and then reviews current tools and approaches to facilitate implementation of CQI. Its final section identifies factors likely to facilitate and inhibit CQI within public health organizations and describes possible solutions.

## PUBLIC HEALTH AND QUALITY IMPROVEMENT

Public health practice and continuous quality improvement (CQI) have an affinity that defies their lack of common ancestry. As a field of practice, public health focuses on the health of communities and populations. Like CQI, public health practice uses a systems perspective in identifying problems and developing interventions—recognizing the multiple inputs, outputs, and processes that affect health at the population level. Also like CQI, public health practice is firmly grounded in scientific methods that allow the measurement of problems and the tracking of system performance over time. Epidemiological investigation, population surveillance, and community health assessment are among public health's core methodologies. Additionally, both CQI and public health practice are based on the premise that meaningful improvements cannot be achieved without the involvement of key stakeholders within the system. In medical care organizations, these stakeholders consist of core clinical and administrative staff and leadership, but for public health organizations they may also include governmental officials, community organizations, the media, and members of the public at large.

When successful, both CQI and public health practice reflect elements of *mass customization* in their strategies for performance improvement. CQI processes in medical care organizations focus on tailoring operations to individual patient needs and expectations, often with the aid of powerful information systems. At their best, public health organizations also tailor their interventions to specific community health needs and risks. Through the process of community diagnosis, these organizations identify clinically-relevant subpopulations within their communities, evaluate health needs and resources within each subpopulation, and design community interventions to address these needs using guidance and direction from the communities themselves (Sharma 2003). Community health information systems are being used to support these activities in a growing number of communities (Starr 1997; Studnicki *et al.* 1997, 2001).

Despite similarities in concept and method, the successful implementation of CQI within public health organizations is not automatic. There are both opportunities and the challenges for public health organizations in applying CQI methods to community health problems. (Kaluzny *et al.* 1992; Hatzell *et al.* 1996) A number of dimensions must be considered—either explicitly or implicitly—when designing and implementing CQI efforts in public health organizations. Then one can use a range of performance assessment and quality improvement tools and processes developed over the past decade for public health organizations. These processes, grounded in core concepts of CQI, offer public health organizations valuable strategies for improving community health. Finally, CQI efforts must overcome a set of implementation barriers commonly encountered within public health organizations. Potential strategies for addressing these barriers are presented together with examples of CQI efforts in both governmental and nongovernmental public health settings to illustrate the benefits and challenges of CQI in these diverse multiorganizational environments.

## CRITICAL DIMENSIONS OF PUBLIC HEALTH QUALITY IMPROVEMENT INITIATIVES

As in other settings, quality improvement efforts in public health organizations must be linked to a core organizational mission. Although the specifics of this mission vary across organizations, a general and widely-recognized statement of the public health mission is given by the Institute of Medicine (IOM):

> The mission of public health is to fulfill society's interest in assuring conditions in which people can be healthy. Its aim is to generate organized community effort to address the public interest in health by applying scientific and technical knowledge to prevent disease and promote health. The mission of public health is addressed by private organizations and individuals, as well as by public agencies. (1988, p. 7)

As this statement indicates, public health performance flows from the efforts of a wide array of organizations, and public health outcomes are defined and evaluated from a societal perspective that reflects "the public interest in health." These concepts of *performance* and *outcomes*—which differ substantially from those often used in the field of medical care—have important implications for how CQI methods are implemented within public health organizations.

The several critical dimensions of CQI implementation examined below are evident in the process improvement efforts undertaken by public health organizations. They determine the focus of the improvement effort, the organizations and individuals involved, and the specific measurement and decision-making strategies to be used.

### Defining the Scope of Public Health Activity

In order to measure and improve performance, public health organizations require a clear definition of core public health activities. Such a definition has historically been the topic of much debate and discussion, and there continues to be substantial variation in how public health organizations define the scope of public health practice. In 1988, the Institute of Medicine (IOM 1988) devised a simple conceptual framework for describing core public health activities that has served as the basis for many recent performance measurement efforts. The IOM framework identifies three core public health functions.

- *Assessment* is the regular and systematic collection, analysis, and dissemination of information on the health of the community, which enables community health needs to be identified;
- *Policy Development* is the exercise of the responsibility to serve the public interest in the development of comprehensive public health plans and policies by promoting the use of scientific knowledge in decision making; and
- *Assurance* is the guarantee to constituents that health services necessary to achieve public health goals are provided to the community by the composite actions of public and private organizations—a responsibility that may be carried out through regulation, contract, or direct service provision.

Subsequent work by the US Centers for Disease Control and Prevention (CDC) and others have led to the identification of specific public health activities that correspond with the three IOM core functions. One such framework, developed by a working group of public health experts convened by the CDC during 1991 and 1992, included 10 *Core Public Health Practices* (Table 14–1, column 1) (Dyall 1995). Several groups of researchers have used these definitions of public health practice to develop surveillance systems for measuring the adequacy of public health practice in local geopolitical jurisdictions (Miller *et al.* 1994a; Turnock et al. 1994). A second framework was developed during the national policy debate over health care reform that took place during the early 1990s. An expert committee convened by the US Department of Health and Human Services (HHS) identified a set of 10 *Essential Public Health Services* ostensibly independent of the IOM core functions and CDC core practices, but conceptually similar to these earlier efforts (Table 14–1, column 2) (Public Health Functions Steering Committee 1994; Baker *et al.* 1994). This framework expands upon the earlier set of public health practices by recognizing explicitly the public health responsibilities involved in assuring access to personal health services and in conducting research (Derose *et al.* 2002a, b). The federal government has tested the Essential Services framework in evaluations of state public health agency expenditures (Eilbert *et al.* 1997) and, more recently, has used the framework to develop national performance standards for state and local public health systems (Corso *et al.* 2000).

---

**Table 14–1** Three Frameworks for Defining Public Health Activity

| Core Public Health Practices[a] | Essential Public Health Services[b] | Essential Public Health Functions[c] |
|---|---|---|
| **Assessment** | | |
| • Assess the health need of the community | • Monitor health status to identify and solve community health problems | • Monitoring the health situation (health status, determinants, risks, and interventions) |
| • Investigate the occurrence of health effects and health hazards of the community | • Diagnose and investigate health problems and health hazards in the community | • Surveillance of communicable and noncommunicable diseases |
| • Analyze the determinants of identified health needs | | |
| **Policy Development** | | |
| • Advocate for public health, build constituencies and identify resources in the community | • Mobilize community partnerships and action to solve health problems | • Public health legislation and regulations |
| • Set priorities among health needs | • Develop policies and plans that support individual and community health efforts | |
| • Develop plans and policies to address priority health needs | | |

[a] Dyall 1995.
[b] Baker, E.L. et al. 1994
[c] Bettcher et al. 1998.

*continues*

**Table 14–1** continued

| Core Public Health Practices[a] | Essential Public Health Services[b] | Essential Public Health Functions[c] |
|---|---|---|
| **Assurance** | | |
| • Manage resources and develop organizational structure | • Inform, educate and empower people about health issues | • Prevention and control of communicable and noncommunicable diseases |
| • Implement public health programs and services | • Enforce laws and regulations that protect health and assure safety | • Health promotion |
| • Evaluate programs and provide quality assurance | • Link people to needed personal health services and assure the provision of health care when otherwise unavailable | • Occupational health |
| • Inform and educate the public | | • Protecting the environment |
| | • Assure a competent work force—public health and personal health care | • Public health management |
| | • Evaluate effectiveness, accessibility, and quality of personal and population-base health services | • Specific public health services (school health, emergency services, and laboratory services) |
| | • Research for new insights and innovative solutions to health | • Personal health care for vulnerable and high risk populations. |

[a.] Dyall 1995.
[b.] Baker, E.L. et al. 1994
[c.] Bettcher et al. 1998.

A third effort to define the scope of public health practice was initiated by the World Health Organization (WHO) in 1997, drawing on the knowledge and experiences of an international collection of public health experts (Bettcher *et al.* 1998). Using a Delphi process with 145 public health administrators, educators, researchers, and practitioners, the WHO study identified and prioritized a list of 37 essential public health functions that fell within nine functional categories (Table 14–1 column 3). One of these categories—prevention, surveillance, and control of communicable and noncommunicable diseases—can be further divided into "surveillance" and "prevention and control" activities to facilitate comparisons with other frameworks.

With straightforward modifications, the frameworks developed by IOM, CDC, HHS, and WHO approximate each other, but it is unlikely that any one of them represents the last word for defining the complex role of public health in modern society. A national survey of state public health agencies conducted in 1997 revealed that many agencies were using the above frameworks in their efforts to measure and improve public health performance, but that few of them used any single approach in an unaltered form (Mays *et al.* 1998b). Many agencies also rely on locally-developed definitions of public health practice. Although the methods are still imperfect, the ability to define the scope of public health activity in measurable terms is a critical first step in supporting quality improvement efforts within public health organizations. Considering the great variability in structure and function of these organizations, it is not surprising that a variety of approaches has emerged for defining and measuring the scope of public health practice.

### Adopting an Organization vs. System Focus

An important distinction exists between performance improvement efforts that focus on the activities of an individual public health organization and those that focus on the collective actions of multiple organizations and individuals. For example, an organization-level CQI effort conducted by a local health department might focus on improving the immunization delivery practices of staff who work in clinics operated by the department. By contrast, a system-level CQI effort might focus on improving immunization practices among the full array of health care providers serving a given community, including private physicians and community health centers as well as public health clinics. Both activities potentially relate to the local health department's mission of improving community immunization rates and reducing the incidence of vaccine-preventable diseases. Organization-level and system-level CQI processes, however, may address markedly different facets of the public health problem under study, and they may require vastly different allocations of resources, skills, legal authority, and political clout.

System-level CQI processes explicitly take into consideration the fact that many public health problems can not be addressed by a single organization acting alone, but rather require collective efforts involving the multiple institutions that currently or potentially influence public health.

Correspondingly, a public health system is defined as the full complement of organizations—both governmental and private—that contribute to the performance of public health activities for a defined population or community (Halverson *et al.* 1996). System-level CQI efforts focus on improving the processes through which these different system components interact in performing core public health activities.

In choosing the appropriate focus for a CQI effort, public health organizations need to consider a variety of factors, including:

- the nature of the public health problem being targeted;
- the internal strengths and weaknesses of the organization;
- the current and potential roles played by external organizations and individuals in the problem under study; and
- the public health organization's current and potential relationships with these external entities.

In some cases, a system-level CQI effort may be ruled out due to insufficient resources and skills or lack of political will in the external environment. In other cases, an organization-level CQI effort may be inappropriate because of the limited effects that internal processes have on the public health problem under study. For example, improving immunization rates only among health department clients may be insufficient to achieve meaningful improvements in community immunization coverage. A system-level CQI effort that targets the immunization practices of all community providers may be needed. In still other cases, an organization-level CQI effort may serve as an important initial demonstration used to generate support for subsequent system-level activities. This strategy follows an approach based on staged successes or "small wins" which has become an essential ingredient of many CQI efforts (Meyerson 2001).

### The Role of Public Health Organizations in the CQI Process

Another critical dimension of CQI implementation involves the roles that public health organizations play in implementing CQI processes. Like other organizational innovations, the adoption of CQI often follows a staged process that includes awareness of a problem, identification of an intervention, implementation of the intervention, and finally institutionalization of the intervention (Glanz *et al.* 1996). Public health organizations may assume roles in any or all of these stages. For organization-level CQI efforts, these stages all occur within the public health organization among its key stakeholders and workforce. For system-level CQI efforts, however, other organizations may play critical roles in the adoption process. Public health organizations may play an *initiating* role for CQI efforts by raising awareness about a public health problem, only to let other organizations assume responsibility for implementing and institutionalizing a CQI process to address the problem. Public health organizations may play a *convening* role in CQI efforts by bringing organizations and individuals together for the purpose of identifying and implementing an intervention. During the process of CQI implementation, public health organizations may choose among several other alternative levels of involvement, including:

- a *governing* role, wherein the public health organization assumes primary responsibility for directing and managing the CQI process;
- a *participatory* role, which entails shared responsibility for managing the CQI process with other organizations; and
- a *contributing* role, which involves providing information, resources, and expertise to a CQI process that is actively managed by other organizations.

The public health organization's role in CQI efforts will depend on its own mission, skills, and resources and those of other organizations having an interest in the public health problems being addressed. By encouraging other organizations to assume key responsibilities in public health CQI efforts, public health organizations sacrifice some measure of control over these efforts. In return, however, public health organizations benefit from the additional expertise and resources contributed by these other organizations, and from the high level of buy-in and commitment maintained by these other organizations. Public health organizations may also gain new knowledge about CQI methods from organizations already skilled in these approaches such as hospitals, managed care plans, medical practices, and clinical laboratories. For example, a private hospital may assume primary responsibility for leading the CQI process aimed at improving the delivery of prenatal care to low income pregnant women. The local public health agency may participate extensively in this process, but the hospital might assume primary responsibility for the core activities of convening and educating local providers, implementing a community-wide outreach and referral service for patients, and evaluating the community's performance in prenatal care delivery.

### Sources of Public Health Authority and Control

A related aspect of CQI implementation involves the sources of public health decision-making authority and control. Governmental public health functions are carried out at federal, state, and local levels with overlapping jurisdictions of authority existing for many public health issues. CQI efforts must be responsive to these different levels of authority and accountability. An important task for public health organizations is to identify the most appropriate and feasible system level for implementing a CQI effort. Some public health problems are most effectively addressed through interventions at state or national levels rather than at the local level. Enhanced legal authority or political will may exist at these higher levels; and superior resources may be available to address the problem. Many public health problems extend beyond the boundaries of a single local community. Moreover, the problem to be addressed may originate in a state or federal policy rather than in an element of local program implementation. For example, environmental health problems such as water quality and hazardous waste disposal often fall into this category because many state governments retain substantial regulatory authority over these issues. Rather than attempting to lead a CQI effort at the local level, local public health agencies may achieve better results by contributing to state-level or federal-level CQI implementation.

Conversely, other public health issues involve primarily local populations, resources, and health needs. Often, these issues can be addressed most effectively through community-level efforts rather than large-scale state or national interventions. For example, the task of improving the accessibility of family planning services within a community may be particularly responsive to a local CQI effort. In this case, the processes of service delivery, outreach, and education are controlled primarily by local community organizations, and are therefore amenable to local improvement efforts. In other cases, local CQI efforts may be implemented because larger-scale state or national efforts are not feasible due to a lack of political will. For example, some local communities have initiated CQI efforts around the task of improving health insurance coverage for the uninsured largely because state and federal initiatives to address this problem have failed to be implemented (Felland and Lesser 2000).

CQI activities may also involve public health organizations at multiple levels of authority. Local CQI efforts may be implemented as components of larger state or national CQI efforts with linkages maintained through communication and information flows among the various levels of public health authority. These approaches are designed to address gaps in performance simultaneously at these multiple levels of authority, and are particularly relevant in cases where performance at one level has substantial influence on performance at another level. For example, the Florida Department of Health maintains a state-level CQI process for improving public health outcomes within the state such as infant mortality, adolescent pregnancy, and the incidence of communicable diseases (Speake *et al.* 1995). As part of this effort, individual CQI processes are implemented at each local public health unit within the state. They identify strategies for improving the delivery of public health services at the community level and generate information about local resource needs and priorities that feed into the state-level CQI process. This information is then used to improve decision making regarding state budget allocations, policy-making, and program development.

The administrative relationships that exist among local, state, and federal public health organizations play important roles in CQI implementation. In states such as Florida, local public health agencies are organized as centralized administrative units of the state public health agency (Frasier 1998). The state agency maintains direct authority for most governmental public health activities within the state and employs most public health workers. In other states, local public health organizations are decentralized and operate under the direct authority of local governments and local boards of health. In still other states, local public health agencies operate under state authority for some public health functions (such as communicable disease control and environmental health protection), and under local authority for other functions (such as health promotion and disease prevention activities and community health assessment). Centralized public health jurisdictions may offer state agencies enhanced authority for organizing and coordinating CQI processes at the local level, while decentralized jurisdictions may offer greater opportunities for incorporating local needs, priorities, and values in the CQI process.

Federal public health agency relationships with state and local public health organizations also play important roles in CQI efforts. Federal agencies interact with state and local organizations primarily through the provision of public health funding, technical assistance, and regulatory oversight. Considerable amounts of federal public health funding are now disbursed through block grants and similar "pass through" arrangements to state health agencies, rather than through categorical grants made directly to local public health organizations. Increasingly, federal agencies are using these funding vehicles to encourage quality improvement initiatives at the state level. For example, the Maternal and Child Health Block Grant administered by the US Health Resources and Services Administration requires state grantees to conduct formal needs assessments and to develop performance objectives and measures for their programs. Other federal agencies are developing similar performance measurement criteria for their public health funding programs, pursuant to requirements under the federal *Government Performance and Results Act of 1993*. These federal efforts provide additional motivation for public health organizations to implement CQI processes.

Federal agencies may also encourage CQI implementation through their regulatory authority. The U.S. Environmental Protection Agency (EPA) uses its regulatory authority to enforce compliance with federal public health standards such as those concerning air quality, water quality, and solid waste disposal. State and local public health organizations that do not meet these standards are required to adopt remediation processes, which offer opportunities for the application of CQI methods (US Environmental Protection Agency 1998).

Federal public health agencies also encourage the implementation of CQI methods through their technical assistance role. CDC's Public Health Practice Program Office provides information and assistance to state and local public health agencies seeking to implement CQI methods. The CDC carries out its technical assistance role in partnership with professional associations such as the National Association of County and City Health Officials and the Association of State and Territorial Health Officials. Through these partnerships, the CDC has been instrumental in developing numerous resources for quality improvement processes, many of which are discussed below. Other federal agencies such as the US Health Resources and Services Administration also provide CQI technical assistance to public health organizations.

## Public Participation and Accountability

Another important dimension of CQI implementation in public health organizations is the extent of public participation and accountability. An essential component of the public health mission lies in responsiveness to community needs, values, and priorities. Some public health organizations ensure this responsiveness through the direct involvement of community representatives in public health decision making and governance. These organizations may operate under governing boards comprised of community representatives, or they may appoint community members to serve on task forces empowered to address specific community health issues. Other public health organizations rely on indirect approaches for ensuring responsiveness and accountability to the public. Many use formal processes for assessing community health needs and identifying public priorities in health. Some organizations also rely on governing boards comprised of publicly-elected officials to reflect public interests and priorities.

These same levels of public participation are often extended to CQI initiatives within public health organizations. Some organizations directly involve community representatives in their quality improvement processes. This approach is used in the projects supported by the W.K. Kellogg Foundation's *Community-based Public Health Initiative* (Mays *et al.* 2000). Each of the seven demonstration projects sponsored through this initiative bring together public health organizations, academic institutions, and community-based organizations to form collaborative processes for identifying community health needs, developing and implementing interventions, and evaluating outcomes. Representatives from community-based organizations, including churches, neighborhood associations, and other local groups, share responsibility for problem identification, intervention, and evaluation with the governmental public health organizations and academic institutions. Steering committees comprised of representatives from each participating organization use consensus-driven processes to make decisions about how to improve public health services within the community. This approach is designed to ensure that improvement processes are focused on issues of high importance for community members, and that they involve organizations and individuals having the greatest knowledge of and experience with community health problems. Although Kellogg support for these projects officially ended in 1996, many of them continue to operate successfully. Another demonstration effort launched jointly by Kellogg and the Robert Wood Johnson Foundation entitled *Turning Point: Collaborating for a New Century in Public Health* also emphasizes community participation in public health improvement processes.

Other public health organizations use CQI processes involving more indirect levels of community participation. They may rely on community representatives to supply information about community health needs and priorities, but may not directly involve them in decision-making processes. For example, many public health organizations invite community participation in their community health assessment processes. They collect information about community perceptions regarding the most pressing public health issues, and elicit opinions about the most promising strategies for addressing these issues. In many of these efforts, direct community participation is limited to the tasks of problem identification, planning, and priority-setting. Decisions regarding what interventions to implement, how to implement them, and how to evaluate them remain the direct responsibility of public health organizations.

The degree of community participation may have important implications for the success of CQI efforts. Direct forms of community participation often ensure that the CQI process maintains a high degree of responsiveness to public health problems as experienced by community members. Moreover, direct community participation in CQI may foster high levels of commitment to problem-solving among community members, thereby increasing the likelihood of successful CQI outcomes. On the other hand, direct participation may add substantial time to the CQI process, since community members must learn about CQI concepts and build trust and familiarity with other participants in the process. CQI processes involving direct community participation may also experience difficulties in reaching consensus about key problems and potential interventions, given the diversity of opinion and perspective likely to exist among participants. Alternative levels of community participation may therefore entail trade-offs in administrative responsiveness, feasibility, and efficiency.

### Measurement and Evaluation

Measurement is an essential element of any CQI process. Public health CQI efforts vary widely in the approaches used to measure performance.

This variation results, in part, from the alternative ways that public health organizations define the scope of public health practice. This variation also stems from the alternative types of indicators that exist for a given public health activity, and the alternative methods for assessing the value of a given indicator. Like performance measures in medical care, public health indicators may reflect the *structural dimensions* of a public health activity, the clinical and administrative *processes* used to implement the activity, and the *outcomes* that result from the activity (Donabedian 1966). Also like those in medical care, public health indicators may reflect elements of technical quality, effectiveness, appropriateness, comprehensiveness, accessibility, efficiency, and equity/disparity.

Methods for assessing the value of a given indicator also vary substantially, but they uniformly entail comparisons (Gerzoff 1997). Some quality improvement initiatives rely on comparisons with *a priori* standards identified by experts, such as the national *Healthy People 2010 Health Objectives for the Nation* identified by the US Public Health Service. These comparisons have the advantage of being relatively simple to carry out once data are available, and of being widely recognizable and understandable. These comparisons, however, have the disadvantage of focusing only on a single target for performance, so that continued improvement is de-emphasized once the standard is met. Some quality improvement initiatives use comparisons over time—also called trend analysis—so that continuous improvement in performance can be detected and measured for a given indicator. This method addresses the problem with *a priori* standards noted above, but it is limited in its ability to value how much improvement is adequate and desirable over a given period of time. Finally, some improvement initiatives rely on benchmark comparisons with other public health organizations, so that performance can be evaluated in relation to similar organizations and/or leading organizations in the field. Combining methods based on *a priori* standards, trend analysis, and benchmarking can be particularly powerful for measuring and motivating continuous improvement in public health performance.

## IMPLEMENTATION OF QUALITY IMPROVEMENT INITIATIVES IN PUBLIC HEALTH

Over the past decade, a wide array of performance assessment and quality improvement activities have been implemented within the field of public health at local, state, and national levels. These efforts reflect the concepts and methods of CQI in varying ways and with varying degrees of success. More importantly, they create opportunities for public health organizations to access models, tools, and insight for their own CQI efforts. Six general types of activities are most prominent in the current landscape of public health improvement efforts:

- community health assessment and planning efforts;
- public health practice guidelines;
- community health report cards;
- public health information networks;
- public health performance measurement systems; and
- performance contracting systems and pay-for-performance metrics.

Each of these activities is examined and compared below.

### Community Health Assessment and Planning Tools

A number of tools have been developed to assist public health organizations in identifying and assessing community health problems within their jurisdictions, and in planning strategies to address these problems. These tools may serve as important foundations and frameworks for implementing CQI efforts within public health organizations.

### *National Health Objectives*

Perhaps the most prominent public health planning tools of the past two decades have been those developed by the U.S. Public Health Service to identify measurable national health objectives. These efforts identified a set of high-priority health issues, formulated national improvement goals for each issue, and specified measurement criteria and data sources to be used in assessing improvement. Objectives were identified for the years from 1980 to 1990 in the document entitled *1990 Health Objectives,* and from 1990 to 2000 in the document *Healthy People 2000: Objectives for the Nation.* The current *Healthy People 2010* document covers the period from 2000 to 2010, and for the first time it includes a chapter of health objectives devoted specifically to public health infrastructure (Table 14–2).

These national objectives have assisted many public health organizations in their improvement processes by identifying a set of priority health issues in need of attention and by offering measurable goals against which performance may be judged. As a CQI tool, however, these objectives are limited in that they may not be sensitive to public health problems of local and regional interest that are not reflected in broad national priorities.

---

**Table 14–2** Three Frameworks for Defining Public Health Activity: Example

**Goal:** Ensure that federal, tribal, state, and local health agencies have the infrastructure to provide essential public health services effectively.

| Number | Objective |
|---|---|

**Data and Information Systems**
| | |
|---|---|
| 23-1 | Improve public health employee access to the Internet |
| 23-2 | Improve public access to information and surveillance data |
| 23-3 | Expand use of geocoding in health data systems |
| 23-4 | Improve health data for all population groups |
| 23-5 | Expand data for leading health indicators, health status indicators, and priority data needs at tribal, state, and local levels |
| 23-6 | Improve national tracking of Healthy People 2010 objectives |
| 23-7 | Ensure timely release of data on objectives |

**Workforce**
| | |
|---|---|
| 23-8 | Adopt competencies for public health workers |
| 23-9 | Expand training in essential public health services |
| 23-10 | Expand continuing education and training by public health agencies |

**Public Health Organizations**
| | |
|---|---|
| 23-11 | Adopt performance standards for essential public health services |
| 23-12 | Formulate health improvement plans |
| 23-13 | Expand access to public health laboratory services |
| 23-14 | Expand access to epidemiology services |
| 23-15 | Adopt model statutes related to essential public health services |

**Resources**
| | |
|---|---|
| 23-16 | Improve data on public health expenditures |

**Prevention Research**
| | |
|---|---|
| 23-17 | Expand population-based prevention research |

U.S. Department of Health and Human Services. 2001. *Healthy People 2010: National Health Objectives for the Year 2010.* Washington, DC: Department of Health and Human Services.

Additionally, these national objectives identify specific performance levels to be achieved rather than establishing a process for continual improvement.

### Health Planning Tools

To complement the national health objectives and address some of their limitations, several additional community health planning tools have been developed in conjunction with the US Public Health Service's efforts. One of the most prominent of these tools, the *Planned Approach to Community Health* (PATCH), was developed by CDC in 1985. The PATCH protocol outlines a standard process for analyzing a few selected health issues, determining their root causes and key intervention points, and planning effective strategies for addressing these issues. Expanding on this effort, the American Public Health Association developed a protocol to assist public health organizations in creating community health planning and monitoring systems that address a comprehensive range of health-related problems. This protocol, named *Healthy Communities Model Standards,* was developed in 1991 and was explicitly designed to link with national health objectives. It provides a process for public health organizations to develop a plan based on measurable public health objectives that target specific public health outcomes, processes, and population groups. Both process and outcome objectives are emphasized in the protocol. The Texas Department of Health, for example, used this protocol in developing performance objectives for local public health departments within the state (Griffin and Welch 1995). Objectives were constructed so that the time frame and extent of improvement could be specified by each local agency, as in the following outcome and process examples:

- The rate of bicycle-related injuries in children ages 5 to 14 in *[name]* County will be reduced from *[number]* per 100,000 in FY *[year]* to *[number]* per 100,000 in FY *[year]*.
- By end of FY *[year]*, secure passage of a local ordinance requiring mandatory use of bicycle helmets.

Another assessment and planning tool, the *Assessment Protocol for Excellence in Public Health* (APEX-PH), was developed by the National Association of County and City Health Officials (NACCHO) with sponsorship from CDC in 1991 to serve as a self-assessment workbook for public health officials. It includes components for assessing the internal capacity of public health organizations as well as the external capacity of other organizations serving the community. The workbook relies on an array of process indicators, including those addressing community health assessment, policy development, financial management, personnel management, program management, and governing board procedures. An expanded version of this protocol, the *Assessment and Planning Excellence through Community Partners for Health* (APEX-CPH) was developed in 1999 to align the APEX-PH indicators with the 10 Essential Public Health Services identified by HHS, and to expand the indicators of community capacity to reflect a broader array of community organizations and activities.

Most recently, NACCHO used components of its earlier protocols to develop a community-wide strategic planning process known as *Mobilizing Action through Planning and Partnerships* (MAPP). The MAPP planning process consists of six related phases that closely follow the plan-do-study-act (PDSA) cycle of CQI, including:

1. Developing organizational capacities and community partnerships to support community-wide planning and health improvement activities;
2. Identifying a shared vision and a common set of values to guide the direction of planning and improvement activities;
3. Conducting four health-related assessments, including: (1) an assessment of community perceptions, values, and assets related to health; (2) an assessment of local public health system capacity and performance; (3) an assessment of community health status; and (4) an assessment of external threats and opportunities for community health;
4. Identifying priority issues to address through community action;
5. Formulating goals and strategies for addressing priority issues; and
6. Implementing and evaluating specific community actions.

Use of the MAPP process is being evaluated in nine local demonstration sites across the country with the goal of identifying successful strategies for implementing the process as a part of community health improvement efforts (National Association of County and City Health Officials 2004).

Other assessment initiatives formally integrate the tasks of collecting and analyzing community health data with the processes of community health planning, priority-setting, and intervention. In many communities, the hospital industry has become actively involved in these activities. Pioneered by efforts in Pennsylvania, Vermont, and Wisconsin, growing numbers of state hospital associations actively encourage their members to conduct community health assessment and improvement initiatives within their service areas (Gordon *et al.* 1996). The Pennsylvania association's process involves a five-step sequence of compiling a community health profile, identifying priorities for community health needs, developing an action plan, implementing community health interventions, and evaluating the interventions. The assessment initiative adopted by the Wisconsin association, like others, draws heavily on the Pennsylvania model as well as the APEX-PH protocol originally developed for public health agencies. Not-for-profit hospitals in California are required by that state's Hospital Community Benefit Program to conduct periodic community health assessments using an established protocol in order to maintain their not-for-profit status. Hospitals must also demonstrate involvement in community health assessment as part of the accreditation process conducted by the Joint Commission on Accreditation of Healthcare Organizations.

## The IOM Model

The proliferation of community health assessment and improvement efforts in the public and private sectors led the Institute of Medicine (IOM) to convene an expert panel to review the many existing processes and recommend a consensus approach for these efforts. The panel identified several essential characteristics of an effective community health assessment and improvement effort, including:

- use of an iterative process that cycles continuously through the tasks of assessment, action, and evaluation;
- use of a team approach, through which decisions are made largely by consensus among community representatives; and
- use of an incremental strategy for improvement, whereby progress is accomplished through a series of small steps rather than through major breakthroughs.

The IOM proposed a model for community health improvement processes consisting of two related cycles of implementation that closely

## Cycle 1: Problem Identifcation and Prioritization

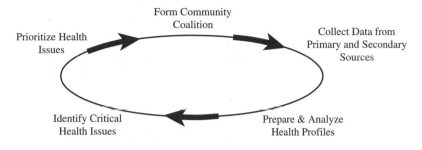

## Cycle 2: Analysis and Implementation

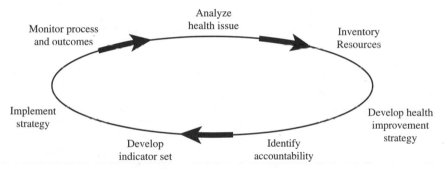

**Figure 14–1**  The Community Health Improvement Process.
Reprinted with permission from Miller CA, Moore KS, Richards TB, and Monk JD.
*A proposed method for assessing the performance of local public health functions and practices,* Copyright (1997) by the National Academy of Sciences, courtesy of the National Academies Press, Washington DC.

reflect the plan-do-study-act process of CQI (Figure 14–1) (Institute of Medicine Committee 1997). The first cycle consists of three main activities: forming a community health coalition; collecting and analyzing data for a community health profile; and identifying high priority health issues. Community efforts can begin with any phase of this cycle. As part of activities in this first cycle, the Institute of Medicine proposed a set of 25 indicators for use in assessing community health status (Table 14–3) (Perrin and Koshel 1997). These indicators are an expanded version of a consensus set of 18 indicators recommended in 1991 by CDC to track progress

**Table 14–3** Community Health Indicators Proposed by the Institute of Medicine

*Sociodemographic Characteristics*

1. Distribution of the population by age and race/ethnicity
2. Number and proportion of persons in groups such as migrants, homeless, and the non-English speaking, for whom access to community services and resources may be of concern
3. Number and proportion of persons aged 25 and older with less than a high school education
4. Ratio of the number of students graduating from high school to the total number of students who entered 9th grade three years previously
5. Median household income
6. Proportion of children less than 15 years of age living in families at or below the poverty level
7. Unemployment rate
8. Number and proportion of single-parent families
9. Number and proportion of persons without health insurance

*Health Status*

10. Infant mortality rate by race/ethnicity
11. Number of deaths or age-adjusted death rates for motor vehicle crashes, work-related injuries, suicide, homicide, lung cancer, breast cancer, cardiovascular diseases, and all causes, by age, race, and gender
12. Reported incidence of AIDS, measles, tuberculosis, and primary and secondary syphilis, by age, race, and gender as appropriate
13. Births to adolescents (ages 10-17) as a proportion of total live births
14. Number and rate of confirmed abuse and neglect cases among children

*Health Risk Factors*

15. Proportion of 2-year-old children who have received all age-appropriate vaccines, as recommended by the Advisory Committee on Immunization Practices
16. Proportion of adults aged 65 and older who have ever been immunized for pneumococcal pneumonia, and the proportion who have been immunized in the past 12 months for influenza
17. Proportion of the population who smoke, by age, race, and gender
18. Proportion of the population age 18 and older who are obese
19. Number and type of U.S. Environmental Protection Agency air quality standards not met
20. Proportion of assessed rivers, lakes, and estuaries that support beneficial uses (e.g. fishing and swimming approved).

*continues*

**Table 14–3** continued

*Health Care Resource Consumption*

21. Per capita health care spending for Medicare beneficiaries

*Functional Status*

22. Proportion of adults reporting that their general health is good to excellent
23. During the past 30 days, average number of days for which adults report that their physical or mental health was not good

*Quality of Life*

24. Proportion of adults satisfied with the health care system in the community
25. Proportion of persons satisfied with the quality of life in the community

Institute of Medicine Committee on Using Performance Monitoring to Improve Community Health. 1997. *Improving Health in the Community: A Role for Performance Monitoring.* Washington, DC: National Academy Press

towards achieving Healthy People 2000 objectives (National Center for Health Statistics 1991). Of course, for any specific community, these general indicators may need to be supplemented with additional measures corresponding to the specific problems and needs of that community. Community improvement strategies may be broad-based simultaneously exploring a number of health issues, as in the APEX-PH model, or they may focus on a small number of specific issues, as in the PATCH model.

Once a specific health issue has been targeted by a community, the health improvement process moves on to the analysis and implementation cycle (Figure 14–1). The steps in this second cycle include: analysis of the health issue; an inventory of health resources; development of a health improvement strategy; discussion and negotiation to establish where accountability lies; development of a set of performance indicators for accountable entities; implementation of the health improvement strategy; and measurement to monitor the outcome of efforts by community organizations.

To help identify risk factors for problematic health outcomes, organizations can use the APEX-PH model and its process for cause-and-effect analysis (National Association of County and City Health Officials 1991).

The State of Florida Department of Public Health and Rehabilitative Services successfully used this type of analysis, in combination with on-site reviews and team meetings, to help communities identify priority public health interventions.

A critical step in the community health improvement process is to formulate appropriate action based on the results of a community health assessment. The IOM uses the term *accountable entities* to refer to stakeholders expected to achieve specific results as part of the community's strategy for addressing a health issue. Traditionally, communities have viewed the local public health agency as the primary accountable entity. As described earlier, solutions to public health problems often require action by multiple groups within a community, and accountability should be recognized as an issue of shared responsibility. An important part of the community health improvement process is to designate the accountable entities, and to establish agreements among entities that specify areas of responsibility, measures of performance, and rewards for successful performance. Performance gaps should trigger problem analysis and a reformulation of each stakeholder's approach to the health issue.

### Public Health Practice Guidelines

Practice guidelines are another quality improvement tool beginning to be used by public health organizations. Like their counterparts in medical care, public health practice guidelines provide scientifically-based, tailored information regarding optimal methods for implementing public health interventions for specific population groups. Guidelines can be used to reduce unnecessary variation in the implementation of public health interventions, and thereby enhance the effectiveness and efficiency of these interventions. The development of practice guidelines has occurred slowly in the field of public health, principally because of the limited availability of scientifically valid information regarding the outcomes and costs of public health interventions. For many of these interventions, the outcomes accrue over long periods of time, making scientific evaluation methodologically difficult and financially costly. Nonetheless, several important sources of public health guidelines exist for assisting organizations in implementing public health quality improvement initiatives. First, organizations may use externally-developed guidelines such as those issued by the U.S. Preventive Services Task Force and CDC. Additionally, a growing number of organizations implement internally-developed guidelines based on evidence collected and analyzed internally.

## Externally Developed Guidelines

One of the most widely-recognized external sources for public health practice guidelines is *The Guide to Clinical Preventive Services,* issued by the US Preventive Services Task Force (1989). Based on an extensive review of scientific evidence, the Task Force constructed guidelines for the provision of over 100 primary and secondary prevention services designed to address more than 70 illnesses and health conditions. The evidence used to develop these guidelines included randomized controlled trials, controlled trials, cohort and case-control studies, multiple time series studies, uncontrolled experiments, and expert opinion. For each intervention, guidelines specify the socio-demographic characteristics of the target population, the timing and sequence of component processes, the contra-indications associated with each intervention, and the health risks and benefits of each intervention. Originally produced in 1989, *The Guide* was updated in 1996 and again in 2001 to reflect new scientific evidence and newly-developed interventions. Evidence from randomized controlled trials serves as the gold standard for guideline development, but *The Guide* continues to draw on expert opinion and nonrandomized studies due to the limited clinical research in many areas of prevention practice.

Expanding on the process for clinical preventive services, the CDC appointed a US Task Force on Community Preventive Services to develop similar guidelines for population-based public health interventions that target communities, schools, and worksites rather than individual patients. Although still under development, The *Guide to Community Preventive Services* offers practice guidelines in the following areas:

- changing risk behaviors;
- reducing specific diseases, injuries, and impairments;
- changing ecosystems, including environmental concerns; and
- cross-cutting public health activities (Pappaioanou and Evans 1998).

Rigorous outcomes studies are limited for these types of interventions; therefore, the guidelines for community preventive services also provide assessments of the volume and strength of the evidence that supports each intervention.

Numerous additional sources for externally-developed public health practice guidelines exist. These include specialized task forces and advisory panels convened by the National Institutes of Health and the CDC, such as the Advisory Council for the Elimination of Tuberculosis, which developed guidelines for the implementation of tuberculosis prevention and control programs (Simone 1995). Professional associations such as the American College of Preventive Medicine are also active in developing and disseminating prevention practice guidelines (Patel and Kinginger 1997; Ferrini 1997).

### Internally-Developed Guidelines

Increasingly, public health organizations are engaging in efforts to develop their own practice guidelines either alone or in combination with other health organizations. These tools are based on evidence and experience amassed by individual organizations in serving specific population groups rather than on the collective knowledge, research, and expertise of national scientific and professional groups. One approach is to begin with a nationally-developed guideline and tailor its specifications to the individual needs and capacities of the organization and the community it serves. This strategy represents an attempt to blend the concepts of *mass customization* with the more general framework of evidence-based process improvement. The Texas Department of Health used this approach in developing its performance measurement process for district health departments (Griffin and Welch 1995), drawing heavily on guidelines established in the American Public Health Association's *Healthy Communities: Model Standards* and the National Association of County and City Health Official's *Assessment Protocol for Excellence in Public Health.* Texas went beyond the generic practices described in these resources by developing specific process objectives tailored to the capacities and policy priorities of its local health agencies.

Some public health agencies adopt practice guidelines developed by other organizations with which they interact. Health plans are key among the organizations helping to disseminate practice guidelines to public health agencies and other health care providers. Public health agencies that contract with plans for the delivery of personal health services adopt many of the same health plan guidelines used by medical care providers (Halverson et al. 1998b). These may include practices for assessing patient health status, delivering clinical preventive services, and making referrals to other health care providers. Agencies participating in health plan provider networks often benefit from the quality improvement processes maintained by these plans which may allow agencies to compare their own performance in a guideline area with that of other providers. The Memphis and Shelby County (TN) Health Department, for example, uses the information it receives from health plans to compare its performance with private providers in areas such as childhood and adult immunization, cervical and breast cancer screening, and asthma and diabetes management. The agency uses documentation of its performance to negotiate favorable contracts with health plans and to demonstrate accountability to local government officials and the public.

At the same time, public health agencies play important roles in disseminating public health practice guidelines to managed care plans and other health care organizations. For example, following a large measles outbreak, the City of Milwaukee Health Department conducted on-site provider education seminars with community physicians—including those in managed care plans—regarding optimal strategies for childhood immunization delivery. More recently, the health department has sponsored workshops on tuberculosis diagnosis and treatment strategies for physicians practicing in managed care plans (Halverson et al. 1997a). Health plan executives in Milwaukee identified the local health department as an important source of information concerning effective prevention practices. In Vancouver, Washington, the Southwest Washington Health District conducts periodic on-site workshops with community physicians concerning optimal ways for storing vaccines—an effort motivated by an earlier health department study that showed widespread use of inappropriate storage techniques.

In some communities, public health agencies have begun to work jointly with other health care organizations in developing community-wide practice guidelines (Mays et al. 1998a). These efforts represent potentially powerful strategies for improving community health through the coordinated actions of multiple stakeholders—including health care providers, purchasers, insurers, and consumers. In one such initiative in Genesee County, Michigan, a local public health agency is working in partnership with a group of hospitals, health plans, employers, community-based organizations, unions, and the local medical society (Mays *et al.*

2000). This coalition has formed working groups to develop a broad range of community practice guidelines in areas such as primary care, clinical preventive services, chronic disease treatment and control, and violence prevention. Once guidelines are developed, each participant works to encourage adoption and implementation within their own and peer organizations.

## Community Health Report Cards

Among the range of performance assessment and evaluation tools, report card systems are emerging as promising strategies for monitoring and improving performance in many areas of health care. Although they vary widely in their structure and content, report card systems typically consist of a set of standardized performance measures that are collected consistently across a group of organizations, individuals, or other entities under study. Using these measures, report card systems employ a metric for comparing and profiling the performance of each entity against its peers on a periodic basis. These systems are distinct from other types of assessment approaches that rely primarily on trend analysis or on comparisons against *a priori* performance standards and goals.

Report cards are being used successfully in other sectors of the health care field to monitor performance and encourage improvement through comparison (Auerbach 1998; Longo *et al.* 1997; Chassin *et al.* 1996; New York Times 1995; National Committee on Quality Assurance 1995; U.S. General Accounting Office 1994; Pennsylvania Health Care Cost Containment Council 1991). Report card methodologies are also being used to assess community-level health issues in some localities (Fielding and Halfon 1997). Report cards offer several distinct advantages over other assessment approaches, including: (1) encouraging continuous improvement in performance rather than establishing specific floors or ceilings for performance; (2) motivating performance improvement through benchmarking and comparisons with peers; (3) generating external pressure for performance improvement when report cards are released publicly; and (4) creating a framework for identifying best practices among the entities under study. In the health field, report card systems are thought to be particularly effective in improving performance among organizations that compete for patients, revenue, or other resources such as hospitals, physician practices, and managed care plans (New York Times 1995).

In these settings, report cards can be used as tools for marketing their services to patients, payers, and purchasers. There exists evidence suggesting that some of these systems have encouraged substantial improvements in health care quality (Auerbach 1998; Longo *et al.* 1997; U.S. General Accounting Office 1994).

The rationale for using report card systems at the community level relies more on coordination and cooperation than competition. By facilitating comparisons of community-level health measures across local areas, report card systems may serve as tools for mobilizing collaborative, interorganizational efforts in community health improvement. Report card systems can be used to profile the aggregate effects of multiple health organizations and interventions within a community, thereby exposing gaps in performance needing remedy. To be sure, local public health agencies and other community health organizations already have an extensive battery of tools, protocols, and planning guides for conducting community health assessment (National Association of County and City Health Officials 1991; Greene 1992; U.S. Agency for Toxic Substances and Disease Registry1992; American Public Health Association 1993). However, by enabling comparisons among peer groups of local communities, report card systems may offer local public health agencies more meaningful and relevant measures of community health performance than other assessment approaches (Gerzoff 1997).

Community health report card systems are attractive tools for organizations other than the local health department. If broadly implemented, these systems may assist state and federal health agencies in targeting health resources and services to areas of greatest need, and in evaluating the community-level effects of health-related interventions. These systems may be able to integrate the reporting requirements and accountability systems of multiple federal and state health programs, thereby reducing reporting duplication and respondent burden while enhancing their utility in program evaluation. Similarly, report card systems may help to inform progress toward performance-based contracting initiatives in public health, which are currently taking shape at both federal and state levels (U.S. General Accounting Office 1997; Nelson *et al.* 1995; Griffin and Welch 1995; Washington State Department of Health 1996.) Under these initiatives, state and local governments may use report card systems to obtain enhanced measures of public health performance at the community level and thereby demonstrate accountability for funds which are appropriated to support public health activities.

A frequent criticism of standardized assessment tools and reporting systems in public health is that they fail to account for the unique ways in which public health is organized and administered at local levels. Local public health officials have raised this issue in relation to community health report cards, questioning the local relevance and utility of a standardized reporting system designed for broad implementation. Additional research and development efforts are needed to identify relevant, reliable, and feasible indicators of community health that can be used to monitor outcomes and practices at the community level (Halverson and Mays 1998). The set of 25 indicators proposed by the Institute of Medicine provides an appropriate starting point for this work (Table 14–2).

## Public Health Information Networks

Community health improvement strategies often face the challenge of acquiring and integrating information from multiple sources in order to adequately monitor practices and outcomes at the community level. Several computerized information management systems have been developed to assist community efforts to collect and display data from multiple sources. Two examples are the Michigan and CDC APEX-PH Information Manager, and the Seattle-King County Department of Public Health VISTA-PH computer software (Vaughn *et al.* 1994; Epidemiology, Planning, and Evaluation Unit, Seattle-King County Department of Public Health 1995). These computer programs allow the integrated display and analysis of secondary data such as demographic information from the U.S. Census, mortality rates, hospitalization rates, birth outcomes, and infectious disease rates. Increasingly, public health organizations are using geographic information system (GIS) technologies to facilitate the display and analysis of spatial patterns in health-related data (Roper and Mays 1999).

A broad range of other public health information systems are being developed at state and local levels to facilitate public health management and decision making. A number of these efforts have been supported by the CDC's *Information Network for Public Health Officials* (INPHO) program. These efforts are working to establish integrated information networks that can support information sharing and communication across public health agencies within the states. Other efforts are carried out through state health data organizations, hospital associations, managed care plans, and health care purchasing coalitions (Mendelson and Salinsky 1997). Public health managers at state and local levels need to be able to identify the information needs of their programs and services, and to understand the array of information resources and systems that may be tapped in addressing these needs.

A prominent example of this is the health information network under development in Indianapolis and Central Indiana through the Indiana Health Information Exchange, a nonprofit corporation formed to share health information among health care providers and public health agencies in the region. Participating hospitals, clinics, laboratories, and state and local public health agencies contribute patient health information to a centralized database that can then be accessed for a variety of authorized purposes including care coordination, disease management, clinical research, and public health surveillance. Among its many purposes, the information network is becoming a core component of the region's bioterrorism preparedness activities by allowing public health agencies to actively monitor patterns of health services utilization and disease incidence across population centers in Central Indiana.

## Public Health Performance Measurement

Proposals for measuring the adequacy of public health system performance in the United States have been offered repeatedly throughout the last century (Turnock and Handler 1997). However, progress in developing sound methods for measuring public health system performance has been slow until relatively recently. A review in 1996 by the Robert Wood Johnson Foundation's Center for Studying Health System Change concluded that, "Unlike the medical care system, there is little research and relatively few measures for studying how well the public health system operates" (Center for Studying Health System Change 1996). More recently, the Institute of Medicine's 2002a review of the nation's public health system called attention to the lack of available data and measures on system performance which has most certainly slowed the development of system improvement activities among public health organizations.

Although far from universal, efforts to measure the performance of public health organizations have grown substantially over the past decade, as public health practitioners faced growing pressures to improve their systems and demonstrate the value of these systems to policy makers, payers, providers, and the public at large. In 1990, the US Department of Health and Human Services formalized the need for public health evaluative efforts in its *Healthy People 2000* objectives for the nation, challenging agencies to "increase to at least 90% the proportion of people who are served by a local health department that is effectively carrying out the core functions of public health." To monitor progress toward this objective, public health researchers, practitioners, and policy makers began to implement approaches for measuring local public health performance.

Existing performance assessment survey instruments include those developed by researchers at the University of North Carolina at Chapel Hill (UNC) (Miller *et al.* 1994b) and by researchers at the University of Illinois-Chicago (UIC) (Turnock *et al.* 1994)—both of which are based upon the Institute of Medicine's three core public health functions, and upon the associated set of 10 public health practices that were identified by a CDC expert work group (Dyall 1995). The performance measurement approach developed by Miller and colleagues has received considerable attention because it focuses on the contribution to public health practice by all providers in a jurisdiction—both public and private—rather than limiting performance measures to the role of the local health department. Eight to ten indicators were developed for each of the 10 practices, yielding a total of 84 indicators. The indicators were included on a self-reported survey instrument designed for administration to local health department directors. The performance scores for the surveyed jurisdictions reported on adequacy of performance for each practice, the proportional contribution to performance by the local health department, and the identification of other providers contributing to the coverage of each practice within the jurisdiction. Performance scores can be presented in graphic form to facilitate analysis and problem identification, as illustrated in Figure 14–2 (Mays *et al.* 2000).

A shortened form of the performance assessment instrument that includes 20 performance indicators from both the UNC and UIC instruments has been used in several national surveys of local public health jurisdictions, including a survey of all jurisdictions serving at least 100,000 residents (Table 14–4) (Mays *et al.* 2004c). Results confirmed that wide variation in performance persists despite various public health improvement efforts implemented at national, state, and local levels during the 1990s (Figure 14–3). On average, 64% of the 20 public health indicators were performed in local public health jurisdictions. The average local health department performed 24% of these services directly, accounting for 67% of the total community effort (Table 14–5). The activities most likely to be performed in the average jurisdiction included investigation of

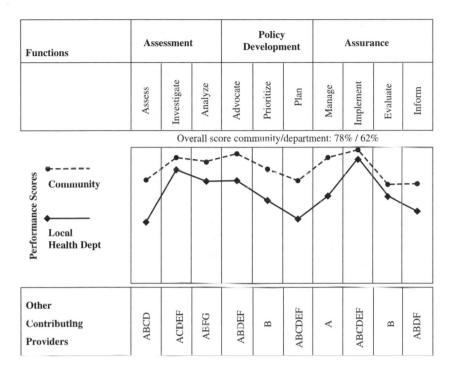

| Functions | Assessment | | | Policy Development | | | Assurance | | | |
|---|---|---|---|---|---|---|---|---|---|---|
| | Assess | Investigate | Analyze | Advocate | Prioritize | Plan | Manage | Implement | Evaluate | Inform |

Overall score community/department: 78% / 62%

| Other Contributing Providers | ABCD | ACDEF | AEFG | ABDEF | B | ABCDEF | A | ABCDEF | B | ABDF |
|---|---|---|---|---|---|---|---|---|---|---|

Other provider codes: A = state agencies; B = local agencies; C = nonprofit agencies; D = hospitals; E = community health centers; F = universities; G = other.

**Figure 14-3** Public Health Performance Profile for a Sample Community and Local Health Department.
Miller CA, Moore KS, Richards TB, and Monk JD. 1994a. A proposed method for assessing the performance of local public health functions and practices. *American Journal of Public Health* 84(11):1743–1749.

adverse health events, provision of laboratory services, implementation of mandated public health programs, and implementation of programs in response to priority health needs. By contrast, the activities least likely to be performed included evaluations of public health programs, analyses of participation in preventive and screening services, and resource allocation planning. Perceptions about the effectiveness of public health activities also varied widely across communities and clustered at lower ranges of the distribution. On average, local health directors rated the effectiveness of their jurisdiction's activities at 35% of the optimum score that would be obtained if all activities fully met community needs.

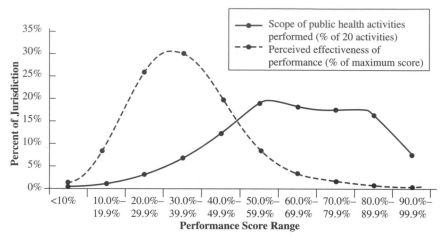

**Figure 14–3** Variation in Local Public Health System Performance of Public Health Activities, United States, 1998

Data from reference Mays, G.P. et al. 2004c. Availability and Perceived Effectiveness of Public Health Activities in the Nation's Most Populous Areas. *American Journal of Public Health,* 94, no.6:1019–1026.

---

**Table 14–4** Twenty Indicators of Local Public Health Performance

1. In your jurisdiction, is there a community needs assessment process that systematically describes the prevailing health status in the community?
2. In the past three years in your jurisdiction, has the local public health agency surveyed the population for behavioral risk factors?
3. In your jurisdiction, are timely investigations of adverse health events conducted on an ongoing basis including communicable disease outbreaks and environmental health hazards?
4. Are the necessary laboratory services available to the local public health agency to support investigations of adverse health events and meet routine diagnostic and surveillance needs?
5. In your jurisdiction, has an analysis been completed of the determinants of and contributing factors to priority health needs, the adequacy of existing health resources, and the population groups most effected?

*continues*

**Table 14–4** continued

6. In the past three years in your jurisdiction, has the local public health agency conducted an analysis of age-specific participation in preventive and screening services?
7. In your jurisdiction, is there a network of support and communication relationships that includes health-related organizations, the media, and the general public?
8. In the past year in your jurisdiction, has there been a formal attempt by the local public health agency to inform officials about the potential public health impact of decisions under their consideration?
9. In your local public health agency, has there been a prioritization of the community health needs that have been identified from a community needs assessment?
10. In the past three years in your jurisdiction, has the local public health agency implemented community health initiatives consistent with established priorities?
11. In your jurisdiction, has a community health action plan been developed with community participation to address priority community health needs?
12. In the past three years in your jurisdiction, has the local public health agency developed plans to allocate resources in a manner consistent with community health action plans?
13. In your jurisdiction, have resources been deployed as necessary to address priority health needs identified in a community health needs assessment?
14. In the past three years in your jurisdiction, has the local public health agency conducted an organizational self-assessment?
15. In your jurisdiction, are age-specific priority health needs effectively addressed through the provision of or linkage to appropriate services?
16. In your jurisdiction, have there been regular evaluations of the effects of public health services on community health status?
17. In the past three years in your jurisdiction, has the local public health agency used professionally recognized process and outcome measures to monitor programs and to redirect resources as appropriate?
18. In your jurisdiction, is the public regularly provided with information about current health status, health care needs, positive health behaviors, and health care policy issues?
19. In the past year in your jurisdiction, has the local public health agency provided reports to the media on a regular basis?
20. In the past three years in your jurisdiction, has there been an instance in which the local public health agency has failed to implement a mandated program or service?

Turnock BJ, Handler AS, Miller CA. 1998. Core function-related local public health practice effectiveness. Journal of Public Health Management and Practice 4(5):26–32.

**Table 14-5** Average Public Health Performance Scores for Local Public Health Jurisdictions

| Indicator | N | Performance Scores | | | |
|---|---|---|---|---|---|
| | | Community Performance | Adequacy of Community Performance[a] | Health Dept. Contribution[a,b] | Health Dept. Contribution as % of Community Performance[a,b] |
| 1 Needs assessment | 335 | 73% | 36% | 21% | 58% |
| 2 Behavioral risk factor survey | 331 | 47% | 22% | 11% | 52% |
| 3 Adverse health events investig. | 336 | 99% | 75% | 57% | 76% |
| 4 Laboratory services | 336 | 96% | 73% | 37% | 50% |
| 5 Analysis of health determinants | 333 | 63% | 30% | 16% | 54% |
| 6 Participation in preventive serv. | 333 | 29% | 13% | 8% | 61% |
| 7 Support and communication | 333 | 79% | 43% | 21% | 48% |
| 8 Inform elected officials | 335 | 82% | 38% | 29% | 77% |
| 9 Prioritization of health needs | 335 | 67% | 35% | 21% | 61% |
| 10 Iplementtion of initiatives | 333 | 83% | 35% | 21% | 61% |
| 11 Community action plan | 333 | 42% | 16% | 9% | 54% |
| 12 Plans to allocate resources | 335 | 27% | 11% | 7% | 63% |
| 13 resources for priority needs | 333 | 50% | 19% | 10% | 54% |
| 14 Self-assessment | 333 | 57% | 32% | 29% | 89% |
| 15 Provision/linkage of services | 332 | 76% | 36% | 19% | 51% |
| 16 Evaluation of services | 333 | 35% | 16% | 12% | 71% |
| 17 Process/outcome measures | 331 | 47% | 22% | 16% | 75% |
| 18 Public information | 334 | 76% | 33% | 20% | 61% |
| 19 Medial information | 335 | 76% | 40% | 31% | 78% |
| 20 Mandated program/services | 323 | 92% | 92% | 92% | 100% |
| Assessment (#1–#6) | 336 | 67% | 41% | 25% | 60% |
| Policy Development (#7–#12) | 336 | 63% | 29% | 18% | 61% |
| Assurance (#13–#20) | 336 | 63% | 36% | 28% | 78% |
| Total Score | 335 | 64% | 35% | 24% | 67% |

Note: Performance scores represent the proportion of communities/departments that perform the selected publichealth activity.
[a] Scores adjusted for perceived adequacy of performane (five point scale)
[b] Scores adjusted for proportion of effort contributed by the local health department (five point scale)
Serving Populations of at Least 100,000 Residents—United States, 1998
Mays, G.P. et al. 2004c. Availability and Perceived Effectiveness of Public Health Activities in the Nation's Most Populous Areas. *American Journal of Public Health*, 94, no.6:1019–1026.

Findings from performance measurement activities such as this are valuable in identifying specific domains of public health practice that should receive priority in quality improvement efforts. By examining the public health contributions made by government agencies and other organizations, this type of measurement effort can also shed light on promising pathways for improving performance. For example, the study described above found that in many communities nongovernmental organizations participate frequently in public health activities but only in a relatively narrow scope of activities, suggesting that there are untapped opportunities for collaboration.

Public health organizations now use a variety of approaches for measuring organizational and/or system-level performance, with some based on the instruments developed at UNC and UIC and others based on locally- or regionally-developed metrics. A survey of the nation's state health agencies during 1997 revealed that fully 88% had some level of involvement in public health performance measurement activities (Mays *et al.* 1998b). A more recent survey found that this number had increased to 96% by 2001 (Public Health Foundation 2002b). One of the most prominent locally-developed initiatives in performance measurement was implemented by the Public Health Division of the Los Angeles County Department of Health Services in 2002 (Derose *et al.* 2003). Through this effort the department sought to address two key limitations of existing measurement instruments such as those developed at UNC and UIC: (1) the reliance on self-reported and subjective assessments of performance; and (2) the exclusive focus on structural and process measures of performance as opposed to outcome measures. The department identified a set of 61 performance indicators based on objective, measurable, and locally-available data that reflect structural characteristics, processes, and intermediate outcomes related to local health department performance (Table 14–6). Although the identified indicators may not be available and relevant for all local health departments, they demonstrate ways in which public health organizations can begin to incorporate more objective and outcomes-based measures into their performance assessment activities.

## Public Health Performance Standards

Successful efforts to measure the performance of public health organizations potentially create a knowledge base that could be used to

**Table 14–6** Examples of Public Health Performance Indicators used in Los Angeles County

**Structural Indicators**
- Ratio of California Children's Services (CCS) patients to CCS nurse providers
- Ratio of California Children's Services (CCS) high-risk patients to CCS skilled nurse providers

**Process Indicators**
- Proportion of confirmatory test results for reportable communicable diseases that hospital and other private labs reported to the health department
- The proportion of people exposed to an acute communicable disease case and contacted by the health department who are not on prophylaxis during relevant disease-specific time period
- Proportion of Class A and B rental housing that is inspected at least 1 time per year

**Intermediate Outcome Indicators**
- Proportion of patients with newly diagnosed active tuberculosis (for whom ≤12 months of therapy are indicated) who complete recommended therapy within 12 months
- Proportion of children who have all recommended immunizations performed on schedule at age 24 months
- Proportion of families eligible for the Child Health Disability Prevention Program who report difficulty obtaining preventive health services for their children

Derose et al. 2003.

---

support the development of performance standards in public health. Performance standards represent expected and/or desired levels of performance in important domains of activity. With this goal in mind, the National Public Health Performance Standards Program (NPHPSP) was launched in 1998 to develop a concrete, measurable set of performance standards for public health systems along with the measurement tools needed to monitor progress. Developed through a partnership between CDC and six national public health organizations, the Performance Standards Program was designed to generate data and information needed to stimulate improvements in performance and support research and evaluation in public health practice. The performance standards and associated measurement instruments were developed around the 10 essential services of public health as identified by the Public Health Functions Steering Committee (1994).

The NPHPSP focuses on public health activities performed by the public health system collectively, including the full range of governmental and private organizations that contribute to such activities. The program uses three main types of instruments to collect information about system performance: (1) a local instrument that assesses performance within county, city, and other local public health jurisdictions; (2) a state instrument that assesses performance of statewide activities; and (3) a governance instrument that focuses specifically on the activities performed by local boards of health. Each of the instruments contains questions that ask respondents to assess the extent to which a range of public health services and activities are performed within their jurisdiction, regardless of whether the local public health agency directly performs these activities. Like the earlier UNC and UIC instruments, these instruments collect self-reported measures of public health performance. Unlike earlier instruments, however, the NPHPSP instruments are designed to be completed by a group of public health professionals who are knowledgeable about local public health activities underway within the community, assembled by the local or state public health agency director. Through this process, group participants are asked to reach consensus about the extent to which specific public health activities are performed within the jurisdiction, and report their consensus response to each question on the instrument.

Each instrument contains questions that correspond to each of the 10 essential services of public health. Each essential service has one to five associated indicators that define specific areas of performance. Each indicator has a model performance standard that specifies the activities that define optimal performance (Table 14-7), along with a summary question that asks about the degree to which the model standard is achieved by the public health system, using an ordinal Likert response scale. These data elements are labeled model standard achievement measures. Additionally, each indicator has an array of specific questions that ask about the extent to which individual activities within the model standard are performed by the public health system, also using Likert scales. These data elements are labeled activity measures. All of the indicators, model standards, and activity measures used on the instruments were developed through an extensive expert panel process that included active participation by public health practitioners, researchers, and policy-makers along with performance measurement experts.

**Table 14–7** Example Indicator, Model Standard, and Activity Measures Used in the National Public Health Performance Standards Program

**Essential Service 1:** Monitor health status to identify community health problems

**Indicator 1.1:** Population-based Community Health Profile

**Model Standard:** The community health profile (CHP) is a common set of measures for the community to prioritize the health issues that will be addressed through strategic planning and action, to allocate and align resources, and to monitor population-based health status improvement over time. The CHP includes broad-based surveillance data and measures related to health status and health risk at individual and community levels including: demographic and socioeconomic characteristics, health resource availability, quality of life, behavioral risk factors, environmental health indicators, social and mental health, maternal and child health, death, illness and injury; communicable diseases; and sentinel events. The CHP displays information about trends in health status along with associated risk factors and health resources. Local measures are compared with peer, state, and national benchmarks. Data and information are displayed in multiple formats for diverse audiences, such as the media and community-based organizations. Data included in the CHP are accurate, reliable, and consistently interpreted according to the science and evidence-base for public health practice.

To accomplish this, the Local Public Health System (LPHS):

Conducts regular community health assessments to monitor progress toward health-related objectives
Compiles and periodically updates a CHP using community assessment data
Promotes community-wide use of the CHP and/or assessment data and assures that the information can be easily accessed by the community

**Summary Measure of Model Standard Achievement:**
1.1    How much of this Model Standard is achieved by the local public health system collectively?

**Selected Activity Measures:**
1.1.1 Has the LPHS conducted a community health assessment?
    1.1.1.1 If so, is the community health assessment updated annually?
    1.1.1.2 Are data from the assessment compared to data from other representative areas or populations?
    1.1.1.3 Does the LPHS use data from the assessment to monitor progress toward health-related objectives?

*continues*

**Table 14–7** continued

1.1.2 Does the LPHS compile data from assessments into a community
     profile (CHP)?
     1.1.2.1 Are the CHP data used to track trends over time?
     1.1.2.2 Does the CHP include data from a local surveillance system?
1.1.3 Does the LPHS have access to community demographic characteristics?
1.1.4 Does the LPHS have access to community socioeconomic
     characteristics?
1.1.5 Does the LPHS have access to health resource availability data?
1.1.6 Does the LPHS have access to quality of life data for the community?
1.1.7 Does the LPHS have access to behavioral risk factor data for the
     community?

CDC. National Public Health Performance Standards Program, Local Public Health Performance Assessment Instrument, Version 1.0. Atlanta, GA: CDC, 2003.

The instruments were pilot-tested in eight states during the program's developmental period, 1999 through 2001. Validity testing conducted in the pilot test states confirmed that the instruments produce measures of performance that are consistent with expert judgments and documentary evidence of performance, and reflect key elements of public health practice as judged by local public health professionals (Beaulieu and Scutchfield 2003). Instruments were subsequently revised and released nationally in June 2002. State and local public health organizations that choose to adopt the national performance standards and their associated measurement instruments can submit their data to CDC through a secure Web-based portal and receive summary measures and comparative feedback based on data collected from other public health jurisdictions.

One of the most powerful incentives for participating in the NPHPSP is the comparative information that it generates that can be used to identify domains of activity that should receive priority in CQI activities. This information can also be used to support practice-based research and evaluation to identify the causes and consequences of variation in public health system performance. Analysis based on the NPHPSP pilot test data, for example, documented wide variation in local public health system performance across the 10 essential service domains, and demonstrated that jurisdictional size and financial resources explained much of the observed variation (Figure 14–4, A-C) (Mays *et al.* 2004a, 2004b).

Participants suggest that an equally powerful incentive for adopting the NPHPSP measures and standards is the group process approach to performance measurement. If successful, this process engages all of the major stakeholders in the public health system and forces them to reach consensus about the status of the system so that, once measurement activities are complete, the group can easily transition into collaborative strategies for action planning and implementation. The program also has significant limitations, including the reliance on self-reported and subjective measures of performance, the need to provide extensive training to group participants on measurement concepts and strategies, and the considerable time commitment required for completion of the measurement instruments. Despite these limitations, more than 16 states have

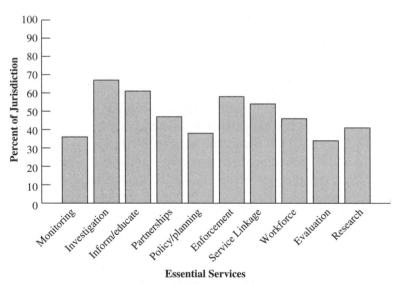

**Figure 14–4A**  Variation in Model Standard Achievement Scores in 7 Pilot States for the National Public Health Performance Standards Program. Data from Mays, G.P. et al. 2004a. Identifying Dimensions of Performance in Local Public Health Systems: Results from the National Public Health Performance Standards Program *Journal of Public Health Management and Practice* 10, no. (3):193–203.

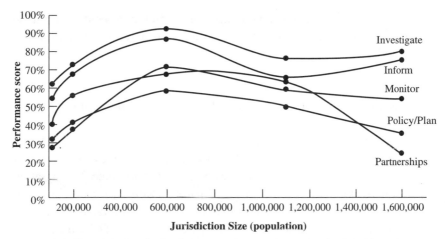

**Figure 14–4B** Variation in Performance Scores Associated with Size of Jurisdiction.
Data from Mays, G.P. et al. 2004a. Identifying Dimensions of Performance in Local Public Health Systems: Results from the National Public Health Performance Standards Program *Journal of Public Health Management and Practice* 10, no. (3):193–203.

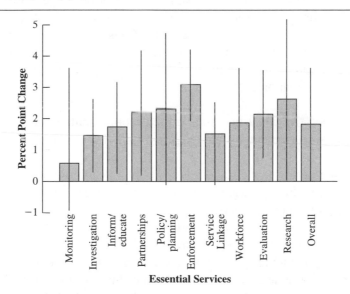

**Figure 14.4C** Change in Performance Scores Associated with a $10 Increase in Per Capita Public Health Funding.
Data from Mays, G.P. et al. 2004b. Getting What You Pay For: Public Health Spending and the Performance of Essential Public Health Services. *Journal of Public Health Management and Practice* 10, no.5:441–9.

implemented the performance standards or are in the process of doing so, and several additional states have passed legislation requiring adoption of these standards.

### Performance Management, Contracting, and Compensation

A national collaborative of public health administrators and scholars formed in 1999 to identify successful models and practices for using CQI tools to improve public health practice. The Performance Management Collaborative was part of the larger *Turning Point Initiative,* an effort sponsored by the Robert Wood Johnson Foundation and the W.K. Kellogg Foundation to strengthen public health system capacity. The collaborative defines performance management as follows:

> Performance management is the practice of actively using performance data to improve the public's health. This practice involves strategic use of performance measures and standards to establish performance targets and goals, to prioritize and allocate resources, to inform managers about needed adjustments or changes in policy or program directions to meet goals, to frame reports on the success in meeting performance goals, and to improve the quality of public health practice. (Public Health Foundation 2002b, p.11)

The collaborative identified four critical components of a successful performance management system (Figure 14–5). These components are:

1. Creating performance standards for public health organizations and systems, including targets and goals and relevant indicators to improve public health practice
2. Developing indicators and collecting measures of the extent to which performance standards are met
3. Documenting and reporting progress over time in meeting performance standards and targets, and sharing this information with relevant stakeholders and the public through feedback mechanisms
4. Implementing processes to improve public health policies, programs and infrastructure based on performance standards, measurements, and reports.

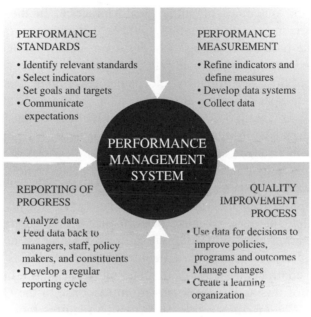

**Figure 14–5** The Turning Point Model for Performance Management in Public Health.
Public Health Foundation. 2002a. *From Silos to Systems: Using Performance Management to Improve Public Health.* Seattle, WA: Turning Point National Program Office at the University of Washington.

Through the Collaborative, seven participating states have worked actively to implement these components in their respective public health systems. The Collaborative has conducted detailed case studies of the experiences of these and other states in implementing performance management practices, and compiled an inventory of tools and resources that have proven useful in implementing these practices. These resources, currently available on the Turning Point Web site, hold considerable promise for strengthening the capacity of public health organizations to engage in quality improvement activities.

One specific set of strategies for performance management—performance–based contracting and compensation arrangements—deserve special attention because of the growing interest in these strategies within the health care and public health arena. Making contract awards and financial payments contingent on measurable attributes of performance could create powerful incentives for improvement both in the processes and outcomes of public health practice. In the domain of medical care, managed care plans pioneered numerous strategies for performance-based contracting with physicians and hospitals, including risk-adjusted capitation payment rates, payment withholds and bonuses based on provider performance, and payment formulae based on performance in specific clinical areas (such as immunization rates) (Robinson and Casalino 2001). More recently, health plans and health care providers have begun experimenting with "pay for performance" compensation arrangements tied specifically to measures of health care quality, including a series of demonstration projects now underway around the country sponsored by the foundation-supported *Rewarding Results* initiative (Marshall and Smith 2003).

In the field of public health, performance-based contracting may have application in several different settings. Federal agencies are beginning to use performance-based contracting principles as part of the grants and contracts they award to state and local public health agencies. Much of this activity is occurring in response to the *Government Performance and Results Act of 1993*, which requires federal agencies to be more accountable for the public funds they administer. Agencies within the US Department of Health and Human Services use "performance partnerships" for selected contracts and grants with state and local health agencies, which require these agencies to establish action plans and measurable performance objectives as part of their contracts with DHHS for federal public health funding (U.S. General Accounting Office 1997).

State and local public health agencies also have begun to integrate aspects of performance-based contracting into their relationships with other health organizations. Some of these efforts are being adopted as part of public health privatization efforts that transfer responsibility for certain public health functions from public agencies to private (or quasi-private) contractors (Halverson *et al.* 1997b). For example, the local health department in Milwaukee, Wisconsin contracts with a network of community health centers to provide specified clinical services to health department clients. Similarly, in Mecklenburg County, North Carolina, the county health department contracts with a hospital-based integrated delivery system for the provision of most personal health services traditionally provided by the health department (Keener *et al.* 1997). Both of these agencies use performance-based contracting mechanisms to ensure the quality of services purchased from private providers.

Several implementation characteristics of performance-based contracting efforts warrant attention. First, these efforts require a clear definition of the public health functions and activities to be carried out under the contract, and a clear delineation of responsibilities to be assumed by each party. Without these elements, contract provisions can be difficult, if not impossible, to enforce. Second, performance-based contracts require accurate, reliable systems for measuring performance. Initiatives based on measures that are self-reported by the contractor introduce a clear moral hazard for "up-coding" these measures in order to receive higher payments. Effective performance-based contracting strategies therefore require substantial investments in measurement systems that are resistant to these types of gaming. Third, performance-based contracting initiatives must be supported by effective plans for enforcing contract provisions and payment rates. Potential barriers to effective contract enforcement include: a lack of alternative contractors that could be engaged if current contractors fail to meet performance expectations and the ability of contractors to use political influence or market power to avoid adverse contract provisions. Public health agencies must anticipate these barriers and incorporate contract mechanisms that offer alternative methods of enforcement.

Several state health agencies have initiated performance-based contracting efforts as part of their public health quality improvement efforts. Rhode Island's Department of Health delivers personal health services and community health services exclusively through contracts with private providers such as community health centers and voluntary health associations. Currently, the state relies primarily on process-based measures of performance in developing and enforcing contracts with private providers. These measures include such elements as waiting times, appointment availability, service volume, and consumer-initiated complaints. The state is in the process of developing strategies to link contracts with measurable public health outcomes—particularly those that are emphasized in the *Healthy People* national health objectives. Similarly, the Utah Department of Health uses performance-based contracting mechanisms in four core areas: services provided under the federal *Preventive Health Services Block Grant;* services provided through the federally-supported *Children with Special Health Care Needs* program; services provided through the federal *Special Supplemental Food Program for Women, Infants, and Children* (WIC) program; and services provided through state HIV and tuberculosis prevention and control programs. Utah develops with each contractor individually-tailored action plans that specify both short-term process objectives and long-term outcome objectives. Objectives are developed through a process that includes input from contractors as well as consumers and links with the national *Healthy People 2000* objectives.

## QUALITY IMPROVEMENT AND PUBLIC HEALTH: KEY IMPLEMENTATION ISSUES

A variety of methods and tools are now available to assist public health organizations in implementing quality improvement initiatives at local, state, national, and international levels. Nonetheless, public health organizations have generally not been as quick to adopt and apply CQI methods successfully as have organizations in other sectors of the health care field (Kaluzny *et al.* 1992; Hatzell *et al.* 1996; Scutchfield *et al.* 1997). Public health organizations face several unique challenges in implementing quality improvement efforts which must be anticipated, recognized, and addressed to ensure success. First, public health organizations frequently confront severe resource constraints that limit their ability to devote human and financial capital to improvement initiatives. Funding streams for public health organizations are often limited and inflexible—consisting mainly of governmental appropriations, categorical grant programs and charitable contributions. Nonetheless, it is critical that public health organizations identify an initial amount of human and financial resources that can be devoted to the improvement effort. A large and permanent funding stream is not essential, since successful improvement efforts often become self-sustaining as early successes lead to resource reallocation and an expanding base of support from core organizational resources. Start-up resources, however, are essential, and may be patched together from sources such as demonstration grants issued by local health care foundations, volunteer labor, and in-kind donations.

Second, governmental public health agencies often function under stringent operational requirements concerning such activities as hiring, salary and benefit determination, purchasing, and contracting. As a result, these organizations seldom have full and immediate control over their own operational processes. Effective quality improvement efforts may require greater administrative flexibility than is typically available within governmental public health organizations. Several strategies may be used to address this constraint. Public health agencies may collaborate with private organizations that have fewer administrative constraints, and allow these private partners to assume responsibility for those tasks that are difficult for a public agency to undertake (Mays *et al.* 1998a). Alternatively, public health agencies may cultivate sufficient political support for their quality improvement efforts in order to secure exemptions from administrative requirements—at least on a temporary demonstration basis. As an extreme example, the public health agency and hospital system in Denver, Colorado successfully achieved local and state approval to convert from a county agency to an independent health care authority chartered by the state government. This change substantially enhanced the agency's ability to undertake quality improvement efforts and other organizational innovations (Mays *et al.* 2000).

Third, adoption of CQI methods is made difficult by the fact that public health practice is inherently a multiorganizational activity, with no single entity within the community being wholly responsible for population-based health processes and outcomes. To be optimally effective in improving community health, CQI methods must be implemented across multiple organizations—a daunting task for many public health organizations. Nonetheless, multiorganizational efforts for community health improvement have become increasingly common in recent years, fueled by marketplace and policy developments that have created shared incentives for improving health at the population level (Lasker 1997; Institute of Medicine 1997; Mays *et al.* 1998a). These developments have also created new opportunities for using CQI methods as part of multiorganizational public health processes. To capitalize on these opportunities, public health agencies must assume a leadership role in identifying shared interests and incentives among community organizations, developing effective mechanisms of communication and information sharing among organizations, and motivating collective action to address shared interests.

A final reason for the limited uptake of quality improvement processes by public health organizations has been the lack of sufficient external pressure to do so (Scutchfield *et al.* 1997). Public health organizations historically have not faced the same pressures—from competitors, consumers, purchasers, and regulators to improve quality, efficiency and value in service delivery—as medical care providers have. Increasingly, public health organizations are no longer protected from these forces. Many agencies now face an environment in which they must actively compete for clients, negotiate complex relationships with public and private organizations, and demonstrate accountability for the public funds they receive from local, state, and federal sources. In the wake of the recent acts of terrorism and bioterrorism and emerging infectious diseases such as SARS, the nation's public health system endures heightened scrutiny from policymakers, the media, and the public at large. The federal government is now spending more than $1 billion annually to strengthen the nation's public health system and improve its capacity to prepare for and respond to public health emergencies. With this new funding comes heightened expectations about performance and a growing demand for public health organizations to demonstrate what the nation has gained from its increased investments in public health. In this environment, growing numbers of public health organizations are turning to quality improvement processes as strategies for surviving and thriving in the evolving health system.

# CHAPTER 15

# Inquiring into the Quality and Safety of Care in the Academic Clinical Microsystem

*Julie J. Mohr, Paul Batalden, and Paul Barach*

A clinical microsystem is a group of clinicians and staff working together with a shared clinical purpose to provide care for a population of patients (Batalden *et al.* 1997; Mohr 2000; Nelson *et al.* 1998). The clinical purpose and its setting define the essential components of the microsystem, which include clinicians, patients, and support staff; information and technology; and specific care processes and behaviors that are required to provide care. Microsystems evolve over time, and they respond to the needs of their patients and providers, as well as to the external pressures such as regulatory requirements. They often coexist with other microsystems within a larger (macro) organization, such as a hospital. This chapter provides additional information about the clinical microsystem and its functioning initially presented in Chapter 11 and suggests a detailed approach for improving the relationships within and across microsystems in the teaching setting as a means of enhancing quality improvement and patient safety research and practice on the front lines of patient care.

## MICROSYSTEM THEORY

The conceptual theory of the clinical microsystem is based on ideas developed by Deming (1986), Senge (1990), Wheatley (1992), and others who have applied systems thinking to organizational development, leadership, and improvement. The seminal idea for the clinical microsystem stems from the work of James Brian Quinn (1992). Quinn's work is based on analyzing the world's best-of-best service organizations such as FedEx, Mary Kay Cosmetics, McDonald's, and Nordstrom. He focused on determining what these extraordinary organizations were doing to achieve high quality, explosive growth, high margins, and wonderful reputations with customers. He found that these leading service organizations organized around, and continually engineered, the front-line relationships that connected the needs of customers with the organization's core competency. Quinn called this front-line activity that embedded the service delivery process the "smallest replicable unit" or the "minimum replicable unit." This smallest replicable unit, or the microsystem, is the key to implementing effective strategy, information technology, and other key aspects of intelligent enterprise.

In the late 1990s, Mohr and Donaldson investigated high-performing clinical microsystems (Mohr 2000; Donaldson and Mohr 2000). This research was based on a national search for the highest-quality clinical microsystems. Forty-three clinical units were identified using a theoretical sampling methodology. Semi-structured interviews were conducted with leaders from each of the microsystems. Analysis of these interviews suggested that eight dimensions, shown in Table 15–1, are associated with effective microsystems. The "microsystem assessment tool" included in Figure 15–1 was first published in 2002 and is based on these 8 dimensions (Mohr and Batalden 2002). Additional research built on the Mohr and Donaldson study conducted 20 case studies of high performing microsystems and included on-site interviews with every member of the microsystem and analysis of individual microsystem performance data (Nelson *et al.* 2002, 2003; Godfrey *et al.* 2003; Wasson *et al.* 2003; Batalden *et al.* 2003a, 2003b; Mohr *et al.* 2003a; Kosnik and Espinosa 2003; Huber *et al.* 2003).

---

**Table 15–1** Eight Dimensions of Microsystems

1. Constancy of purpose
2. Investment in improvement
3. Alignment of role and training for efficiency and staff satisfaction
4. Interdependence of the care team to meet patient needs
5. Integration of information and technology into work flows
6. Ongoing measurement of outcomes
7. Supportiveness of the larger organization
8. Connection to the community to enhance care delivery and extend influence.

## CLINICAL MICROSYSTEM ASSESSMENT TOOL

**Instructions:** Each of the "success" characteristics (e.g. leadership) is followed by a series of three descriptions. For each characteristic, *please check* the description that *best describes* your current microsystem and the care it delivers *OR* use a microsystem you are *MOST* familiar with.

| Characteristic and Definition | Descriptions | | | |
|---|---|---|---|---|
| **Leadership** — **1. Leadership:** The role of leaders is to balance selling and reaching objective goals, and to empower individual autonomy and accountability, through building knowledge, respectful action, reviewing and reflecting. | ☐ Leaders often tell me how to do my job and leave little room for innovation and autonomy. Overall they don't foster a positive culture. | ☐ Leaders struggle to find the right balance between reaching performance goals and supporting and empowering the staff. | ☐ Leaders maintain constancy of purpose, establish clear goals and expectations, and foster a respectful positive culture. Leaders take time to build knowledge, review and reflect, and take action about microsystems and the larger operation. | ☐ Can't Rate |
| **2. Organizational Support:** The larger organization looks for ways to support the work of the microsystem and coordinate the hand-offs between microsystems. | ☐ The larger organization isn't supportive in a way that provides recognition, information, and resources to enhance my work. | ☐ The larger organization is inconsistent and unpredictable in providing the recognition, information and resources needed to enhance my work. | ☐ The larger organization provides recognition, information, and resources that enhance my work and makes it easier for me to meet the needs of patients. | ☐ Can't Rate |
| **Staff** — **3. Staff Focus:** There is selective hiring of the right kind of people. The orientation process is designed to fully integrate new staff into culture and work roles. Expectations of staff are high regarding performance, continuing education, professional growth, and networking. | ☐ I am not made to feel like a valued member of the microsystem. My orientation was incomplete. My continuing education and professional growth needs are not being met. | ☐ I feel like I am a valued member of the microsystem, but I don't think the microsystem is doing all that it could to support education and training of staff, workload, and professional growth. | ☐ I am a valued member of the microsystem and what I say matters. This is evident through staffing, education and training, workload, and professional growth. | ☐ Can't Rate |
| **4. Education and Training:** All clinical microsystems have responsibility for the ongoing education and training of staff and for aligning daily work roles with training competencies. Academic clinical microsystems have the additional responsibility of training students. | ☐ Training is accomplished in disciplinary silos, e.g. nurses train nurses, physicians train residents, etc. The educational efforts are not aligned with the flow of patient care, so that education becomes an "add-on" to what we do. | ☐ We recognize that our training could be different to reflect the needs of our microsystem, but we haven't made many changes yet. Some continuing education is available to everyone. | ☐ There is a team approach to training, whether we are training staff, nurses or students. Education and patient care are integrated into the flow of work in a way that benefits both from the available resources. Continuing education for all staff is recognized as vital to our continued success. | ☐ Can't Rate |
| **5. Interdependence:** The interaction of staff is characterized by trust, collaboration, willingness to help each other, appreciation of complementary roles, respect and recognition that all contribute individually to a shared purpose. | ☐ I work independently and I am responsible for my own part of the work. There is a lack of collaboration and a lack of appreciation for the importance of complementary roles. | ☐ The care approach is interdisciplinary, but we are not always able to work together as an effective team. | ☐ Care is provided by a interdisciplinary team characterized by trust, collaboration, appreciation of complementary roles, and a recognition that all contribute individually to a shared purpose. | ☐ Can't Rate |
| **Patients** — **6. Patient Focus:** The primary concern is to meet all patient needs—caring, listening, educating, and responding to special requests, innovating to meet patient needs, and smooth service flow. | ☐ Most of us, including our patients, would agree that we do not always provide patient centered care. We are not always clear about what patients want and need. | ☐ We are actively working to provide patient centered care and we are making progress toward more effectively and consistently learning about and meeting patient needs. | ☐ We are effective in learning about and meeting patient needs—caring, listening, educating, and responding to special requests, and smooth service flow. | ☐ Can't Rate |

© Julie J. Mohr, MSPH, PhD. November 2001, Revised 2/21/03

Side A

*Please continue on Side B*

*continues*

**Figure 15–1** Microsystem Assessment Tool.

## CLINICAL MICROSYSTEM ASSESSMENT TOOL
### - continued -

| | Characteristic and Definition | Descriptions | | | |
|---|---|---|---|---|---|
| **Patients** | **7. Community and Market Focus:** The microsystem is a resource of the community; the community is a resource to the microsystem; the microsystem establishes excellent and innovative relationships with the community. | ☐ We focus on the patients who come to our unit. We haven't implemented any outreach programs in our community. Patients and their families often make their own connections to the community resources they need. | ☐ We have tried a few outreach programs and have had some success, but it is not the norm for us to go out into the community or actively connect patients to the community resources that are available to them. | ☐ We are doing everything we can to understand our community. We actively employ resources to help us work with the community. We add to the community and we draw on resources from the community to meet patient needs. | ☐ Can't Rate |
| **Performance** | **8. Performance Results:** Performance focuses on patient outcomes, avoidable costs, streamlining delivery, using data feedback, promoting positive competition, and frank discussions about performance. | ☐ We don't routinely collect data on the process or outcomes of the care we provide. | ☐ We often collect data on the outcomes of the care we provide and on some processes of care. | ☐ Outcomes (clinical, satisfaction, financial, technical, safety) are routinely measured, we feed data back to staff, and we make changes based on data. | ☐ Can't Rate |
| | **9. Process Improvement:** An atmosphere for learning and redesign is supported by the continuous monitoring for care, use of benchmarking, frequent tests of change, and a staff that has been empowered to innovate. | ☐ The resources required (in the form of training, financial support, and time) are rarely available to support improvement work. Any improvement activities we do are in addition to our daily work. | ☐ Some resources are available to support improvement work, but we don't use them as often as we could. Change ideas are implemented without much discipline. | ☐ There are ample resources to support continual improvement work. Studying, measuring and improving care in a scientific way are essential parts of our daily work. | ☐ Can't Rate |
| **Information and Information Technology** | **10. Information and Information Technology:** Information is THE connector – staff to patients, staff to staff, needs with actions to meet needs. Technology facilitates effective communication and multiple formal and informal channels are used to keep everyone informed all the time, listen to everyone's ideas, and ensure that everyone is connected on important topics. *Given the complexity of information and the use of technology in the microsystem, assess your microsystem on the following three characteristics: (1) integration of information with patients, (2) integration of information with providers and staff, and (3) integration of information with technology.* | | | | |
| | **A. Integration of Information with Patients** | ☐ Patients have access to some standard information that is available to all patients. | ☐ Patients have access to standard information that is available to all patients. We've started to think about how to improve the information they are given to better meet their needs | ☐ Patients have a variety of ways to get the information they need and it can be customized to meet their individual learning styles. We routinely ask patients for feedback about how to improve the information we give them. | ☐ Can't Rate |
| | **B. Integration of Information with Providers and Staff** | ☐ I am always tracking down the information I need to do my work. | ☐ Most of the time I have the information I need, but sometimes essential information is missing and I have to track it down. | ☐ The information I need to do my work is available when I need it. | ☐ Can't Rate |
| | **C. Integration of Information with Technology** | ☐ The technology I need to facilitate and enhance my work is either not available to me or it is available but not effective. The technology we currently have does not make my job easier. | ☐ I have access to technology that will enhance my work, but it is not easy to use and seems to be cumbersome and time consuming. | ☐ Technology facilitates a smooth linkage between information and patient care by providing timely, effective access to a rich information environment. The information environment has been designed to support the work of the clinical unit. | ☐ Can't Rate |

Side B

**Figure 15–1**  Microsystem Assessment Tool  continued

As we continue to move beyond conceptual theory and research to application in clinical settings, the emerging fields of chaos theory, complexity science, and complex adaptive systems have influenced how these concepts have been applied to improving microsystems (Arrow *et al.* 2000; Peters 1987; Plsek and Greenhalgh 2001; Plsek and Wilson 2001). This is evident in the work seeking to bring together microsystems from around the world to learn and share best practices. (Updates on these efforts are available at http://clinicalmicrosystem.org.) Please refer to Chapter 11 of this book for more about microsystems research as one of several generic approaches to clinical process improvement.

## IMPROVING QUALITY AND SAFETY WITHIN THE ACADEMIC CLINICAL MICROSYSTEM

The clinical microsystem—as a unit of research, analysis, and practice—is an important level at which to focus patient safety interventions. Most patients and caregivers meet at this system level and it is here that real changes in accepted patient care can (and must) be made. Academic clinical microsystems—microsystems that exist within academic health centers—face the challenge of a dual mission to provide excellent patient care and excellent professional development/learning. While academic clinical microsystems clearly have these dual missions, in fact, all clinical microsystems are about both patient care and professional formation.

Errors and failure occur within the microsystem and ultimately it is the functioning microsystem that can stop, prevent or mitigate errors and failure from causing patient harm. Safety is a property of the clinical microsystem that can be achieved only through a systematic application of a broad array of process, equipment, organization, supervision, training, simulation, and teamwork changes. The case included in Table 15–2 illustrates a patient safety event in an academic clinical microsystem and how the resulting analysis can allow a microsystem to learn from the event. Throughout the story, as told from the perspective of a senior resident in pediatrics, there are many system failures. Many methods are available to explore the causal system at work (Vincent 2003; Vincent *et al.* 1998; Dekker 2002; Reason 1995) and they all suggest the importance of holding the entire causal system in our analytic frame, not just seeking a "root" cause. One method that we have

**Table 15–2** Interview with a 3rd Year Pediatrics Resident

**Resident:** I had a patient who was very ill. We thought that an abdominal CT would be helpful and it needed to be infused. He was 12 years old and was completely healthy up until three months ago and since then has been in our hospital and 2 other hospitals, pretty much the entire time. He has been in respiratory failure, he's had mechanical ventilation—including oscillation, he's been in renal failure, he's had a number of mini strokes, and when I came on service he was having diarrhea—3 to 5 liters/day—and we still didn't know what was going on with him.

He was a very anxious child. Understandably. it's hard for the nurses, and for me, and for his mother to deal with. He thought of it as pain, but it was anxiety and it responded well to anxiolytics.

When I came in that morning, it hadn't been passed along to nursing that he was supposed to go to CT that morning. I heard the charge nurse getting report from the night nurse. I said, "You know that he is supposed to go for a CT today." She was already upset because they were very short staffed. She heard me and then said that she was not only the charge nurse, but also taking care of two patients, and one had to go to CT. She went off to the main unit to talk to someone. Then she paged me and said, "If you want this child to have a scan you have to go with him." I said, "OK." Nurses are the ones who usually go. But it didn't seem to be beyond my abilities . . . at the time.

So, I took the child for his CT and his Mom came with us. We gave him extra Ativan on the way there, because whenever he had a procedure he was extra anxious. When we got there, they weren't ready. We had lost our spot from the morning. My patient got more and more anxious and he was actually yelling at the techs "Hurry up!" We went in the room. He was about 5 or 6 hours late for his study and we had given him contrast enterally. The techs were concerned that he didn't have enough anymore and they wanted to give him more through his G-tube. I said, "That sounds fine." And they mixed it up and gave it to me to give through his G-tube and I went to his side and unhooked—not registering that it was his central line—I unhooked his central line, not only taking off the cap but unhooking something and I pushed 70 cc's of the gastrografin in. As soon as I had finished the second syringe I realized I was using the wrong tube. I said, "Oh no!" Mom was right there and said, "What?" I said, "I put the stuff in the wrong tube. He looks OK. I'll be right back, I have to call somebody."
I clamped him off and I called my attending and I called the radiologist. My attending said that he was on his way down. The radiologist was over by the time I had hung up the phone. My patient was stable the whole time. We figured out what was in the gastrografin that could potentially cause harm. We decided to cancel the study. . . . I sent the gastrografin—the extra stuff in the tubes—for a culture just in case he grew some kind of infection and then we would be able to treat it and match it with what I had pushed into the line. I filled out an incident report. I called my chiefs and told them.... They said, "It's OK. He's fine, right?" I said, "Yes." They came up later in the evening just to be supportive. They said, "It's OK. It's OK to make a mistake."

*continues*

**Table 15–2** continued

**Interviewer:** What was your attending's response?

**Resident:** The attending that I had called when I made the mistake said, "I'm sorry that you were in that situation. You shouldn't have been put in that situation." Another attending the next day was telling people, "Well, you know what happened yesterday," as if it were the only thing going on for this patient. I thought it was embarrassing that he was just passing on this little tidbit of information as if it would explain everything that was going on. As opposed to saying, "Yes, an error was made, it is something that we are taking Into account." And he told me to pay more attention to the patient. Yes, I made the mistake, but hands-down I still and always did know that patient better than he did. I just thought that was mean and not fair. And the only other thing I thought (that) was not good was the next morning when I was prerounding some of the nurses were whispering and I just assumed that was what they were whispering about. I walked up to them and said, "I'm the one who did it. I made a mistake. How is he doing?" I tried to answer any questions they had and move on.

**Interviewer:** How did the nurses respond when you said that you made a mistake?

**Resident:** The nurse that had sent me down with him told me "It's OK, don't worry about it." The others just listened politely and didn't say anything.

**Interviewer:** How did the mother respond to you the next day?

**Resident:** The next day, I felt really bad. I felt very incompetent. I was feeling very awkward being the leader of this child's care—because I am still at a loss for his diagnosis. And after the event, when the Grandma found out—she was very angry. I apologized to the Mom and I thought it would be overdoing it to keep saying, "I am so sorry." So, the next day I went into the room and said to the Mom, "You need to have confidence in the person taking care of your son. If my mistake undermines that at all, you don't have to have me as your son's doctor and I can arrange it so that you can have whoever you want." She said, "No. No, it's fine. We want you as his doctor." Then we just moved on with the care plan. That felt good. And that felt appropriate. I couldn't just walk into the room and act like nothing had happened. I needed her to give me the power to be their doctor. So, I just went and asked for it.

---

found to be useful for systematically looking at patient safety events builds on William Haddon's overarching framework (1972) on injury epidemiology.

As the first Director of the National Highway Safety Bureau (1966 to 1969), Haddon was interested in the broad issues of injury that result from the transfer of energy in such ways that inanimate or animate objects are damaged. The clinical microsystem offers a setting in which this injury can be studied. According to Haddon, there are a number of strategies for reducing losses:

- Prevent the marshaling of the energy
- Reduce the amount of energy marshaled
- Prevent the release of the energy
- Modify the rate or spatial distribution of release of the energy
- Separate in time and space the energy being released and the susceptible structure
- Use a physical barrier to separate the energy and the susceptible structure
- Modify the contact surface or structure with which people can come in contact
- Strengthen the structure that might be damaged by the energy transfer
- When injury does occur, rapidly detect it and counter its continuation and extension
- When injury does occur, take all necessary reparative and rehabilitative steps.

All these strategies have a logical sequence that is related to preinjury, injury, and post injury.

The Haddon Matrix is a 3 × 3 matrix with factors related to an auto injury (human, vehicle, and environment) heading the columns and phases of the event (preinjury, injury, and postinjury) heading the rows. Figure 15–2 shows how the Haddon Matrix can be used to analyze an auto accident (Haddon 1972). The use of the matrix focuses the analysis on the interrelationship between the factors (in this matrix version the human, vehicle, and environment) and the three phases (pre-event, event, and postevent). A mix of countermeasures derived from Haddon's strategies outlined above, are necessary to minimize loss. Furthermore, the countermeasures can be designed for each phase—pre-event, event, and postevent. This approach confirms what we know about adverse events in complex environments—it takes a variety of strategies to prevent and/or mitigate harm. Understanding injury in its larger context helps us recognize the basic nature of "unsafe" systems and the important work of humans to mitigate the inherent hazards (Dekker 2002).

**Factors**

| Phases | Human | Vehicle | Environment |
|---|---|---|---|
| Preinjury | Alcohol intoxication | Braking capacity of motor vehicles | Visibility of hazards |
| Injury | Resistance to energy insults | Sharp or pointed edges and surfaces | Flammable building materials |
| Postinjury | Hemorrhage | Rapidity of energy reduction | Emergency medical response |

**Figure 15–2** Haddon Matrix Used to Analyze Auto Accident.
Reprinted with permission from *Healthy Communities: New Partnerships for the Future of Public Health* © 1996 by the National Academy of Sciences, courtesy of the National Academies Press, Washington, D.C.

We can also use the Haddon matrix to guide analysis of patient safety scenarios. To translate this tool from injury epidemiology to patient safety, we have revised the matrix to include phases labeled "pre-event, event, and postevent" instead of "preinjury, injury, and postinjury." The revised factors, "patient–family, health care professional, system, and environment," replace "human, vehicle, and environment." Note that we have added "system" to refer to the processes and systems that are in place for the microsystem. "Environment" refers to the context that the microsystem exists within. The addition of system recognizes the significant contribution that systems make toward harm and error in the microsystem. Figure 15–3 shows a completed matrix using the pediatric case. The next step in learning from errors and adverse events is to develop and execute countermeasures to address the issues in each cell of the matrix.

Table 15–3 builds on the research of high-performing microsystems and provides specific actions that can be further explored. This list provides an organizing framework and a place to start applying patient safety concepts to microsystems. It also provides linkages to the macrosystem's ongoing organization-centered and issued-centered quality efforts, which can either support or conflict with this approach.

### Microsystems and Macrosystems

Health care organizations are composed of multiple, differentiated, variably autonomous microsystems. These interdependent small systems exhibit loose and tight coupling (Weick and Sutcliffe 2001). Several assumptions are made about the relationship between these microsystems and the macrosystem:

1. Bigger systems (macrosystems) are made of smaller systems;
2. These smaller systems (microsystems) produce quality, safety, and cost outcomes at the front line of care; and
3. Ultimately, the outcomes from macrosystems can be no better than the microsystems of which they are formed. (Nelson *et al.* 2002)

This suggests that it is necessary to intervene within each microsystem in the organization if the organization as a whole wants to improve. A microsystem cannot function independently from the other microsystems it regularly works with or its macrosystem. From the macrosystem perspec-

| | | Factors | | | |
|---|---|---|---|---|---|
| | | Patient/Family | Health Care Professional | System | Environment |
| **Phases** | Pre-event | Consent (process, timing) Anxiety (play therapy) Patient lines Mother's presence | Not familiar with procedure Lack of MD-RN communication Focus on anxiety and not on procedure Assumed roles, made assumptions Arrogance/respect | Several lines in patient Silos | RN shortage Scheduling delays Manufacturing (performance shaping factors, human factors) Lack of process for risk analysis |
| | Event | Anxiety (pt & parent's) No shared expectations No active participation | Fatigue Aware of limitations Training | Work hours Protocols Standardization Double checking | Work hours for residents Rushed No other clinician |
| | Postevent | Lack of explanation Disclosure Who should talk to family? | Guilt Lack of confidence Loss of face | Lack of understanding of errors/systems Lack of supportive environment for resident Incidence report M&M Analysis of event | Regulatory |

**Figure 15–3** Completed Patient Safety Matrix.

tive, senior leaders can enable an overall patient safety focus with clear, visible values, expectations, and recognition of "deeds well done." They can set direction by clearly expecting that each microsystem will achieve alignment of its mission, vision, and strategies with the organization's mission, vision, and strategies. Senior leadership can offer each microsystem the flexibility needed to achieve its mission and ensure the creation of strategies, systems, and methods for achieving excellence in healthcare, stimulating innovation, and building knowledge and capabilities. Finally,

**Table 15–3** Linkage of Microsystem Characteristics to Patient Safety

| Microsystem Characteristics | What This Means for Patient Safety |
| --- | --- |
| 1. Leadership | • Define the safety vision of the organization<br>• Identify the existing constraints within the organization<br>• Allocate resources for plan development, implementation, and ongoing monitoring and evaluation<br>• Build in microsystems participation and input to plan development<br>• Align organizational quality and safety goals<br>• Engage the Board of Trustees in ongoing conversations about the organizational progress toward achieving safety goals<br>• Recognition for prompt truth-telling about errors or hazards<br>• Certification of helpful changes to improve safety |
| 2. Organizational support | • Work with clinical microsystems to identify patient safety issues and make relevant local changes<br>• Put the necessary resources and tools into the hands of individuals |
| 3. Staff Focus | • Assess current safety culture<br>• Identify the gap between current culture and safety vision<br>• Plan cultural interventions<br>• Conduct periodic assessments of culture<br>• Celebrate examples of desired behavior, e.g., acknowledgement of an error |
| 4. Education and Training | • Develop patient safety curriculum<br>• Provide training and education of key clinical and management leadership<br>• Develop a core of people with patient safety skills who can work across microsystems as a resource |
| 5. Interdependence of the Care Team | • Build PDSA* into debriefings<br>• Use daily huddles to debrief and to celebrate identifying errors |
| 6. Patient Focus | • Establish patient and family partnerships<br>• Support disclosure and truth around medical error |

*continues*

**Table 15–3** continued

| | |
|---|---|
| 7. Community and Market Focus | • Analyze safety issues in community and partner with external groups to reduce risk to population |
| 8. Performance Results | • Develop key safety measures<br>• Create feedback mechanisms to share results with microsystems |
| 9. Process Improvement | • Identify patient safety priorities based on assessment of key safety measures<br>• Address the work that will be required at the microsystem level |
| 10. Information and Information Technology | • Enhance error reporting systems<br>• Build safety concepts into information flow (eg, checklists, reminder systems.) |

*PDSA, Plan-Do-Study-Act.

**Table 15–4** Questions Senior Leaders Could Ask About Patient Safety

❑ What information do we have about errors and patient harm?
❑ What is the patient safety plan?
❑ How will the plan be implemented at the organizational level and at the microsystem level?
❑ What type of infrastructure is needed to support implementation?
❑ What is the best way to communicate the plan to the individual microsystems?
❑ How can we foster reporting—telling the truth—about errors?
❑ How will we empower microsystem staff to make suggestions for improving safety?
❑ What training will staff need?
❑ Who are the key stakeholders?
❑ How can we build linkages to the key stakeholders?
❑ What stories can we tell that relate the importance of patient safety?
❑ How will we recognize and celebrate progress?

senior leaders can pay careful attention to the questions they ask as they nurture meaningful work and hold the microsystems accountable to achieve its strategic mission to provide safer care. Table 15–4 provides a set of accountability questions that senior leaders might ask as they work to improve safety and quality of the organization.

### Promoting System Resilience Across and Between the Microsystems

Microsystems usually coexist with multiple other microsystems within the organization. Patients are aware of the gaps and handoffs between microsystems as they navigate the healthcare system, e.g., as they transfer from inpatient care back into the community. Patients are aware of the challenges of "synthesizing" knowledge across the various microsystems they encounter. Models developed by Zimmerman and Hayday (1999) for understanding and encouraging work on the relationships across microsystems offer insight into the generative work of interdependence. Understanding the dynamics of effective organizational relationships can be helpful in thinking about how to foster relationships between microsystems within the same organization and across differing organizations. These cross-microsystem relationships are fundamentally related to improving handoffs but this inquiry can also provide opportunities for learning about systemic problems within the institution and interventions to improve quality and safety.

An effective collaborative relationship is based on the underlying assumption that collaboration is a more effective approach to achieve a goal than multiple individual efforts. Weick (1993, 1995) suggests that leaders today need to develop groups that are also respectful of the interactions that hold the group together. Resilient groups have respectful interactions that are founded on three major elements: (1) trust—a willingness to base beliefs and actions on the reports of others; (2) honesty—reporting so that others may use one's observations in developing and enhancing their own beliefs; and (3) self-respect—integrating one's perceptions and beliefs with the reports of others without depreciating them or oneself (Weick 1996).

Four aspects of the relationship can help generate creative responses to the diagnosed challenges facing entities needing to work better together (Zimmerman and Hayday 1999). These elements are: (1) the separateness or differences of the two microsystems; (2) the talking–listening–tuning opportunities that the two microsystems have; (3) the action opportunities that the two entities have; and (4) the reasons they have to work together. Balanced attention to each aspect enables creative work.

Conditions also must be present for relationships across organizations to develop (Kaluzny 1985). For voluntary interactions—which may be quite different than those mandated by an external power—several conditions must be met. There must be an internal need for resources, a commitment to an external problem, and the opportunity to change. In addition, there must be a consensus on the external problem(s) facing the organizations as well as a consensus on the specific goals and services for developing a joint effort. The 1999 Institute of Medicine report, *To Err is Human* (Institute of Medicine 2000), brought patient safety to the forefront of the agenda as well as set the stage for discussing specific goals and strategies for achieving those goals.

Mitchell and Shortell (2000) provide a synthesis of the literature on the success of community health partnerships that suggests several factors that influence the success of interorganizational relationships. (See Table 15–5.) Context refers to the environment in which the partnership exists—the internal and external stakeholders, their historical relationships and influence, the presence or absence of human and financial resources, the political environment, public sentiments, and the current challenges facing the community. Strategic intent—a similar concept to a consensus on the external problem(s) facing the organizations—refers to the reasons the interorganizational relationship is formed. A diversified resource base helps assure that the collaborative is able to pursue the strategic intent without getting sidetracked by pursuing the goals of a single funding agency. Membership heterogeneity refers to the balance of the participating members in regard to the number and types of participants. Informal as well as formal communication mechanisms assure that the collaborators meet their own goals and are held accountable to demonstrate their progress internally and externally.

---

**Table 15–5** The Successful Interorganizational Relationship

1. Context
2. Strategic Intent
3. Resource Base
4. Membership Heterogeneity
5. Coordination Skills
6. Response to Accountability

## Partnership Synergy

The Center for the Advancement of Collaborative Strategies in Health (CACSH) at The New York Academy of Medicine focused on strengthening the ability of partnerships to assess and achieve the unique advantage of collaboration—what they term "partnership synergy." CACSH conducted a study, as described in Exhibit 15.6, to create and operationalize a framework for assessing partnership synergy and for identifying its likely determinants (Lasker *et al.* 2001).

According to CACHS, *effective leadership* facilitates productive interactions among partners by bridging diverse cultures; performing boundary-spanning functions; and revealing, as well as challenging, assumptions that limit thinking and action.

*Partnership efficiency* refers to making good use of partners' time, in-kind resources, and financial resources. The effectiveness of a *partnership's administration and management* also has an impact on partnership synergy, although this effect is not statistically significant. Administration and management activities, such as coordination of communication among partners and partnership activities, and the preparation of materials that inform partners, are the "glue" that makes it possible for multiple, independent people and organizations to work together. Analysis results indicate that the sufficiency of nonfinancial resources influences, although nonsignificantly, partnership synergy. Nonfinancial resources such as skills and expertise, information, and connectivity to target populations play a unique role; synergy is largely built from these resources, and it is only by combining them in novel ways that partners can potentially create something that enables them to accomplish more than they could on their own.

---

**Table 15–6** Six Dimensions of Partnership Synergy

1. Effectiveness of leadership
2. Effectiveness of administration and management
3. Sufficiency of intangible resources
4. Partnership efficiency
5. Challenges related to partner involvement
6. Challenges related to the community

## CONCLUSION

Clinical microsystem concepts have evolved from systems theory and primary research on characteristics of high performing clinical units. Deconstructing error and failures at the level of the front lines of health care can benefit from the use of one of the several multidimensional models. After diagnosis has suggested better work across discrete elements within or across microsystems, a variety of approaches for enhancing cooperative work are available. Such understanding and corrective efforts can be made to embed quality and safety into the microsystem. Leaders can set the stage for making safety a priority for the organization in both quality of care and professional development, and they can both attract and encourage individual microsystems to create innovative strategies for improvement.

# CHAPTER 16

# Quality: From Professional Responsibility to Public Policy and Back Again[1]

*Curtis P. McLaughlin and Arnold D. Kaluzny*

Public perceptions of who is responsible for quality are shifting from individual professionals and institutions to those responsible for developing and implementing public policy. All three have valid roles in quality improvement, but there seems to be increasing emphasis on quality as a public policy issue. Politicians of all political affiliations at all levels of government have responded with their solutions and recommendations, particularly in the area of information technology and its impact on health care quality.

## POLITICAL INITIATIVES

The primitiveness of health care's information technology infrastructure is well documented and includes low investment levels, inability of systems to interact, failure to share information among providers, failure to use existing data on processes and outcomes to develop better practices, waste and duplication, and the tragic errors introduced by the use of handwritten paper systems. To address these concerns, attention has been focused on technology. People are especially interested in two major applications—computerized physician order entry (CPOE) and the

---

[1] Portions of this chapter have been adapted from C.P. McLaughlin, A.D. Kaluzny, D.C. Kibbe and R. Tredway, Changing Roles for Primary-Care Physicians: Addressing Challenges and Opportunities. *Healthcare Quarterly,* 8(2): 70–78. Copyright Longwoods Publishing Corporation 2005.

electronic health record (EHR). The CPOE is a primary concern of the Leapfrog Group (see Chapter 10) and has been implemented in a number of large hospitals with mixed results (Berger and Kichak 2004, Kuperman and Gibson 2003). EHR has been set as a goal of the federal government by the year 2014, offering support for demonstration systems and hinting that it is willing to pay for and demand such services for federal employees. While the approach has inherent challenges, it also provides some exciting opportunities. The purpose of this chapter is to (1) examine some of the challenges faced as quality improvement enters the realm of public policy through its emphasis on technology, and (2) explore the opportunities that technology offers primary care physicians within the changing marketplace of health care.

The technological approach is effective in theory, but difficult to implement in practice. It suffers most of the barriers that other quality improvement efforts face, namely:

- Technological change may or may not be linked to the business case for quality improvement. Various hospitals have instituted CPOE and encountered implementation problems because physicians felt that the required data entry reduced their productivity without compensation (Kolata 2004a). Moreover, clinical decision-making and information is decentralized within a community. Most information systems in health care are stand-alone, supporting a single application area such as radiology, pharmacy, or clinical laboratories. The challenge is to provide access to an integrated data base relevant to a given patient for decision making within any clinical setting anywhere (Lohr 2004a). There are major "gauge breaks" between them that require special interface equipment and programs. While some equipment vendors favor a seamless system, others strongly favor dedicated systems, at least in the short run.
- Rewards and impacts fall differently on different players. Physician opposition to CPOE is an example. The systems must fit into how the office works. One complaint reported in a number of places is the difficulty in handling typographical errors and corrections efficiently. Furthermore, these costs to the physician are not offset by savings to the physician. The savings accrue to the hospital, the insurer, and the patient instead. These failures of the market must be addressed in the health care environment of administered pricing.

Figure 16–1 shows one estimate of the allocated savings once community-wide health information networks are in place. Note that the biggest savings occur to "Providers," which involves a whole group of different, often unrelated, entities such as physician practices, hospitals, and nursing homes. Walker *et al.* (2005) estimate the ultimate net value of a fully standardized health information exchange and interoperability at $77.8 billion per year. Baker's response (2005) in the same issue of *Health Affairs* suggests that their estimate is overly optimistic but notes, as do James (2005) and Brailer (2005), that such a system is a requirement of major improvements in the quality of health care delivery.

- Economics of scale and scope differ from setting to setting. Large institutions, especially those that also at risk through their insurance arms, can afford to invest heavily in the technology, but that is hardly relevant in terms of most rural hospitals or primary care practices. Some institutions like the American Academic of Family Physicians' Center for Information Technology are trying to address the scale problems of small practices, but it may be difficult in the time frame that politics will allow.

- Risk shifting leans most heavily on those least able to bear it. Leatherman *et al.* (2003) suggest that capitation is one way to take care of the fact that fee-for-service care does not compensate for quality. Capitation does push the risk to the physician practice level, but it has often failed because of lack of a sufficient pooling of risks necessary to offset the effects of a few catastrophic cases.

- Proposals often ignore basic physician–patient relationships. An electronic health record (EHR) that is accessible throughout the health care community is being pushed by many public policymakers. President Bush's *Health Information Technology (HIT) Plan* calls for most Americans to have EHRs within the next ten years (see Case 8). This is backed by a plan to:

  - double funding to $100 million for HIT demonstration projects; and
  - create a new sub-cabinet position, National Health Information Technology Coordinator, to guide the development of information standards, take steps to support and encourage health care technology in public and private delivery systems, and coordinate partnerships between public and private sector stakeholders to speed adoption of HIT.

### Net Benefits Distribution*

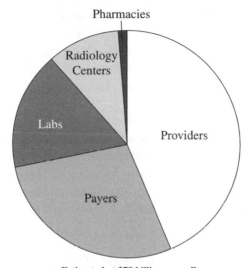

**Estimated at $78 billion annually**
*Public Health Department value not shown

### Allocation of Rollout Costs

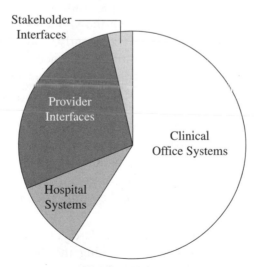

**Estimated at $276 billion over 10 years**

**Figure 16–1** Impacts of Health Care Information Exchange and Interoperability. Pan E, Johnston D, Walker JD, Adler-Milstein J, Bates DW, Middleton B. *The Value of Healthcare Information Exchange and Interoperability.* Boston, MA: Center for Information Technology Leadership, 2004. Adapted with permission.

Also implicit in the HIT plan is the assumption that the record would be in the possession of the patient or be accessible to any legitimate provider over the Internet. That would severely affect any one physician's information monopoly. Overall, that monopoly may be illusory anyway. Medicare beneficiaries see on average 6.4 unique providers per year, resulting in exposure to medical errors. About 18% of medical errors are attributable to inadequate information availability (Marchibroda 2004).

Supporters of EHR and other technological approaches for health care quality improvement and cost reduction measures seem prone to ignore the mediating and continuity-maintaining roles of the primary care physician as well as the professional quest to maintain autonomy. This occurs across the political spectrum from the White House to Senator Hilary Clinton to Newt Gingrich and Patrick Kennedy. Senator Clinton wrote in *New York Times Magazine*

> Now it is possible to imagine all of a person's health files stored securely on a computer file—test results, lab records, X-rays—accessible from any doctor's office. It is easy to imagine, yet our medical system is not here. . . .
>
> Why rely solely on the doctor's brain to store that information? Computers could crunch the variables on a particular patient's medical history, constantly update the algorithms with the latest scientific evidence and put that information at the clinician's fingertips at the point of care. (Clinton 2004, p. 30)

- Capital requirements fall heaviest on those least able to pay. The bulk of the physician practices in the United States have only a few practitioners. They provide net incomes which have been shrinking as payers have reduced rates and controlled utilization. Providing information technology in each of these may require investments that these practitioners can ill afford.
- Methods of coordination and standardization are not consistent with market philosophy. Overcoming the "gauge breaks" along the information tracks between providers and subsystems of care requires prompt setting of technical standards and development of integrated systems that are mandated throughout the provider community

- The challenge is to provide an integrated information system to meet the requirements of the decision making process of clinicians throughout the provider community. However, doing so might well close out those who are already successful vendors of stand-alone systems and developers of proprietary systems that are already on the market, but not interoperable. There will be profound resistance to mandating specific systems, standards, or investments from independent provider groups or individuals. This has already been demonstrated by the ability of medical staff to reject various technological modifications when they are perceived as having a negative impact on their personal interests. (Kolata 2004a)

## RESPONDING IN A MARKET ECONOMY

Technology *per se* will not guarantee quality nor assure the use of evidence-based best practices. This will require implementation of additional interventions that are less culturally and politically acceptable. Porter and Teisberg (2004) have suggested a number of these interventions:

- Nondiscriminatory Insurance Underwriting: something like the high-risk pools used for automobile insurance in some states and consolidated pools for small businesses and individuals. These would be effective, if coupled with:
- A National List of Minimum Coverage: making a standard set of minimum necessary benefits available to all insureds such as that used by the Federal Employees Health Benefits Program.
- Measures to make the Market more perfect:
  - Transparent pricing and simplified billing
  - Accessible information on provider outcomes
  - No restrictions on choice
  - Market differentiation of providers based on performance and service.
- Reduced malpractice lawsuits with comparable reductions in insurance costs and defensive medicine cases.

Others have suggested (1) greater use of evidence-based best practices; (2) major changes in payment mechanisms to make providers more responsive to outcomes and to longer-run patient interests including quality; and (3) reintermediation of a responsible primary care provider individual or organization into the delivery of care. All of these are means of converting the externalities of the social and economic arguments for quality into internalities for providers and patients.

## HEALTH CARE DISINTERMEDIATION: AN EXPANDING FORCE

In recent years, the market economy has been driving wedges between the patient and an overall responsive provider. Physicians and others are experiencing the effects of direct public access to information by lucrative segments of their patient (client) population (Murray *et al.* 2003; Baker *et al.* 2003). Patients come in with a set of printouts or notes from direct-to-consumer drug advertising and may be perceived as demanding a prescription for that product. A less visible example is the patient who checks a Web site and decides that a doctor visit is not warranted. Increasingly patients are receiving advice directly from their insurers through personalized Web pages and from drug companies, pharmacy chains, advocacy groups, government agencies, and a host of other would-be providers. The quality impacts of this information are mixed. The educated patient may make better choices or may be stressed and confused by the information which may or may not be valid.

While disintermediation is most evident in the pharmaceutical arena, it is appearing throughout the health care delivery system (McLaughlin and Kaluzny 2002; McLaughlin *et al.* 2005). Legislation, especially states' medical practice acts, still limits the ability of others to take over the physician's control of many transactions like prescribing drugs or performing surgery, so the situation does not really parallel the fate of stock brokers and travel agents, but similar pressures exist. Table 16–1 illustrates various activities that alternative providers and organizations are using to sidestep the traditional information control and transaction control previously exercised by primary care physicians. However, with the loss of information control and transaction control, the relationship experiences a loss of a quality controller as well. A surprisingly large variety of actors have a stake in directly influencing the behavior of patients and they are not hesitating to use new technologies to exert their sometimes conflicting influences.

As presented in Table 16–1, information which was once the sole province of the physician is delivered to patients by pharmaceutical companies, scanning centers, insurers, case management firms, employers, pharmacists, hospitals and others. What is more surprising is that many of these actors are also gaining influence over the transaction phase, by mak-

**Table 16-1** Disintermediation Activities and Actors Affecting the Primary Care Physician

| Actor | Activities Affecting Information Control | Activities Affecting Transaction Control |
|---|---|---|
| Pharmaceutical companies | Direct-to-Consumer (DTC) advertising Websites | Moving patent-expired drugs over the counter (OTC) |
| Screening centers | Direct-to-consumer advertising Direct patient reporting | No referral required Direct patient pay |
| Nurse practitioners, physician assistants | Independent practice | Independent practice |
| Psychologists | Independent practice | Gaining prescribing Authority |
| Insurers | Deep portals for enrollees Case management | Forcing drugs OTC Case management |
| Case management firms | Taking over patient management Self-care advice service | Patient advocacy in community |
| Pharmacy benefits management firms | Formulary feedback to patients | Multitiered copays |
| Employers | Educational programs and Web portals | Screening programs |
| Academic medical centers | Newsletters–Web sites Telemedicine programs | Telemedicine programs |
| Government agencies | Web sites–Advertising Screening recommendations | Preferred drug lists Screening programs |
| Patient/disease advocacy groups | Web sites–Advertising Screening recommendations | Screening programs |
| Pharmacists | Counseling centers | Screening programs |
| Hospitals | Protocols shared with patients and their families Formularies | Formularies Screening programs |

McLaughlin, Kaluzny, Kibbe and Tredway 2005

ing drugs available over the counter, bypassing the referral process, gaining prescribing authority in circumscribed areas, running screening programs, and influencing patient behaviors through case management, co-payment systems, and formularies.

Even within clinical medicine itself, efforts are underway to influence the traditional care process, characterized by referrals and professional prerogatives. Perhaps this is best illustrated by the emergence of telemedicine when used by one provider to avoid another's geographic monopoly. As described by Stan Davis in his 1987 book, *Future Perfect:*

> . . . telemedicine represents a threat, rather than a blessing, to many physicians. Like other forms of electronic transactions, including banking and shopping, telemedicine will eliminate middlemen and introduce competition where none has existed before. Whether we focus on its advantages or disadvantages, telemedicine eliminates the barriers of time and space, and medicine will never be the same. (1987, p. 8)

### Transaction: Forcing OTC Status

An attempt to bypass primary care physician's transaction control was visible on May 11, 2001, when a Food and Drug Administration (FDA) scientific advisory panel held a hearing on whether or not three nonsedating antihistamine drugs—Claratin, Allegra, and Zyrtec—would be moved from prescription-only status to over-the-counter (OTC) use. The impetus for this change did not come from the drug companies. All three manufacturers and the professional society representing allergists were against the move. These drugs were still protected by patents and generic versions were not yet available. The impetus came from Wellpoint, a health insurer, who cited multimillion-dollar savings to insurers and patients. The allergists' spokesperson emphasized the need for a "mediating" physician who could provide a differential diagnosis between allergies, sinusitis, and other medical problems. The advisory committee voted 18-5 to recommend OTC status for Claritin and 19-4 for the other two drugs (Michaels 2001). The FDA's hearing focused on the first condition, whether or not the consumer had adequate knowledge for effective decisions. If so, then OTC status would enable the second condition—independent means for completing the transaction.

While this hearing did not lead directly to an OTC ruling, it probably hastened the OTC availability of Claritin once its patent protection expired. Since the OTC drug became available, many drug benefit programs have moved all three drugs to Tier III status, using higher copayments to steer patients away from the prescription versions.

### Removing the Mediating Physician from the Transaction: Introducing Other Actors

Specialists sometimes choose to work around or ignore the primary care physician and deal direct with the consumer. While some HMOs have tried to interpose a primary care physician as a gatekeeper, new technologies have enabled the specialists to seek expanded roles. The typical urban newspaper contains numerous ads by plastic surgeons, alternative medicine clinics, and others. Whole body scanning centers will tout electron beam tomography of the heart to detect coronary artery disease, emphysema, vascular disease, prostate disease, ovarian disease, endocrine disease, and kidney and gall stones, calling such studies "Preventive Medicine for the 21st Century." These advertisements were aimed at the consumer, not referring colleagues. The information requested when making an appointment at one site asked for "name of referring physician—if necessary," while another did not even request that information. Like advertising elsewhere in health care, the messages have become ever more aggressive. Ultimately, those pushing full body scans ran afoul of regulations concerning false advertising. Then came opposition from professional societies and insurers citing excessive false positives and most centers closed (Kolata 2005).

Nurse practitioners and physician assistants substitute one intermediary for a more expensive one. Where labor substitution efforts are involved, specialized training programs may be required to transfer knowledge and skills from the physician to the entering class of professionals. For example, the 2002 New Mexico law allowing psychologists to prescribe drugs independently for mental health patients requires 450 hours of course work; a 400-hour, 100-patient practicum; and passing a national certification examination, plus a two-year apprenticeship period under the supervision of a physician (American Psychological Association 2002).

Other actors support disintermediation with personalized information systems. Insurers provide personal internet access portals for enrollees. Academic medical centers and hospitals provide newsletters, Web sites and telemedicine programs and offer copies of their clinical pathways and protocols to patients and their families. Pharmacists and drug chains develop screening and counseling centers, while government agencies and disease-oriented consumer groups offer screening programs, Web sites and direct-to-consumer advertising. Payers intervene even more directly through case management, formularies, preferred drug lists and a host of other controls. They also exert indirect controls by giving patients information on community resources, formulary restrictions, and best practices, while market-oriented reinforcements are applied through deductible and copayment systems.

## Reintermediation

Advertising can have an important educational impact, empowering the patient to make better choices. The greater availability of information is a trend favoring improved quality. However, that information is often biased and may even be inaccurate or at the least conflicting. Unless there is some professional input to mediate commercial interests, the market is unlikely to fully support the highest levels of quality in the long run. As Solberg *et al.* note in Chapter 12:

> The net result of all of these changes has been to focus attention and pressure on clinicians, especially those in primary care. They are feeling both stressed and unappreciated as they have to run faster to keep up while being constantly told that what they do isn't good enough. At the same time, it is becoming clearer that if we are to address the cost and quality conundrums we face, clinicians must not only be involved, they must take the lead in making change happen. (See Chapter 13.)

Those who argue for publicly available performance data for high cost, high impact services like open-heart surgery or cancer treatment are on the right track. However, those big-ticket items account for only a third of costs and a tenth of patient visits. What about the maintenance of quality in the other two-thirds, especially the other third involving chronic diseases and their prevention in an aging population. Our attempts to do so through gatekeepers and HMOs have not been very successful because patients do not want closed physician panels nor constrained physician access. Integrated delivery systems that combine the insurance function with the delivery of office, hospital, and home care by employed providers still seem to have considerable promise, but they seem acceptable only to a subset of communities, providers, and patients. Over time such organizations seem to have provided good leadership in improving the quality of care, especially in the chronic disease management and prevention areas (see Chapter 12).

Many patients sense the need for a physician relationship that integrates care, guarantees access in person and electronically, and is responsive to personal preferences and situation. Some who can afford it today, even pay a premium for the boutique practices that limit enrollment and promise care and attention to the individual. Furthermore, there is no guarantee of enhanced technical quality despite the extra compensation. However, such attentiveness is beyond the financial means of most of us. What is called for is for the future practice of medicine to leverage the technology that is becoming more economical and more available to enhance both quality and to reintermediate the process of care that professionals who fulfill many roles for the patient (including dealing with uncertainty, integrating signs and symptoms for diagnosis, knowing the science, selecting a course of action, doing procedures and providing support) provide. Only a few roles are affected by direct patient access to information and to tests and procedures. The primary loss through disintermediation is the monopoly on knowing the science. The other roles still exist.

## Identifying Opportunities for Interaction and Personalization

Today's practitioner must deal with both art and science, but with the latter's role ever expanding. For example, a specific genetic test for a disease leaves little to chance or intuition. It also may limit the range of practice options. However, the availability of information technology in medicine offers many new opportunities to enhance the doctor–patient relationship.

Patients are bombarded with health-related information in newspapers, magazines, direct mail, television ads, and increasingly from insurers and other interested parties via the Internet. In the face of this onslaught, the on-going relationship with the physician is under heavy pressure. Yet the task of integrating and interpreting all this information, configuring a care routine adapted to the needs and preferences of the patient and orchestrating its delivery still requires a craft person to add art where the science is lacking (Masys 2002).

To counter those who want to bypass the physician or to motivate the patient to change the routing of their information exchanges, physicians must focus on the linkage to the patient—reinvigorating the relationship with one's clients—recapturing their trust and desire to have a linkage that is reliable, up-to-date, and responsive to their needs as they see them. This requires a two-way relationship in which consumers are free to come to the provider and give the provider explicit permission to bring new concepts and opportunities to their attention. When the patient is seriously ill and in the hospital, that permission is implicit. With nonacute care encounters the physician must seek consumer permission to provide service as a way of maintaining or enhancing a longer-term market relationship (Godin 1999).

Models are available from other service providers. Think about the systems operated by small animal vets, dentists, and auto dealers' service departments. If you do not follow their advice, they come after you. They provide both episodic treatment and preventive care and they share responsibility for the latter part with you. It is an element of your relationship with them that you give them permission to do so.

## THE FUTURE: SHIFTING ROLES

Medicine is a premier profession but, unlike law and the ministry, it has developed a systematic connection to science and technology. Elliot Freidson, in his classic work *The Profession of Medicine* (1970a), presents an extended analysis of medicine as a profession that assumes a dominant position over a division of labor so that it gains control over the determination of the substance of its own work. He points out that

> . . . unlike most occupations, it is autonomous or self-directing and is permitted as a result of its trustworthiness over time the privilege to change the definition and shape of problems as experienced and interpreted by the layman . . . the layman's problem is recreated as it is managed—a new social reality is created. (p. xvii)

Greenwood (1957), however, notes that the opposite of the professional relationship is "the consumer is always right" and that advertising by professionals undermines that authority by conceding consumer sovereignty.

While patients are taking a more proactive role about health and wellness, the physician remains an important source of information and provider of tests, prescriptions, and procedures. The patient, however, now looks to a much wider range of sources of information and products. New information technology has rapidly expanded the consumer's access to information and the consumer's accessibility to new content providers.

## The New System and the Role of the Physician

The genetic revolution and the Internet will create an explosion of information that will make it even more impractical for individual physicians to master, let alone control, the information that must be accessed on behalf of one's patients. Patients with chronic illness often acquire extensive knowledge about their condition, but this aggressive search and learning behavior may now extend to more acute situations. Individual physicians and their health care organizations must respect the patient's role in this changing environment and develop complementary new role definitions in alignment with it.

Although care organizations have undertaken the industrialization of health care (Rastegar 2004; Britten 2001), these changes provide opportunities to explore countermeasures for physician practices. Concepts such as evidence-based medicine and mass customization offer providers exciting possibilities for redefining the doctor–patient relationship within the changing health care system (McLaughlin and Fitzgerald 2001). Old roles make way for newer ones as medical science advances.

The physician fulfills many roles for the patient, including dealing with uncertainty, integrating signs and symptoms for diagnosis, knowing the science, selecting a course of action, doing procedures and providing support. The primary loss through disintermediation is the monopoly on knowing the science. The other roles still exist. The remainder of this chapter outlines alternative ways of rethinking the physician roles in this setting and suggests a number of ways to transition primary care practice into new reintermediating roles consistent with developing technological opportunities.

## Projecting Modernity

Patients with their wireless Web access, personal digital assistants, and picture phones are not likely to be content sitting in a physician's office just to receive information. Neither are today's medical students with their reliance on access to expert systems and wireless reference links going to respect their colleagues who are not using these and other contemporary tools. Consumer satisfaction, a component of quality, is going to rest both on bedside manner and on convenient access to mediated information.

### Interaction Alternatives: The Case of the Chronically Ill Patient

Table 16–2 illustrates a series of steps in the interaction between a primary care physician's practice and a chronically ill patient that provides an opportunity to re-establish and enhance the physician–patient relationship in an era of disintermediation. Many of these can be influenced by those outsiders who would disintermediate the process, but they can also be refined by the physician or practice to develop stronger, longer-term doctor–patient relationships.

**Table 16-2** Illustrative Alternatives for Reintermediated Delivery

| Stage of Process | Offering Information | Obtaining Permission |
|---|---|---|
| Educate and instruct | Disease symptom and treatment information | Arrange to send data on asthma triggers daily over Internet |
| Set expectations | Consider, develop and review asthma action plan | Enroll patient in feedback and monitoring scheme |
| Understand instruction | Ask patient to demonstrate use of electronic equipment | Arrange for follow-up on use over phone |
| Adherence compliance | Provide motivational plan | Patient self-monitoring and diary to review on visits |
| Behavior modification | How-to's and FAQs on use of prescribed devices | Follow up in case of emergency room visit |
| Prescription | Education on effective use by referral to diabetes educator | Follow up at Rx renewal time |
| Monitor, support & retain | Return appointment Call-in line Responses to e-mails | Remote monitoring of blood sugar or weight to follow compliance |

*Source:* McLaughlin, Kaluzny, Kibbe and Tredway 2005

## Patient Education and Instruction

Many physicians acknowledge that an increasingly important role of the physician is that of educator, but also point (often with some guilt) to the lack of time for it. Yet there are many ways to support the learning process, although physician face time is known to be a most effective intervention. More and more patients will be leaving their physician's offices with literature and/or printouts about their recurrent problems. This will go beyond the brochures in the waiting room. It may be a monograph or a printout adapted to the patient's ability to comprehend the process. It may be retrieved from a file folder, printed in the office, or ordered out of a central repository to arrive a short time later.

At the same time the physician or the office staff may obtain permission to send up-to-date reminders about the current medical condition. One example would be to provide daily information on the asthma triggers expected the next day, so that patients can respond by adjusting his or her choice of or frequency of treatment.

### Setting Expectations

Individuals perform better in response to expectations that they helped set. Physicians have a role in helping patients develop expectations for how they will respond to a disease episode or to the results of self-administered tests. This could begin with information about an opportunity like developing an asthma action plan and following through on its development. The permission step can be reinforced by having the patient fill out and sign an enrollment form, perhaps including an information release form, for a monitoring and feedback arrangement customized to that action plan.

### Understanding Instruction

Patients may or may not listen to their physician. To assess comprehension, one can ask patients to demonstrate verbally or physically how they understand instructions given or agreements reached. Permission can also be solicited for telephone follow-up (emulating disease management programs) to ascertain whether the instructions were understood or followed.

## Adherence and Compliance

This is a major issue in health care, one which physicians can influence markedly. Again the physician can develop a motivational plan for the patient, i.e., how they will respond if they do or do not follow instructions. A possible permission step is to provide the patient with a diary for that disease that documents one's failures and successes. At the very least, the patient may agree that the physician will review it on a return visit.

## Behavior Modification

While printed information is a weak determinant of behavior, the practice can do things like giving the patient information about equipment that they are to use with how-to illustrations or answers to frequently-asked questions to reinforce new, more appropriate behaviors. The physician might also obtain patient assent to a follow-up call, if the patient ends up in the local emergency room, presumably after inappropriate behavior.

## Prescriptions

Physicians usually tell patients how to use a new prescription, but the physician can also specify reinforcing steps. For diabetics this could include a visit with a certified diabetes educator to deal more extensively with dietary and other relevant behaviors. The practice may also obtain permission to follow up as prescription renewal time approaches. An example would be an anti-hypertensive drug where the patient is not aware of symptoms, only side effects, and hence likely not to renew. Physicians specify a period for which a prescription is valid, but patients must then track them down for the renewal. The practice has data on when it should run out, but takes no part in finding out whether the patient is taking it and wants to renew it. Think of the opportunity for relationship in following up on the results of prior visits. How did that prescription work? Do you have any questions? Can we be of further service?

*Monitoring, Supporting, and Retaining*

The standard approach to monitoring, supporting and retaining patients is the return appointment. However, physicians often report that they have no system for knowing if the patient fails to return and certainly do not know why. Greater access through call-in lines and times and e-mail responsiveness could help with this. On the permission side one can arrange with the patient to forward to the physician data on recorded weight for congestive heart failure or blood sugar readings for diabetes with the idea that the physician will review these occasionally to see whether the patient is complying with the prescribed regimen and permitting the physician to reach out and request an office visit.

## Costs and Expectation Risks

Balancing customization, convenience, and efficiency is a major task of any service provider, but a critical one for physicians.

> Individual permission is essential for a doctor, lawyer, or any professional. But because it is so personal, it carries a number of risks. . . .
>
> Bad service or a bad interaction can cancel this sort of permission forever. A trusted chiropractor who uses a new technique that causes sudden discomfort discovers that he has lost a patient forever. . . .
>
> Personal permission is the most powerful form of permission for making major shifts in a consumer's behavior. Frequent flier miles won't get someone to consent to open-heart surgery, no matter how many free trips are offered. But a doctor with the consumer's trust can make a difference. (Godin 1999, p. 122)

There are costs to steps that reintermediate patients. However, the costs of not using them are losses of patients to those who aggressively compete for patient time, attention, and dollars. The physician has a tremendous asset in the patient's trust, but it can be broken, either by inaction or by failing on the promises implied by initiating the activities cited above. If the patient faithfully records airflow capacity every day and knows that the data has been aggregated and transmitted to the physician, the physician must stand ready to acknowledge the patient's performance on the next visit. If the physician gives the patient permission to e-mail questions and fails to respond, that patient is unlikely to return. All of these steps imply not only patient behaviors but also physician responsibilities that can add to existing burdens.

### Developing a Support System

Customization is neither easy nor cheap, but it will be effective in the competitive marketplace of the future. Michael Hammer, the reengineering guru, argues that after-sales customer service is the next competitive battleground in both goods and services. It is a place where most organizations can differentiate their offerings from their competitors. Two of the attributes among many of successful after-sales customer service systems are (1) fact-based planning and management, and (2) interorganization coordination and collaboration (Hammer and Co. 2001). Individual physicians or small practices are not going to introduce systems for information dissemination, monitoring, feedback, and support on their own. They are going to have to collaborate with one or more of those other actors in their environment, using Internet resources, instrumentation, and common interests in patient health and welfare. Each will have to find out which aspects of the system support their objectives and meet their pocketbooks and proceed from there. However, those that choose not to participate now may be forced to become followers later. Many of the systems that will enhance the customized relationship with the patient are already being espoused by the Institute of Medicine's *Crossing the Quality Chasm* report (IOM 2001) and the Agency for Healthcare Research and Quality's program on "Patient Centered Care: Customizing Care to Meet Patient Needs" (AHRQ 2001).

In the case of asthma patients, there are potentials for systems development among physicians, pharmaceutical companies, health maintenance organizations, patients, and monitoring equipment and software vendors. Together they have an opportunity to implement a number of the steps outlined above. The physician must enroll and train the patient; the patient or the pharmaceutical company must acquire and pay for the peak flow meter and the data entry device; and a data warehousing and storage organization must receive the data and send a periodic summary to the physician, the pharmaceutical company, and the patient. Then each must be prepared to use that information effectively in order to continue the relationship and justify the time, effort, and money spent. These will be complex undertakings but ones well worth considering.

## CONCLUSION

Disintermediation is an ongoing process with profound implications for the clinical practice of medicine and the challenges involving information technology will further affect the provider community. While one can lament the erosion of prerogatives that traditionally characterize the profession and the physician–patient relationship, this change also provides an opportunity to realign that relationship with the realities of a changing health care system and provide both customer satisfaction and technical quality. Doing so activates frequently overlooked parts of the Donabedian quality matrix, especially access and continuity of care. Meeting this challenge requires a two way interaction, a new partnership in which the physician reintermediates and recaptures patient trust and motivates desire to maintain a relationship that provides up-to-date information and responds to patients' needs as they evolve. While this partnership will be framed by the realities of the health care system as an economic marketplace, health care managers need to be ever alert to the special challenges involved, as described by Dr. Avedis Donabedian as he reflected on being a patient in the last stages of his own illness.

> Health care is a sacred mission. It is a moral enterprise and scientific enterprise—not fundamentally a commercial activity. We are not selling a product. We don't have a consumer who understands everything and makes rational choices. (2001, p. F12)

He goes on to conclude that "things won't improve until something is done about the design of the system." Designing that system is still a challenge and a responsibility of the provider community. Recapturing patient trust and maintaining a relationship that responds to patient needs, as they evolve, in an information-rich environment is a good place to start, especially given the new potentials of information technology becoming practical for the typical practice (Scherger 2004). Failure of the provider community to meet the challenge and the responsibility is well summarized by Margaret O'Kane, President of the National Committee for Quality Assurance (NCQA):

> We are at a moment in time when leaders in the physician and hospital communities need to acknowledge that our delivery system is no longer sufficiently well organized to deliver the benefits of current scientific knowledge. To have the vast array of medical knowledge deployed in a system that is well behind even twentieth-century advances in management science and technological development is inexcusable. And to have progress in the advancement of quality driven by payers and consumers demands that the validity of current constructs of professionalism be questioned. (2004, p. 280.)

# PART V

# Illustration

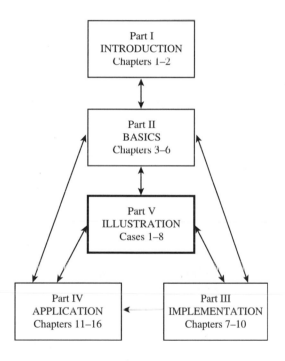

# CASE 1

# Intermountain Health Care

*Richard M. J. Bohmer, Amy C. Edmondson,*
*and Laura R. Feldman*

Dr. Brent James, executive director of Intermountain Health Care's
(IHC's) Institute for Health Care Delivery Research, explained to a group
of IHC's clinical leaders gathered around the conference room table that
the more often physicians and nurses complied with IHC's Clinical
Integration care delivery protocols, the more patient-care quality improved. He summarized his thoughts: "Anytime I get physicians to use
them, I'm basically tracking them into an evidence-based, standardized
line of clinical thought." One nurse appeared reluctant and—perhaps
overstating her case to emphasize that each patient was unique and could
not be treated in an assembly line manner—exclaimed, "We're not making widgets here!" Unexpectedly, James countered, "Oh yes we are!"

Clinical Integration referred to an organizational structure and network of
tools, including paper and electronic protocols and a centralized patient
database that organized the delivery of clinical care at IHC Health Services.
Clinical Integration was presented as a set of care- and productivity-
enhancing tools that would "Make it easy to do it right." For example,

diabetes management was most effective among patients whose physicians had full electronic clinical-decision support; not inconsequentially, those physicians were directly employed by IHC.

Even though no one—neither practitioners employed by IHC nor non-employee physicians who admitted patients to IHC facilities—was required to adhere strictly to the Clinical Integration care-delivery protocols, critics saw an insidious element to them, calling them a Taylorist[1] system that stripped away the autonomy of those who practiced the craft of medicine. James acknowledged that following the protocols increased the interdependence between the physician and the health care team, but believed that Clinical Integration was a crucial component of IHC's affordable and high quality clinical care. James reflected:

> The big strategic issue I face is how to bring the affiliated [non-employee] physicians on board. Some of the affiliated physicians vociferously hate our evidence-based care-delivery protocols. Using the protocols moves previously independent physicians into *de facto* group practice. They see such group practice, where they are directly and transparently accountable for their treatment decisions, as a loss of traditional physician autonomy, prestige, power, and income. . . . But you see, I can protect their money, and they will retain autonomy—although at a professional, not an individual level. But, they have to be willing to function as part of a group.

## INTERMOUNTAIN HEALTH CARE: STRUCTURE

Intermountain Health Care was established in 1975 by volunteer trustees as a nonprofit system of fifteen hospitals in the state of Utah. Most of the hospitals were established after 1905 (when LDS Hospital in Salt Lake City was founded) by local communities in partnership with the Church of Jesus Christ of Latter-day Saints (LDS). When the LDS Church decided that the operation of health care facilities was no longer critical to

---

[1]Referring to the ideas of Frederick Taylor, author of *The Principles of Scientific Management* (1911). Taylor had a profound influence on U.S. manufacturing practices, preferring discrete, highly controlled tasks to the craft-based practices that had preceded the assembly line. An analogous phrase to Taylorism in medical practice is the derogatory term "cookbook medicine."

its religious mission, IHC was created as a secular, nonprofit organization to own the hospitals on behalf of the community.[2]

In 1983, IHC transitioned from being exclusively a hospital company and became an insurer. The provider arm was known as IHC Health Services. (Exhibit 1–1 describes IHC's insurance business.) By 2001, IHC Health Plans directly enrolled 460,000 members or about 40% of the Utah commercial market.[3] (Exhibit 1–2 provides more detail on the population of Utah.) IHC Health Services was an award-winning vertically integrated health care organization, recipient of Healthcare Forum's Witt Award in 1991 and the NC-QHC Quality Health Care Award in 1996. IHC was named by *Modern Healthcare* as the premier organization of its kind for three consecutive years.

### Facilities

By 2002, IHC Health Services comprised more than 150 facilities, including 22 hospitals; 25 health centers; and over 70 outpatient clinics, counseling centers, and group practice offices located across Utah and southeastern Idaho. IHC had invested $1.9 billion over nine years for renovation and expansion of existing facilities and for construction of a new flagship campus for the Salt Lake Valley, scheduled to open in 2006.

### Information Technology

IHC was nationally recognized for its information systems, the backbone of which was the Health Evaluation through Logical Processing system (HELP) for inpatient care, and Clinical Workstation (CW) for use in outpatient clinics and physician offices.[4] HELP was a clinical information

---

[2]IHC's mission stated "Excellence in the provision of health care services to the communities in the Intermountain region" and the vision promised "The best clinical practice delivered in a consistent and integrated way; lowest appropriate cost to the population we serve; a service experience, supported by systems and processes, that focuses on the patient and enrollee; a genuine caring and concern in our interactions with patients, enrollees, families, and one another."

[3]While IHC did not track race or income within their Health Plans population, they estimated their enrollees mirrored the general employed population of Utah.

[4]When first introduced thirty years ago, hospital computing systems were almost exclusively billing and financial functions; clinical computing systems, which manage medical data, were much less common. Forerunners in clinical computing systems were the HELP system at IHC, the Regenstrief Medical Record System at the Regenstrief Institute (Indiana University), and the Brigham Integrated Computing System at Brigham and Women's Hospital (Boston). For more detail on clinical information systems see the *International Journal of Medical Informatics,* 54 (1999): 3.

**Exhibit 1–1**    Intermountain Health Care: Insurance

**IHC Health Plans**    IHC entered the insurer market in 1983 at the behest of Dr. David Burton, an internal medicine doctor leading a private emergency medicine group that covered Cottonwood and AltaView Hospitals. While running the group, he anticipated the role insurance companies were going to come to play in the United States. Burton presented a business plan pro forma to the board and IHC management to start IHC Health Plans and was appointed CEO for its first three years of operation.

In 2001, IHC offered five traditional HMO health plans. Three of the plans were available as a POS-HMO (Point of Service) option under the PLUS moniker. The POS was similar to a Preferred Provider Organization (PPO), a form of health insurance in which the enrollee paid a higher premium and had to meet a larger deductible in exchange for access to an expanded set of physicians. By contrast, enrollees in the traditional HMO paid less for a basic and more restrictive package of health care services. IHC Med, a traditional HMO (also available as Med PLUS), was touted as the most economical plan with a 600-physician panel of PCPs and specialists. SelectMed and SelectMedPLUS featured 1,500 PCPs and specialists. IHC Care (also available as IHC Care PLUS) was a large panel HMO with a network of 2,600 PCPS and specialists. There was a step-wise increase in the out-of-pocket cost—and a pool of physicians from which to choose—from IHC Med to SelectMed to IHC Care. Health Choice was a nonpanel option that allowed enrollees to receive care outside the panel at a lower level of coverage. IHC Access was for Medicaid enrollees who were required to select a physician from a set provider list. The Health Plans boasted a longer tenure per enrollee (5–6 years average) compared to a national average of 1–2 years.

**Competition**    In 2001, IHC Health Plans enrolled 40% of the insured population of Utah. Blue Cross Blue Shield, Altius, and United HealthCare were the other major market players with 425,000, 180,000, and 150,000 enrollees respectively. A second tier of smaller insurers included Public Employees (85,000 enrollees), Educators (73,000), CIGNA (60,000), Mailhandlers (52,000), Aetna (48,000), and Deseret Mutual (45,000). Beyond the second tier were many smaller insurers with fewer than 20,000 enrollees; most enrolled fewer than 10,000. IHC management wanted the Health Plans to maintain a 40%–60% market share of the insured population.

**Pricing of the insurance product**    Consistent with their nonprofit status the Health Plans maintained break-even prices against which second-tier insurers could compete and were willing to accept a loss in the short-term in order to be a permanent player in the Utah insurer market. As a consequence, the Health Plans forced their competitors' prices down. The Health Plans aimed to encourage competition based on quality, not cost, in order to create a positive pressure to raise the standard of health care.

Source: Casewriter.

**Exhibit 1–2**  The Population of Utah in 2000

|  | Utah | United States |
|---|---|---|
| Population, 2001 estimate | 2,269,789 | 284,796,887 |
| Population, percent change, April 1, 2000–July 1, 2001 | 1.6% | 1.2% |
| Population, percent change, 1990 to 2000 | 29.6% | 13.1% |
| Persons under 5 years old | 9.4% | 6.8% |
| Persons under 18 years old | 32.2% | 25.7% |
| Persons 65 years old and over | 8.5% | 12.4% |
| White persons[a] | 89.2% | 75.1% |
| Black or African American persons[a] | 0.8% | 12.3% |
| American Indian and Alaska Native persons[a] | 1.3% | 0.9% |
| Asian persons[a] | 1.7% | 3.6% |
| Native Hawaiian and Other Pacific Islander[a] | 0.7% | 0.1% |
| Persons reporting some other race[a] | 4.2% | 5.5% |
| Persons reporting two or more races | 2.1% | 2.4% |
| Persons of Hispanic or Latino origin[b] | 9.0% | 12.5% |
| White persons, not of Hispanic/Latino origin | 85.3% | 69.1% |
| Female persons | 49.9% | 50.9% |
| High school graduates and higher, persons 25 years and over | 87.7% | 80.4% |
| Bachelor's degrees and higher, persons 25 years and over | 26.1% | 24.4% |
| Housing units | 768,594 | 115,904,641 |
| Homeownership rate | 71.5% | 66.2% |
| Households | 701,281 | 105,480,101 |
| Persons per household | 3.13 | 2.59 |
| Households with persons under 18 | 45.8% | 36.0% |

*continues*

**Exhibit 1–2**  continued

|  | Utah | United States |
|---|---|---|
| Median household money income, 1997 model-based estimate | $38,884 | $37,005 |
| Persons below poverty, 1997 model-based estimate | 10.0% | 13.3% |
| Children below poverty, 1997 model-based estimate | 12.5% | 19.9% |
| *Employment Status* |  |  |
| Population 16 years and over | 1,600,279 | 217,168,077 |
| In labor force | 69.0% | 63.9% |
| Employed civilian labor force | 65.3% | 59.7% |
| Unemployed civilian labor force | 5.0% | 5.8% |
| Not in labor force | 31.0% | 36.1% |

Sources: U.S. Census Bureau: State and County QuickFacts. Data derived from Population Estimates, 2000 Census of Population and Housing, 1990 Census of Population and Housing, Small Area Income and Poverty Estimates, County Business Patterns, 1997 Economic Census, Minority- and Women-Owned Business, Building Permits, Consolidated Federal Funds Report, 1997 Census of Governments, available at http://quickfacts.census.gov/qfd/states/49000.html, accessed July 30, 2002; U.S. Census Bureau, Census 2000 Summary File 3, Matrices P30, P32, P33, P43, P46, P49, P50, P51, P52, P53, P58, P62, P63, P64, P65, P67, P71, P72, P73, P74, P76, P77, P82, P87, P90, PCT47, PCT52, and PCT53, available at http://factfinder.census.gov/bf/_lang=en_vt_name=DEC_2000_SF3_U_DP3_geo_id=01000US.html, accessed September 25, 2002.

[a]Includes persons reporting only one race.

[b]Hispanics may be of any race, so also are included in applicable race categories.

system first conceptualized in the early 1960s as an automated diagnostic tool for physiologic monitoring.[5] Over time, the system evolved to provide practitioners clinical-decision support. In the early 1970s, pharmacists entered prescriptions into the system to screen for drug-drug, drug-lab, and drug-radiology interactions. In the early 1990s, an electronic medical record (EMR) was introduced enabling ICU patient monitoring, surgery

---

[5]H.R. Warner, A.F. Toronto, L.G. Veasey, R.A. Stephenson, "A mathematical approach to medical diagnosis: application to congenital heart disease." *Journal of the American Medical Association.* 177 (1961): 177–183.

scheduling, and transcription. By 1994, the Antibiotic Assistant, one of several clinical-decision support modules built within HELP, could essentially "read" a patient's medical history and suggest appropriate antibiotics and dosage schedules for patients suffering from infections.[6] In early 2001, IHC added Results Review, a function that gave physicians Web-based online access to appointment books, patient consult notes and charts, and patients' laboratory results. By 2001, the EMR allowed users to perform structured queries and in three clicks of the mouse go from reviewing a patient's clinical data to the pertinent medical literature. In 2001, the system featured 18,000 workstations and 16,000 clinical users. (See Exhibit 1–3 for a diagram of IHC's information system.)

## Regions

IHC Health Services was organized into four regions: Urban North, Urban Central, Urban South, and Rural. Each Urban Region was centered around a large tertiary "collector" hospital, with a series of smaller feeder hospitals and outpatient facilities. Each urban region coordinated with geographically associated rural region facilities. Regions were led by a regional vice president, one or a team of medical hospital directors, and one or a team of medical directors representing the facility-based physician groups. Regional senior management teams included a chief medical officer, medical directors from each of the Clinical Integration Clinical Programs, and a variety of staff with financial and data management expertise.

## Physician Rings

Professional staff at IHC Health Services were arranged in three rings. Ring 1 included about 1,200 practicing primary care and specialist physicians, 400 of whom were salaried IHC employees (60%+ of the 400 were primary care physicians) working under the auspices of the IHC Physician Division. The Physician Division had 1,457,000 outpatient encounters in 2001 and accounted for about half of all outpatient and inpatient care delivered

---

[6]R.S. Evans et al. "A computer-assisted management program for antibiotics and other anti-infective agents." *New England Journal of Medicine* 338 (1998): 232–238.

**Exhibit 1–3**   IHC's Clinical Information System

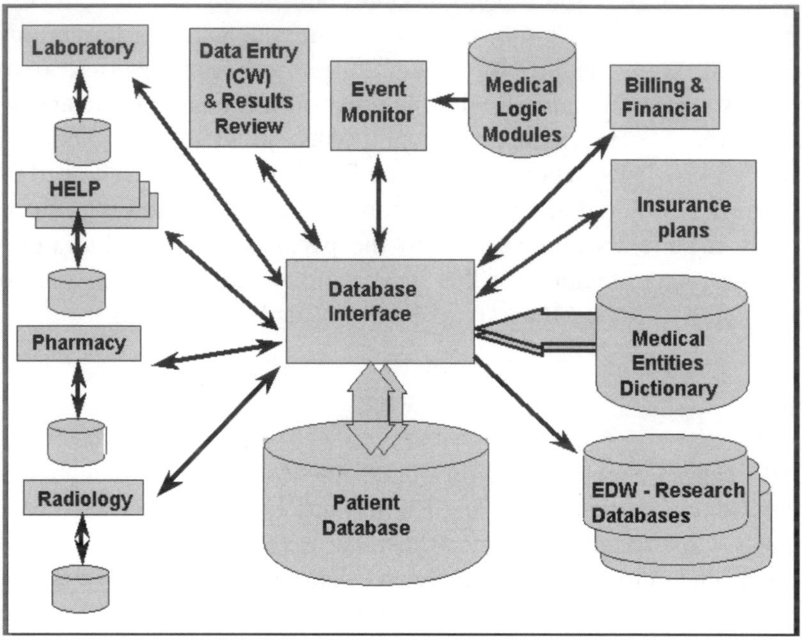

*Note: Cylinders represent databases.*

All inpatient and outpatient clinical information resided together in the IHC Clinical Data Repository (CDR or "lifetime patient record"). The CDR included a series of key subfunctions essential to the operation of an EMR, such as an electronic master patient index (EMPI), and a database of shared field definitions (the Vocabulary Server, or VOCSER). These data interacted with medical knowledge—compiled from the medical literature, physician consensus, and best practice guidelines and protocols—to provide real-time clinical decision support in applications such as the Antibiotic Assistant. An electronic data warehouse (EDW) pulled together all clinical data, as well as financial transaction data, insurance claims data, patient outcomes data, and all other information used across the entire enterprise, into condition-specific data marts. The data marts, in turn, generated clinical and administrative management information to drive management within the IHC system. In effect, the CDR was the core information resource for the whole system, and HELP (inpatient), Clinical Workstation (outpatient), and Results Review were tools used to view and update that shared resource.

Source: Intermountain Health Care.

within IHC during 2001.[7] An additional 800 "affiliated" or "non employed" physicians completed Ring 1. Although the 800 were private community-based practitioners, 80% of their patients were insured by IHC Health Plans or received care at IHC institutions. An analysis of patient volume performed by Dr. David Burton, IHC's Vice President for Health Care Delivery Research, found that 94% of all patients (inpatient and outpatient) treated at IHC facilities were under the care of one of the 1,200 Ring 1 physicians. Ring 2 comprised a small group of 50–100 "splitter" physicians, who derived between 40% and 60% of their practices from IHC-associated patients. Ring 3 totaled more than 1,500 additional physicians who were only loosely associated with IHC, admitting patients to IHC facilities, referring patients to IHC-employed physicians, or occasionally treating IHC-insured patients.

Practitioner groups within the Physician's Division—most often in the form of regionally-based multi-specialty clinics—were fairly common. The two largest multi-specialty groups employed about 150 Physician Division physicians. There were half a dozen specialty groups; Greg Poulsen, MBA, vice president for Strategic Planning and Research, anticipated more would be formed in the future. Physician's Division primary care practitioners were spread among 30 locations.

IHC Health Services frequently contracted out to other insurers who were too small (with fewer than 30,000 enrollees) to create their own physician network. A subset of tightly aligned, independent insurance plans, accounting for more than 500,000 additional commercial insurance lives, used IHC's facilities and physician networks almost exclusively. IHC gave those insurance plans the same footing and rates as its own internal health plans.

## Compensation

The compensation structure for employed physicians was divided into four parts: salary (30%), fee for service (FFS) payments (40–50%), and a performance-based bonus (10%). Although specific criteria for the bonus varied from group to group (i.e., clinic to clinic), it generally

---

[7]The provider garnered 65% prospective payments (33% for Medicare, 11% for Medicaid, 15% for IHC Health Plan enrollees, and a small savings from self-pay, or charity care) from its enrollees, compared to an average of 30–35% on the East Coast.

reflected group-level financial performance and clinical quality indicators. The fourth component, "profit sharing" for overall organizational profitability, sometimes bumped physician salaries above 100%. The 800 affiliated physicians were paid by a discounted FFS system and did not have performance incentives. None of the 1,200 physicians worked under capitation.

## Governance

In 1993, IHC invited physicians to participate more fully in the operation and governance of the organization. Half of the 28 member IHC board of trustees were selected from Ring 1 physicians; the remaining seats were occupied by volunteer members of the community and IHC senior management. In addition, about 300 community members served on the boards of local facilities.

## BRENT JAMES, MD, M.Stat

Brent James, a surgeon and biostatistician by training, was Executive Director of Intermountain Health Care's Institute for Health Care Delivery Research (IHCDR, or the Institute) and served as IHC's Vice President for Medical Research and Continuing Medical Education. He came to IHC in 1986 from the Harvard School of Public Health, where he taught biomedical computing and biostatistics. James returned to Utah (he received his undergraduate, medical, and masters degrees from the University of Utah) because he believed IHC had one of the finest data systems in the country. Presented with the task of leading a clinical research program at IHC, James became intrigued by the quality of health care services.

The Institute—employing 15 staff, roughly one-half of whom were trained as biostatisticians and analysts—was founded in 1990 to support James' work around organizing for clinical management. It was co-located with IHC senior administration in a downtown Salt Lake City facility. The Institute was a hub for internal research on the management of clinical medicine. Another arm of the Institute ran 2-, 9-, and 20-day training sessions on quality management and clinical quality improvement for physicians and health care system administrators within IHC and from around the world. James' calendar was always booked: in addition to conducting research, honoring speaking engagements, and serving on several national task forces on health care quality, he facilitated all the classes offered by the Institute.[8]

## HISTORY OF CLINICAL CARE MANAGEMENT AT IHC

Nationally lauded as a leader in clinical quality improvement among delivery systems, IHC's approach to clinical-care management changed course in 1995 when then IHC Executive Vice President Bill Nelson (now CEO) challenged James to fuse his "science projects"—Nelson's pet term for the proliferation of clinical and managerial quality improvement projects across IHC over the past nine years—into a comprehensive clinical management model. James explained, "There was a sentinel moment when we realized that our business was clinical medicine." He continued, "A big hindrance to quality improvement in health care centers around deployment . . . you tend to get these silo projects that just don't spread." Clinical process management would replace the previous piecemeal approach to improvement in health care delivery.

### Early Interest in Quality Improvement

Reflecting on his tenure at IHC, James noted that IHC had begun to tinker with the concept of clinical-care management in 1986, with a series of investigations called QUE (Quality, Utilization, and Efficiency) studies, which was classic health services research examining variation in clinical practice. While conducting the QUE studies, James attended a lecture by Dr. W. Edwards Deming, known as the father of TQM, who introduced a "crazy" idea: Deming argued that higher quality could lead to lower cost.[9] James returned to Salt Lake City and tested Deming's cost-quality

---

[8]James served on the Institute of Medicine's National Roundtable on Quality, and its subsequent Committee on Quality of Healthcare in America, and contributed to their nationally heralded reports, *To Err Is Human* (1999) and *Crossing the Quality Chasm* (2001).

[9]Deming (1900–1994) founded Total Quality Management, a widely used method of statistical process control to ensure consistency in production industries. Credited for invigorating the Japanese economy following WWII, he received the Second Order Medal of the Sacred Treasure from the Emperor of Japan in 1960.

hypothesis in pre-existing IHC clinical trials: "We just started to add cost outcomes to our traditional clinical trials and proved it true within a few months." James realized that it was due to a "godsend" that he was able to collect cost outcomes: in the early 1980s Steven Busboom in finance and Poulsen in business strategic planning had decided they had to be able to measure the cost of clinical care. Busboom and Poulsen built an activity-based cost accounting system and implemented it across all facilities in the IHC system. James was able to attach costs to individual clinical activities and then build a cost profile of different strategies for managing a particular clinical condition.

Senior management within IHC felt they could realize Deming's maxim by allowing their physician population to self-manage. In 1986, Dr. Steve Lewis, a pulmonary intensivist and IHC's Senior Vice President for Medical Affairs, lead the formation of The Great Basin Physician Corporation, similar to a Preferred Provider Organization (PPO) structure for community physicians within IHC. According to James, the model's emphasis on self-governance and protocols for care "helped pull the physicians together, but it never really materialized. It sort of died quietly on its own."

*The Quality Movement*

As a follow-up to the 1991 annual management conference, IHC CEO Scott Parker sent a memo with the subject line "Is quality improvement important for IHC?" Eighty percent of the respondents, representing IHC's top 200 managers, said "Yes." Many referenced IHC's mission statement in their responses. Parker consulted James as to what sort of action they should take, and James suggested all managers should attend IHC's internal quality improvement training where they could "rub shoulders with rank and file." James reasoned that such a clear indication of top-management support could deliver a very positive quality message to all IHC employees. Parker declined; instead, he asked James to conduct a special session of the IHC Facilitator Workshop Series (totaling 8 days over 4 sessions) for the top 40 managers in IHC. Parker mandated attendance and was present himself in all sessions. James presented a concept (e.g., the use of protocols to control care delivery, how service quality affected the business, and models of leadership and participation) and then opened the floor for discussion. He said to the group: "Here's a central concept. Does it apply to IHC? How would it look as it plays out within

IHC? What things would we need in place?" Later, James commented, "Here's the crazy thing: we never reached any formal conclusions. But it's fair to say that the shared vision that we came away with from that series of meetings has informed our decision making ever since."

The clinical counterpart to the Facilitator Workshop series, developed in 1992, offered senior physician leadership the opportunity to learn about clinical quality improvement. Participants in the 20-day, biannual Advanced Training Program in Health Care Delivery Improvement (ATP) workshops were required to do a clinical-improvement project, such as implementation of an evidence-based best practice protocol for diabetes mellitus, or reduction of postoperative wound infections in elective surgical cases. In James' words, "[the] ATP acted as a magnet to draw what today I would call early adopters. Physicians and nurses would come out of the ATP as absolute quality zealots, convinced that this was something the profession needed to do."

*The Project Phase*

Enthusiasm for clinical management swelled between 1992 and 1995 as more clinical and managerial staff were exposed to ATP and the Facilitator Workshop Series. On the administrative side of IHC, literally thousands of improvement projects were undertaken to reduce costs and solve facilities-management problems. (For example, one project streamlined installation and maintenance of IHC's extensive telecommunications network.) In 1995, at Nelson's request, James identified 65 clinical protocols that had been developed and implemented, producing about $20 million in net annual savings in a clinical operating budget of about $1.5 billion, as well as significant gains in clinical quality. (See Exhibit 1–4).

**Developing a Strategic Plan**

The second attempt at physician self-management was in 1993, when a newly hired senior vice president for medical affairs tried to establish a clinical management structure by hiring physician leaders and providing them with management tools. By the time he was called away to serve a mission for the LDS Church, several million dollars had been spent without any significant changes in management practice.

**Exhibit 1–4**  Performance Improvement Outcome Data

Savings from Clinical Projects, 1995

| Clinical Project | Cost Structure Improvement, ($ Millions) |
|---|---|
| Fast-track extubation in TICU | $5.5 |
| Long-term ventilator management | 4.7 |
| HFOV (RDS in premature newborns) | 3.7 |
| Shock Trauma Respiratory ICU (12 protocols) | 2.5 |
| Antibiotic Assistant | 1.2 |
| Pediatric ICU (8+ protocols) | .7 |
| Infection prophylaxis in surgery | .6 |
| Adverse drug event prevention | .5 |
| Community-acquired pneumonia | .5 |
| Ventilator support for hypoxemia | .5 |
| Group B strep sepsis of newborn | .3 |
| Subtotal | 20.7 |
| + 30 additional successful clinical projects without cost savings analysis | ? |

Source: Intermountain Health Care.

James felt that in order to build a successful clinical management system there had to be an overarching guidance structure. He approached Burton, himself just returned from a three-year LDS Church mission, and began to form a strategic quality plan for IHC. James reflected on previous attempts to have physicians manage clinical operations:

> In each of the [two prior] programs, we found physicians willing to manage. We trained them in management skills, gave them the financial data we used for the administrative operations, and then asked them to go manage physicians. In retrospect, it was the wrong data—or, at least, not enough of the right data. It was financial data organized for facilities management. At best, it was health plans claims data that gave a full financial history of a patient's care without the associated clinical detail. But even that didn't even come close. That's the reason we failed the first two times we tried to introduce clinical management.

James continued: "You manage what you measure . . . Doctors manage patients, not money. The data [that we provided them] didn't have anything to do with those tasks, as physicians and nurses saw them." The key to engaging physicians in clinical management was to make it meaningful by aligning data collection to work processes. This represented a pivotal shift in mental model and in practice. James explained: "Managers think in terms of cost-per-facility, which, in health care, translates to cost-per-unit [e.g., ICU, phlebotomy, or surgery]. By contrast, doctors think in terms of resources, or tests and treatments required for a specific condition."

*Families of Care*

The strategic plan developed by Burton and James organized IHC Health Services into (1) clinical conditions, (2) clinical support services, (3) service quality (internally referred to as Patient Perceptions of Quality), and (4) administrative support processes.

When looking at clinical conditions, Burton and James used four criteria to identify key work processes and families of care that comprised the bulk of care provided at IHC facilities. They identified key processes according to patient volume, intensity of care (cost per day), variability, and what were termed "socially important conditions" (e.g., conditions common in ethnic minorities and women). They found that 62 of over 600 clinical work processes accounted for 93% of inpatient clinical volume and about 30 processes (15 chronic, 15 acute) comprised about 85% of outpatient clinical volume. They named the resulting series of clinical process-based families "Clinical Programs," and used them to group the most common Diagnosis Related Groups (DRGs) for which hospitals sought third-party payment.[10] Burton and James identified eight families of care for hospital-based procedures, then added a ninth clinical program (the Primary Care Clinical Program) to cover the 30 conditions most commonly managed in the outpatient setting. Each clinical program comprised a series of high-priority, tightly related clinical-care processes.

---

[10]DRGs, or Diagnosis Related Groups, are standard codes used by health care providers for billing purposes. Developed for use by Medicare in 1983, DRGs represent prospective payment based on diagnosis (regardless of resources actually utilized), assuming a given diagnosis will require a basic packet of resources, tests, and days in the hospital.

For example, the nine most common clinical treatment processes performed in the Cardiovascular (CV) Clinical Program (to treat ischemic heart disease or congestive heart failure) represented 18.5% of IHC's inpatient and outpatient expenditures in 1997. (See Exhibit 1–5 for a list of the eight referral care clinical programs and the CV clinical processes.)

The strategic plan used a similar method to identify key work processes in the other three areas. For example, Clinical Support Services included non-condition-specific clinical work processes. Major divisions in Clinical Support Services reflected traditional facility management groupings such as pharmacy operations, pathology, procedure rooms (e.g., anesthesiology, operating rooms, and labor and delivery rooms), imaging, ICUs, and nursing units. Respiratory therapy, for example, was found to have five key processes among the more than 40 routinely performed: (1) oxygen therapy, (2) aerosolized bronchodilators, (3) chest physical therapy, (4) incentive spirometry, and (5) support for ventilator management, which accounted for more than 90% of all work performed by that group.

The strategic plan, called "Clinical Integration," was approved by the IHC board of trustees in 1996 and represented a major shift for IHC. Its aim was to establish quality (defined as process management with measured outcomes) as IHC's core business approach and to extend full management accountability to IHC's clinical functions. The plan unfolded over the next four years. In 1997, Burton and James tested, on a pilot basis, whether it was possible and practical to build clinical-outcomes-tracking data systems representing the two largest clinical activities within IHC: Pregnancy, Labor, and Delivery, which represented 11% of all inpatient care within IHC, in the Women and Newborn Clinical Program and ischemic heart disease (10% of all inpatient care delivery within the system, in the Cardiovascular Clinical Program).

In 1998, they began to use outcomes data to hold IHC-associated employed and non employed professionals accountable for their clinical performance and to enable IHC to set and achieve clinical improvement goals. In 1999, the strategic task was to align financial incentives. To avoid passing on all the savings generated by clinical improvement to the payers, Burton and James found it necessary to build and test strategies to harvest part of those savings back to IHC Health Services and IHC's associated independent physicians, thereby making clinical management financially stable. Finally, in 2000, the board of trustees instructed IHC's senior management to roll Clinical Integration out across all operational functions.

**Exhibit 1–5** Referral Care Clinical Programs

**IHC Referral Care Clinical Programs as percent of hospital cost**

| Clinical Program[a] | Hospital Inpatient and Outpatient Cost | % of Total Cost | Cumulative % |
|---|---|---|---|
| Cardiovascular | $129,442,947 | 18.5 | 18.5 |
| Neuromusculoskeletal | 128,675,965 | 18.4 | 36.9 |
| Surgical Specialties | 116,646,327 | 16.7 | 53.6 |
| Women and Newborn | 114,984,231 | 16.4 | 70.0 |
| Medical Specialties | 94,773,645 | 13.5 | 83.5 |
| Pediatric Specialties | 44,552,204 | 6.4 | 89.9 |
| Behavioral Health | 17,185,283 | 2.5 | 92.3 |
| ICU + Trauma | 31,079,870 | 4.4 | 96.7 |
| Unassigned | 22,759,375 | 3.3 | 100 |
| Total | 700,099,847 | 100 | 100 |

[a]Note: the 9th clinical program was for Primary Care medicine, the domain of general practitioners. Based on 1997 Case Mix Database; cost data organized by APR-DRG.

**Cardiovascular Clinical Program Family of Processes**

| Process | DRGs | Hospital Inpatient and Outpatient Cost | % of Total Cost | Cumulative % |
|---|---|---|---|---|
| *Ischemic heart disease* | | | | |
| CABG et al. | 106–108, 110–111 | $34,228,000 | 28.9 | 28.9 |
| Dx cath, PTCA, stents, etc. | 112, 124–125 | 24, 213,792 | 20.5 | 49.4 |
| Acute chest pain | 121–123, 132–133, 140, 143 | 9,293,639 | 7.9 | 57.2 |
| *Congestive heart failure* | | | | |
| Valves | 104–105 | 13,417,746 | 11.3 | 68.5 |
| CHF | 87, 127 | 5,348,209 | 4.5 | 73.1 |
| Transplant | 103 | 4,243,428 | 3.6 | 76.7 |
| Arrhythmias/ pacemakers | 116–118, 129, 138–139, 141–142 | 9,015,295 | 7.6 | 84.3 |

*continues*

**Exhibit 1–5**   continued

| Process | DRGs | Hospital Inpatient and Outpatient Cost | % of Total Cost | Cumulative % |
|---|---|---|---|---|
| *Congestive heart failure,cont'd* | | | | |
| Peripherial vascular surg | 5, 130–131, 478–479 | 8,374,590 | 7.1 | 91.4 |
| Resp Ca/ pulmonary surg | 75–77, 82–84, 94–95 | 7,343,294 | 6.2 | 97.6 |
| Other Cardiovascular | 120, 126, 144–145 135–136, | 2,879,647 | 2.4 | 100 |
| Total | — | 118,857,706 | 100 | 100 |
| Source: | Intermountain Health Care. | | | |

## CHANGE INFRASTRUCTURE

To facilitate the transition from a traditional management structure focused on managing the facilities within which clinical care took place, to one oriented around clinical quality and clinical processes, Burton and James built a clinical administrative structure to be the clinical counterpart of the administrative structure at each level in the organization.

### Clinical-Care Management

*Guidance Councils*

In 1998, pilot Guidance Councils were established for the Cardiovascular Clinical Program (initially focused on management of ischemic heart disease) and the Women and Newborn Clinical Program to coordinate program goals, management strategies, and data collection across an integrated system.

The Guidance Councils were built around physician/nurse leadership dyads based in IHC's three urban regions. In each region, a Clinical Pro-

**Exhibit 1–6**   Guidance Council Structure

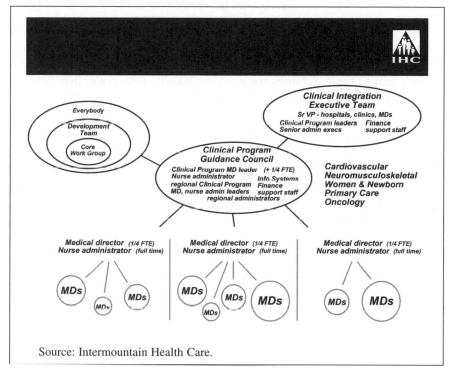

Source: Intermountain Health Care.

gram physician leader was selected from practicing physicians. IHC
bought one-quarter of their time for Clinical Program leadership activities, and provided additional training in quality management, leadership,
and financial skills. A full-time nurse manager dealt with routine administrative matters and provided a direct link to clinical staff. The physi-
cian/nurse dyads within each region had two major responsibilities: meeting with clinical-care delivery groups that executed any of the key clinical
processes in their Clinical Program and meeting with line administrative
management structures in the region. (For more details on program governance see Exhibit 1–6.)

Monthly Guidance Council meetings always included a report on current level of performance, progress toward meeting clinical goals, and the
identification of barriers toward realizing the goals. Guidance Councils
were authorized to approve guideline updates.

*Development Teams*

Within each of the Guidance Councils were one or more permanent Development Teams that focused on select clinical processes.[11] Guidelines, or protocols for specific procedures, were created by Development Teams, sent to the front lines for implementation, data collection, and review, and updated as results traveled back up the pyramid. Exhibit 1–7 shows one such protocol.

Each Development Team comprised a physician leader, nurse, and physician team members drawn from front-line care deliverers who would actually implement any protocols the team developed, and a "core work group" of three or four expert physicians dedicated to following research around that specific key clinical process. IHC reimbursed all Development Team members for time spent working on the team. (Many were independent, community-based practitioners.) IHC also supplied staff support for the development teams to (1) help design outcomes tracking systems (with assistance from the Institute's statisticians, as well as representatives from IHC's Electronic Data Warehouse group) using a set of formal design tools; (2) generate educational materials for professionals and for patients; (3) design and implement electronic medical record and clinical decision support systems (through IHC's Medical Informatics group); and (4) plan and support operational implementation at the front line.

Specialist physicians serving on core work groups had salaried time to fill four specific roles: (1) provide expertise to develop the initial evidence-based best practice protocol; (2) keep the protocol current over time by applying new findings from the medical literature, from similar practice groups in other institutions, and by closely tracking and leading discussions based on IHC's internal outcome and protocol variation data; (3) detail front-line practitioners on "state-of-the-art care" for their particular protocol through regular CME sessions; and (4) operate a specialty clinic for patients who could not be well-managed within the primary care setting. The pyramidal structure facilitated transference of

---

[11]For example, in 2001 the Primary Care Clinical Program had Development Teams in place for Diabetes, Adult Asthma, Pediatric Asthma, Lower Respiratory Infection (Community Acquired Pneumonia plus Acute Bronchitis), Otitis Media, Chronic Anticoagulation, Depression, Congestive Heart Failure (also part of CV Clinical Program), Ischemic Heart Disease (also part of CV Clinical Program), and Low Back Pain (also part of Neuromusculoskeletal Clinical Program).

**Exhibit 1–7**   Clinical Protocol for Cardiovascular Care

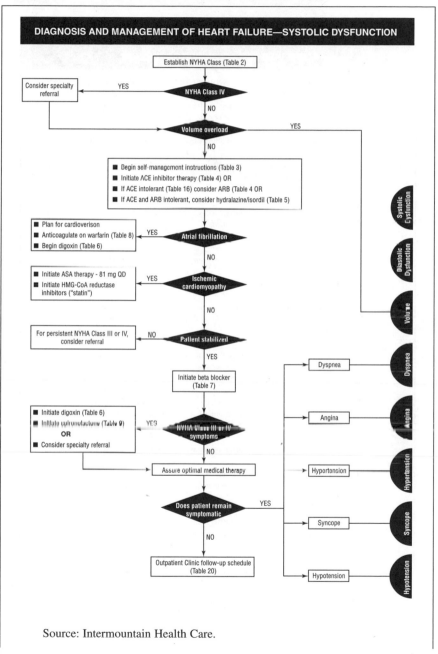

Source: Intermountain Health Care.

*continues*

**Exhibit 1–7**  continued

---

## GUIDELINES FOR ACE INHIBITOR THERAPY

1. **ANGIOTENSIN CONVERTING ENZYME INHIBITORS (ACEI):** Proven to improve symptoms, decrease hospitalizations, and decrease mortality in patients with heart failure. May be safely initiated even with systolic blood pressure as low as 90 mmHg. Risk of hypotension increased with hypovolemia; consider decreasing diuretic dose prior to ACE inhibitor initiation or titration.

2. **MEDICATIONS:** (Lisinopril is preferred in stable patients given its daily dosing schedule)

   a. **\*Lisinopril (Prinivil®, Zestril®):** Target 20mg daily, start at 2.5 mg daily, increase by 5 mg every week until target dose reached.
   *Max dose: 40mg daily.*

   b. **\*Enalapril (Vasotec®):** Target 10mg twice a day, start at 2.5mg twice a day, increase by 2.5mg per dose every week until target dose reached.
   *Max dose: 40mg daily.*

   c. **\*Captopril (Capoten®):** Target 50mg three times a day, start at 6.25mg three times a day, increase by 6.25 to 12.5mg per dose every 2 weeks until target reached.
   *Max dose: 300mg daily.*

   d. **\*Quinapril (Accupril®):** Target 20mg twice a day, start at 5mg daily, increase by 5mg per dose every week until target dose reached (divided doses when daily dose >10mg).
   *Max dose: 40mg daily.*

   e. **Ramipril (Altace®):** Target 5mg twice a day, start at 1.25-2.5mg daily, increase by 2.5mg every week until target dose reached (divided doses when daily dose >10mg).
   *Max dose: 20mg daily.*

3. **LABS:** Basic Metabolic Panel weekly until target dose achieved. Monitor for elevations in potassium (>5.0) and decrease potassium supplementation (if applicable) or modify target dose of ACE inhibitor.

4. **CONTRAINDICATIONS:** Shock, angioneurotic edema, or significant hyperkalemia >5.5 mm/L.

5. **PRECAUTIONS:** Renal impairment (creatinine >3.0), mild hyperkalemia >5.0 mm/L, dialysis, hypovolemia (consider decreasing diuretic dose if applicable), cerebrovascular disease, renal artery stenosis, hypotention (systolic BP <90mmHg).

6. **ADVERSE REACTIONS:** Dizziness, headache, fatigue, diarrhea, upper respiratory symptoms, cough, nausea, hyperkalemia, orthostatic hypotension, renal impairment, angioneurotic edema.

7. Therapy should continue for life.

---

*\*IHC Formulary*

Source: Intermountain Health Care.

best practice and most recent developments in the field to front-line practitioners.

Similar to the work performed by the Development Teams, processes occurring within the clinical support services were analyzed, standardized, and specified. For example, twelve key processes defined the care delivered in the Shock Trauma Respiratory ICU (a Level 1 trauma unit). The standardization of key processes extended to all clinical pathology laboratories across all IHC inpatient and outpatient settings. An electronic laboratory reporting system, based on standard reporting language, made all results quickly available at any location within the system, regardless of its point of origin.

*Protocol Development*

James identified three sources of ideas for developing and updating protocols: the medical literature, variance in outcomes data, and "spontaneous neat ideas." In the first situation, for example, the Development Team for cardiovascular care scoured the medical literature (or guidelines published by professional societies, such as the American College of Cardiology) and found that IHC's rates of appropriate use of discharge medications for cardiovascular disease—57% for beta blockers—while significantly better than national average performance of 41%, or even the average major academic hospital of 49%, was still well below theoretic perfect performance of 100%. In response, the CV team created a check sheet with indications and contraindications for patient discharge medications. In the new system, the nurse wrote the order on the medication sheet and presented it to the physician for approval and signature. Exhibit 1–8 shows improvement in appropriate use of discharge medication following implementation of the new protocol.

In the second example, aggregated variance data were used to update protocols. Development Teams would look for statistically significant patterns of variance in process and outcome, with the view that they presented opportunities to improve the protocols. In 1995, in the course of analyzing outcomes data, a physician in family medicine recognized a split among the physician population in choice of antibiotics for Community Acquired Pneumonia (CAP). Part of the variance was attributed to a debate between two macrolides: clarithromycin and azithromycin. The development team conducted a literature review, which suggested no

**Exhibit 1–8**　Protocol for Discharge Medication

2000 Hospital Discharge Medicine Goals:
Patients discharged from the cardiovascular (or main medical) unit(s)
achieve at least 90% compliance with appropriate discharge medications:
  1. Ischemic Heart disease (aspirin, HMG agent; beta blocker post-
     Myocardial Infarction (MI))
  2. Heart failure due to Left Ventricular dysfunction (ACE inhibitor)
  3. Atrial fibrillation (Coumadin)

Percent eligible patients treated at discharge with appropriate
  medications, 2000

|  | Before Protocol | After Protocol | National Rate |
|---|---|---|---|
| Beta blockers | 57% | 91% | 41% |
| ACE/ ARB inhibitors | 63 | 94 | 62 |
| Statins | 75 | 95 | 37 |
| Antiplatelet | 42 | 99 | 70 |
| Wafarin | 10 | 90 | |

Mortality and Readmissions within one year of discharge

|  | Mortality | | Readmissions | |
|---|---|---|---|---|
|  | Before Protocol | After Protocol | Before Protocol | After Protocol |
| Chronic Heart Failure (n519,083) | 22.7% | 17.8% | 46.5% | 38.5% |
| Ischemic Heart Disease (n543,841) | 4.5 | 3.5 | 20.4 | 17.7 |

Source:　　Intermountain Health Care

difference in efficacy. Dissatisfied with the medical literature, the group launched a randomized controlled trial and found improved outcomes were associated with azithromicin or a second class of antibiotics called quinolones, and specifically, levoflocacin. The protocol was written to indicate azithromicin or levoflocacin as default antibiotics for the outpatient management of CAP.[12]

---

[12]Following this, significant resistance (as high as 20%) to azithromicin developed among inpatients treated for CAP within IHC, leading to further modifications to the protocol.

**Exhibit 1–9**   CAP Outcomes Tracking

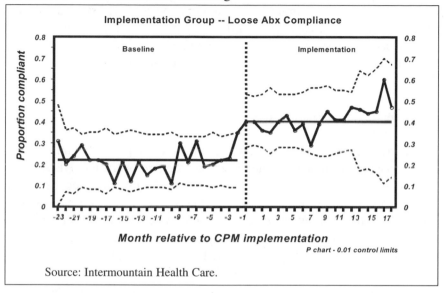

Source: Intermountain Health Care.

Finally, as James explained, "Sometimes people just come up with a neat idea," a result of many years of practice and the accumulation of subtle observations about patient care. James cited LDS Hospital internist Dr. Alan Morris as an example: "Morris has all sorts of hunches that he tests. His ICU is a little learning lab. At one point he had three trials running, all using his standard ventilator hypoxemia protocol as the control arm."

To assess the effectiveness of protocols and other clinical management strategies, James and his colleagues developed an outcomes tracking system based on a "drill down" mentality. Starting with key clinical processes, they iteratively refined the set to identify the most pertinent measures. They took care to develop a set of balanced measures, including medical outcomes,[13] patient perceptions of functional status, service quality, and cost. (See Exhibit 1–9 for an example of outcomes tracking for CAP.) James explained, "The aim was to develop data that showed appropriate intermediate and final outcomes within those categories aligned

---

[13]*Medical outcomes* is defined as appropriateness of referral and procedures (indications guidelines), complications, and achievement of therapeutic goals developed among inpatients treated for CAP within IHC, leading to further modifications to the protocol.

along the clinical processes of care." The pilot programs allowed James and Burton to test the Clinical Program Guidance Council structure for organizing families of care, developing flow charts, setting annual clinical goals (focused on one aspect of care), and gathering data on current practice while simultaneously working to standardize and improve it.

## Integrated Management Structure

Having built a new clinical management structure parallel to the existing line management, James planned to merge the two over time. His strategy for merging the two structures was to encourage interdependence so the groups would realize "they have to be joined at the hip." Both branches of the parallel structure reviewed clinical goals and assessed outcome data according to their level of focus (i.e., individual physician, practice group, or region). Exhibit 1–10 provides more detail.) James continued:

> We build it up parallel, give the medical management structure tight links and shared goals with the traditional administration, and then let the two management structures collapse together, into a single structure. We hope that over time they will experience and see the redundancy and ask themselves, "Why are we holding two meetings?" and merge of their own accord.

IHC's integrated management structure was cemented in 1998 when the format of the annual board-level goals was revised to include two or three goals per clinical program. (Exhibit 1–11 lists goals for the CV program.) James stated that one-third of board meeting time was devoted to clinical outcomes, which was far above the norm; the remaining two-thirds were focused on service quality performance and a traditional financial performance review.

Finally, IHC senior management's existing withhold-incentive-pay system was changed to reflect the new balanced priorities. The board established a median salary for each senior management position based on a survey of other not-for-profit delivery systems similar in size to IHC. Twenty-five percent of the median salary was withheld from senior management but could be won back by meeting goals. Prior to Nelson assuming the role of CEO, nearly all goals were financial, but he changed the salary withheld so that one-third was based on medical-outcome goals,

**Exhibit 1–10**  Parallel Administrative Structure

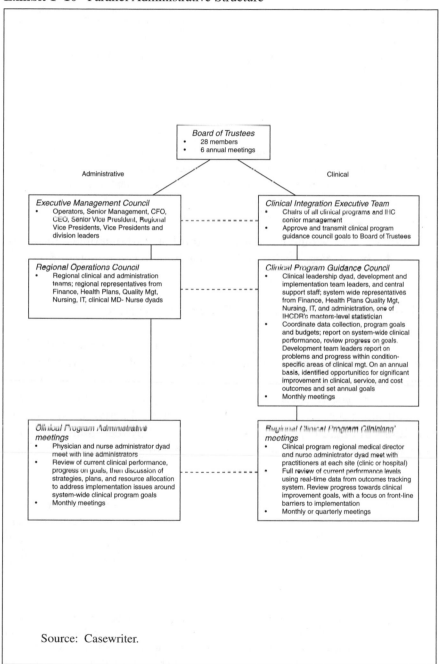

**Board of Trustees**
- 28 members
- 6 annual meetings

Administrative

Clinical

**Executive Management Council**
- Operators, Senior Management, CFO, CEO, Senior Vice President, Regional Vice Presidents, Vice Presidents and division leaders

**Clinical Integration Executive Team**
- Chairs of all clinical programs and IHC senior management
- Approve and transmit clinical program guidance council goals to Board of Trustees

**Regional Operations Council**
- Regional clinical and administration teams; regional representatives from Finance, Health Plans, Quality Mgt, Nursing, IT, clinical MD- Nurse dyads

**Clinical Program Guidance Council**
- Clinical leadership dyad, development and implementation team leaders, and central support staff; system wide representatives from Finance, Health Plans Quality Mgt, Nursing, IT, and administration, one of IHCDR's masters-level statistician
- Coordinate data collection, program goals and budgets; report on system-wide clinical performance, review progress on goals. Development team leaders report on problems and progress within condition-specific areas of clinical mgt. On an annual basis, identified opportunities for significant improvement in clinical, service, and cost outcomes and set annual goals
- Monthly meetings

**Clinical Program Administrative meetings**
- Physician and nurse administrator dyad meet with line administrators
- Review of current clinical performance, progress on goals, then discussion of strategies, plans, and resource allocation to address implementation issues around system-wide clinical program goals
- Monthly meetings

**Regional Clinical Program Clinicians' meetings**
- Clinical program regional medical director and nurse administrator dyad meet with practitioners at each site (clinic or hospital)
- Full review of current performance levels using real-time data from outcomes tracking system. Review progress towards clinical improvement goals, with a focus on front-line barriers to implementation
- Monthly or quarterly meetings

Source:  Casewriter.

**Exhibit 1–11**   2001 System Goals for Cardiovascular Clinical Program

Exceed national standards for timeliness of reperfusion for ST-Elevation
  MI's
Prescribe appropriate hospital discharge medicines for CAD, heart failure,
  atrial fibrillation
Stabilize readmission rate after hospitalization for ischemic syndromes
Achieve CV surgical mortality rate lower than national standards
Achieve average extubation time after CV surgery of 7.5 hours or lower
Improve CV surgical costs
Implement evidence-based indications/ guidelines for 13 CV procedures
Inpatients with heart failure document LV ejection fraction and provide diet,
  smoking cessation, weight, and medication management instructions

Source: Intermountain Health Care.

one-third on service outcomes, and one-third on cost outcomes. In James' words, this had "a very positive effect on getting the administrators to look at the clinical side of things."

## CLINICAL CARE MANAGEMENT: OPERATIONS

Most health care delivery systems ran two parallel, redundant, data systems. Clinicians (i.e., physicians and nurses) maintained a medical record, while administrators tracked financial measures for billing and facility management. The financial information was captured, in large part, from the clinical process. Data were moved from clinical activities to financial operations through, (1) chart abstraction, and (2) by recording all billable clinical services (e.g., a dose of a drug, an imaging examination, or use of a procedure room).[14]

James noted that "such parallel data systems violate a key principle of data management—to obtain accurate data, collect data once, at its point of origin." Moreover, such redundancy was wasteful. At one point, IHC estimated that as much as 15% of its single largest business expense, salary for operational staff, was devoted to entering data into the billing/ financial tracking system.

---

[14]Chart abstraction in most hospitals was notoriously inaccurate and a potential source of significant management problems relative to fraud and abuse in health care payment. The average hospital took more than three months to prepare a final bill, with every bill seeing a large number of corrections and changes after the fact. One study of bill accuracy estimated that over 50% of all final hospital bills contained at least one significant error.

## The Patient Care Management System

The Patient Care Management System (PCMS) was conceived in 1997 when Burton and James asked themselves if it would be possible to organize nursing services by task and then structure an electronic clinical data collection system accordingly. James explained, "It's that old idea of work processes that has worked so well in industry. PCMS is a new thing for health care but it's not new to Alcoa Aluminum." Part of the impetus for the PCMS was to reduce redundant data collection. Once nursing services (and all support services) were defined by type of task they could create one data system for clinical charting that would automatically generate billing data. The PCMS would also embed clinical protocols in a clinical workstation (a computer).

Burton and James' team identified four subcategories of nursing tasks: assessment, intervention, monitoring, and patient comfort and education. These categories were derived from a hierarchy of clinical reasoning that began with a functional problem list (making a diagnosis) to a goal list (how should the problem be controlled), and finally, a task list (actions to achieve the goal).

For example, a patient presenting with an acute myocardial infarction (heart attack) would be entered into the computer system with left ventricular myocardial infarction (the functional problem). A window with a series of sub problems would pop up on the screen. Some of the sub-problems, such as decreased coronary blood flow and oxygenation, were automatically generated, while an optional series of other problems could be checked off by the physician. Identification of the functional problem and sub problem would trigger a list of goals, including pain management and restoring blood flow through the heart. Each goal was directly linked to a series of orders or tasks, including follow-up patient monitoring tasks, to be performed by physicians and nursing staff. (See Exhibit 1–12 for an example of clinical care management interventions for diabetes.) The PCMS incorporated decision support into the order set so that the system could automatically calculate, for example, morphine dosing for pain control.

In 2001, IHC partnered with the Mayo Clinic and Stanford to develop the protocols (goal and task lists for major diagnoses) and with the health care information-systems firm IDX Systems Corporation to develop the software platform. IHC planned to go live on a pilot basis at Primary Children's Hospital, two floors of LDS Hospital, and the medical surgery floor at American Fork Hospital in April of 2003.

**Exhibit 1–12**  Examples of Clinical-Care Management Intervention

15 Mar 99                                                                ID# 12345

## Clinical Workstation Diabetes Worksheet

| PATIENT NAME | SEX | DOB | |
|---|---|---|---|
| DOE, JOHN Q. | M | 05/21/1933 | - Diabetes Mellitus [250] |

**Active Medications**

1. - Glucophage (metformin hcl), 500mg, tablet, 1 tablet bid

| HgbA1c (<=7.0) | | LDL (<100) | TriG(<200) | BP (<135/85) | |
|---|---|---|---|---|---|
| 02/10/1999  6.6% | 02/10/1999 | 113 mg/dl | 211 mg/dl | 02/10/1999 | 136/84 mmHg |
| 11/29/1998  6.9% | | | | 11/29/1998 | 130/80 mmHg |
| 10/11/1998  7.5% | | | | 10/11/1998 | 130/78 mmHg |

| UA Protein | uAlb/Cr (<30) | 24° Urine Albumin (<30) |
|---|---|---|
| 10/11/1998  Negative | 10/29/1998   9.55 | |

| Dilated retinal exam | Pedal sensory exam |
|---|---|
| 10/11/1998   Robert Christiansen, MD | 10/11/1998   Normal |

15 Mar 99                                                                       1

### Clinical Workstation Diabetes Action List

**Physician Name:** XXXXXX, XXXXXX X (Internal Medicine)

| | | | Examinations Presently Due | | | |
|---|---|---|---|---|---|---|
| Pt. Name | IDX-MRN | A1c | Lipid Panel | Urine Protein | Retinal Exam | Sensory Exam |
| XXXXX, XXXXXX X | XXXXXXX | 15DEC1998 | 13FEB1998 | 13FEB1998 | | |
| XXX, XXXXXX X | XXXXXXX | | | | 9MAR1998 | |
| XXXXXX, XXXXX | XXXXXXX | 12SEP1998 | | | 11MAR1998 | 11MAR1998 |
| XXXX, XXXXXXXX X | XXXXXXX | 9AUG1998 | | 14MAR1998 | | |
| XXXXXXXX, XXXXXX | XXXXXXX | 11MAR1998 | 11MAR1998 | 11MAR1998 | | 11MAR1998 |
| XXXXXXXXX, XXXXX | XXXXXXX | | 08MAR1998 | 08MAR1998 | 11MAR1998 | |
| XXXXX, XXXXXXXXX | XXXXXXX | | 24FEB1998 | 24FEB1998 | 9MAR1998 | |
| XXXXXXXXXX, XXXXX | XXXXXXX | 4DEC1997 | 4DEC1997 | 4DEC1997 | 22DEC1997 | 4DEC1997 |
| XXXXX, XXXXXX X | XXXXXXX | 29NOV1998 | | 3MAR1998 | | |
| XXXX, XXXXX X | XXXXXXX | 14AUG1998 | | | | |
| XXXXX, XXXXX X | XXXXXXX | 12AUG1998 | | | | |

Source: Intermountain Health Care.

**Clinical Information Systems**

James believed that IHC could "make it easy to do it right" by embedding protocols in the PCMS and making them the default option for care. The next step, after successful paper-based pilots of the PCMS, was to automate patient medical records and make them dynamic electronic documents that could interact with the electronic PCMS. To achieve this level of standardization, James turned to IHC's IT system, and more specifically, the EMR.

*The Electronic Medical Record*

Two heuristics governed James' strategy to encourage physician usage of the EMR: (1) every stage paid for itself, and (2) it had to fit into the flow of practice. James explained, "The rule is you can't destroy clinical productivity." A major strength of the EMR was that usage was largely intuitive and each step in the adoption process prepared the user for the next. (See Exhibit 1–13.) James elaborated:

> When one of our physicians got to this point [using the EMR for clinical charting] we didn't have to even tell him about [the order function]. He found it on his own and it was literally a week to go from electronic charting to online medication orders. The EMR doesn't require that you rethink the structure of the medical record—it's enough to ask you to move from paper to computer.

In addition to encouraging PCMS compliance, the EMR had several features for specialists—for example, the Antibiotic Assistant and automated ventilator settings—that supported the decision making associated with routine care.

*Antibiotic Assistant*

One of IHC's more popular decision support tools was the Antibiotic Assistant.[15] Given a list of possible sources of infection, Antibiotic Assistant applied a protocol to perform a customized epidemiologic

---

[15]Antibiotic Assistant was available across all of IHC's major facilities, including outpatient clinics.

**Exhibit 1–13**  EMR Roll-out

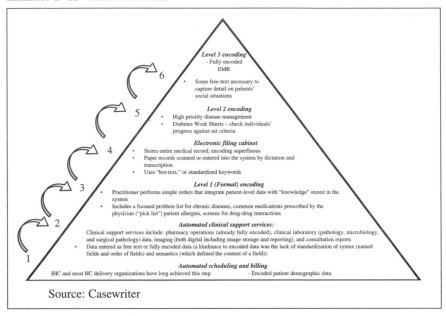

Level 3 encoding
- Fully encoded EMR
- Some free-text necessary to capture detail on patients' social situations

*Level 2 encoding*
- High priority disease management
- Diabetes Work Sheets – check individuals' progress against set criteria

*Electronic filing cabinet*
- Stores entire medical record; encoding superfluous
- Paper records scanned or entered into the system by dictation and transcription
- Uses "hot-text," or standardized keywords

*Level 1 (Formal) encoding*
- Practitioner performs simple orders that integrate patient-level data with "knowledge" stored in the system
- Includes a focused problem list for chronic diseases, common medications prescribed by the physician ("pick list") patient allergies, screens for drug-drug interactions

*Automated clinical support services:*
Clinical support services include: pharmacy operations (already fully encoded), clinical laboratory (pathology, microbiology, and surgical pathology) data, imaging (both digital including image storage and reporting), and consultation reports
- Data entered as free text or fully encoded data (a hindrance to encoded data was the lack of standardization of syntax (named fields and order of fields) and semantics (which defined the content of a field))

*Automated scheduling and billing*
IHC and most HC delivery organizations have long achieved this step          - Encoded patient demographic data

Source: Casewriter

assessment of a patient, producing (1) a list of "most likely" causative pathogens, and (2) a list of the most appropriate antibiotic regimens to treat that set of possible sources of infection, including such factors as allergies, drug-drug interactions, and ideal patient-specific dosing. The program incorporated current antibiotic sensitivities in the hospital population. Dr. Colin Grissom, an academic attending in the ICU at LDS Hospital, stated, "I use this as a guide. I generally make my own decisions, but the great thing about it is the drug information."

*Ventilator Settings*

A second function of the EMR, available in the ICU of LDS Hospital, advised physicians and nurses about optimal ventilator settings customized to a particular patient. Additionally, it standardized the procedures followed by respiratory therapists for taking patients off the ventilator. For example, one ventilator weaning rule stipulated that a patient should always be taken off in the morning so that they could be off the ventilator during daytime hours, when more physicians were in-house.

## Encouraging Physician Buy-in

Two features attracted physicians to the EMR: increased productivity and protocol override.

### *Increased Productivity*

Physician use of the automated Diabetes Work Sheet bumped up a typical outpatient visit from Level 1 to Level 4,[16] allowing physicians to document and appropriately bill $75 for a visit instead of $35. (Use of the Work Sheets, shown in Exhibit 1–12, also boosted a patient's abilities to self-manage and reduced the incidence and prevalence of diabetes-related complications.) Additionally, entering data into the system during a patient consult meant that fewer resources were spent on transcription. In one study, a group of six physicians decreased their average transcription cost per relative value unit (RVU) from $2.50 to $.20.[17] Clinical note-taking was facilitated by the default options on each screen which represented the most common care strategy.

### *Override Capability*

James' vision for the PCMS hinged on the idea that one "designed for the common and managed the uncommon cases individually."[18] He clarified, "No protocol fits *every* patient, and no protocol perfectly fits *any* patient." All physicians were granted override capability; if they did not want to follow the recommended orders automatically generated for a particular patient, they were prompted to type their reason for varying into the system. IHC designed this function not as a way to track instances of physician "disobedience" but to learn from exceptions. There were two

---

[16]The workload associated with a consultation was graded into four levels based on a relative value scale. For more detail see W.C. Hsaio, "The Resource-Based Relative Value Scale: Toward the development of an alternative physician payment system." *Journal of the American Medical Association* 258(6), (1987): 799–802.

[17]S.D. Narus and P. D. Clayton, "Clinical Information Systems at Intermountain Health Care," *Decisions in Imaging Economics, Special Projects Supplement,* February 2002.

[18]Institute of Medicine, *Crossing the Quality Chasm.* Washington, D.C.: National Academy Press, 2001, p. 128.

options for variation from the protocol: the protocol was wrong and it should be modified; or the protocol was correct but the patient presented with significant complications so the protocol was not applicable. To James, the latter situation was "random noise."

## REALIZING THE BENEFITS OF CLINICAL MANAGEMENT

By the mid-1990s, IHC clinical-improvement projects routinely showed significant cost savings, but system administrators kept complaining that they were not seeing concomitant improvements in their operating budgets; net operating income was not improving, even though documented cost reductions suggested that they should be. The puzzle was resolved when James was preparing results of a new protocol for community acquired pneumonia (CAP). (See Exhibit 1–14.) For the first time, James ran reimbursement as well as cost figures and found that if a CAP patient had a major complication, it changed their DRG. The most common switch was from DRG 89 (uncomplicated CAP) to DRG 475 (ventilator support). DRG 475 paid about $16,400 per case; by contrast, reimbursement for DRG 89 was $4,600, with an average real cost to the facility of $5,400. The protocol saved money by changing physicians' choice of antibiotics to treat CAP, resulting in significantly lower complication and mortality rates. While costs had dropped by about $1.2 million, Medicare reimbursement, secondary to the shifts in DRG categories, had dropped by almost $1.7 million. James presented this finding—outstanding clinical outcomes and distressing financial news—to IHC's top 25 managers. He remembered:

> I took them down through all the clinical changes, how the protocol worked, change in complication and mortality rates, the cost data and, finally, the reimbursement data. Then I apologized, basically. It turned out all the savings floated back to CMS, leaving us holding the bag for the cost of the project and a net loss of [Medicare] reimbursement. Bill Nelson, our CEO, publicly chastised me for apologizing, but it's one of the few times that it felt good to be scolded. He said, "You will not apologize for better patient outcomes." What he was really doing was using this to deliver a message to the rest of the managers. Bill said, "I expect clinical management like that to be done. It's our job as administration to figure out how to balance the finances."

**Exhibit 1–14**   Community Acquired Pneumonia Protocol Compliance, 1994–1995

|                                  | 1994<br>Before Protocol | 1995<br>With Protocol |
|----------------------------------|:----------------------:|:---------------------:|
| Percent patients admitted        | 39                     | 29                    |
| Average length of stay (days)    | 6.4                    | 4.3                   |
| Time to antibiotic (hours)       | 2.1                    | 1.5                   |
| Average cost per case ($)        | 2,752                  | 1,424                 |

Source: Intermountain Health Care.

Building on that initial experience, IHC developed three strategies by which the clinical management system could harvest savings back from payers and boost revenues: (1) picking projects based on their ability to bring back savings to the health care provider; (2) contracting strategies to insurers that sold on the basis of true price, not discount; and (3) "shared benefit" contracts under which IHC Health Services (the delivery organization), IHC Health Plans (the payer), and Clinical Program physicians equally split quality-derived savings. James explained:

> The first strategy is not very attractive—you end up leaving too many good projects on the table. Under the second strategy, you start to sell [health care delivery services to insurers] on the basis of true price, not on the size of the discount. In most commercial medical markets in the country today, you get the contract based on the size of your discount. In essence, you tell a purchaser, "Last year we gave you a 9% discount from billed charges. This year, we propose to give you only a 7% discount—but because of our clinical improvement, you will still be ahead financially." The third strategy is the best of all, because all of the key players have some skin in the improvement game.

In 1999, Burton and Sidney Paulson, Health Plans CEO, piloted the third strategy as a three-way risk and benefit-sharing arrangement between physicians, IHC, and the insurer if a given clinical program came in below their actuarial projections by demonstrating improvements in care.[19] However, the physician population was wary of the proposal: while

---

[19]The shared benefit approach routed distribution of the savings through the insurance arm of the organization—IHC Health Plans—so that the final approach could meet federal fraud and abuse standards.

IHC originally proposed that the physicians, as a group, accept 20% of the risk, the physicians ultimately accepted a smaller upside benefit to avoid any direct downside risk. The health plan and IHC Health Services split the downside risk evenly. James estimated that within the Primary Care Clinical Program pilot, the annual payout per physician was about $3,000. James anticipated expansion of risk sharing to specialty physicians as they implemented the outcomes tracking system. In 2002, IHC's senior management began "marketing" Clinical Integration and its shared-benefit cost models to their larger insurance partners. Prior to that, it had been used only for the health plans' large employer segment—large, self-insured employers who purchased all insurance services through IHC Health Plans.

## THE LONG-TERM PLAN

Reflecting on the Clinical Integration meeting and the nurse's alarm about standardizing care, James realized that he had been hosting an internal debate on this topic for years. Would physicians adopt best practices on their own, or must best practice be paired with measurement and accountability systems? In addition to thinking about incentives, about what constituted "best practice," and about how to develop systems that would simultaneously increase the quality of care and decrease cost, James listed progress on the implementation of the clinical care management system. In mid-2002, five of the Clinical Programs (CV, Neuromusculoskeletal, Women & Newborn, Oncology, and Primary Care) were in use; the remaining four would be up by 2007. Four of 500 conditions (acute myocardial infarction, bronchitis, CAP, and total hip replacement) in the PCMS were running, albeit on paper. The IT department hoped to have 35 conditions charted by the end of 2002 and 75 by the end of 2003, at which point the PCMS would go live.

James realized that it would take at least ten years to fully consolidate the clinical management structure and get all components of Clinical Integration running; however, that period was negligible compared to how long it would take to get IHC's physicians to subscribe to the concept. He commented:

> Dr. W. Edwards Deming once said, "If you want to convert the culture of an organization, and that organization contains *n*

people you first need to convert the square root of n." Well, he should have added, "You specifically need the early adopters." It's not just *any* square root of n. I've got about 1,200 core physicians, so the square root is somewhere between 30 and 40. There was a palpable change in the medical staff when we crossed that number. It wasn't just Brent James, partially tainted by being over in the administration offices, saying that physicians as a profession needed to do this. It was a long list of respected physicians who could say, "Guys, I've done this in my practice and it really makes sense. It's better care for our patients, a better lifestyle for me, and more productive."

## CASE ANALYSIS

This case shows the effect of consistent clinical leadership over time when influenced by industrial leaders in continuous quality improvement (CQI) like Dr. Deming. Note the length of time that it has taken to have a major impact on the effectiveness of the institution. Dr. James is a recognized leader in clinical quality improvement at the national level, a fellow of the Institute of Medicine, and a contributor to its influential reports.

## ASSIGNMENT QUESTIONS

### Introduction

1. How has Dr. James gone about introducing the concepts of Deming's "total quality management" into the health care environment?
2. How effective has this effort been overall? What has been its measurable impact at IHC?

### Basics

3. What are the fundamental attitudes toward variability in clinical practices exhibited in this case?

    4. How does Intermountain Health Care illustrate the role of the "shadow organization" in clinical CQI? Why has this aspect of the organization undergone so many changes over time?

    5. Compare and contrast the CQI effort at IHC with the models of team building in Chapter 6. How would you describe the current stage of team development at the end of the case?

## Implementation

    6. How has IHC set itself up to be a learning organization?

    7. What have been the contextual variables affecting the implementation of CQI at IHC?

## Application

    8. IHS provides a wide range of services at its many locations and facilities? What can you learn from their experience about the application of CQI concepts in multisite and diverse organizations?

## CLASS EXERCISE

Use the Internet to follow up on any changes in the clinical quality program at Intermountain Health Care (www.ihc.com/xp/ihc). Then interview quality improvement leaders and implementers at institutions in your area to ascertain how their clinical quality improvement efforts have been proceeding? How have they paralleled or differed from the IHC approach? Have the results been similar or different? Why?

# CASE 2

# Quality in Pediatric Subspecialty Care

*William A. Sollecito, Peter A. Margolis, Paul V. Miles,
Robert Perelman, and Richard B. Colletti*

The American Board of Pediatrics (ABP) is one of 24 certifying boards of the American Board of Medical Specialties (ABMS). ABP awards certificates in the 13 pediatric subspecialties listed in Exhibit 2-1. Certification provides assurance to the public and the profession that a pediatrician has successfully completed an accredited educational program and possesses "the knowledge, skills, and experience requisite to the provision of high-quality care in pediatrics." Historically, certification was based on individual knowledge rather than actual performance in practice. Evidence has shown significant variation in medical care, even among board-certified physicians, indicating that medical knowledge alone is not sufficient to ensure high quality of care. In response to this evidence, the ABMS voted to create a more continuous process of recertification. By 2010, 85% of U.S. physicians will be required to participate in ongoing maintenance-of-certificate programs to document competency in performance, practice, and systems-based thinking in addition to the current requirements for medical knowledge, communication skills, and professional behavior.

As a component of this evolving certification process, ABP launched the Quality in Pediatric Subspecialty Care (QPSC) initiative in the fall of 2003 "to improve the health care delivery system for children with complex medical conditions." Based on previous studies of how to apply CQI principles in individual pediatric practices, ABP decided to use a mass customization approach and extend the lessons learned to each pediatric subspecialty incrementally. The common elements of CQI and mass customization are the sharing of existing knowledge and experiences among peers to achieve mutually agreed-upon improvement goals, using data-

**Exhibit 2–1**   13 Pediatric Subspecialties

| | |
|---|---|
| • Adolescent Medicine | • Hematology-Oncology |
| • Cardiology | • Infectious Diseases |
| • Critical Care | • Neonatology |
| • Developmental and Behavioral Pediatrics | • Nephrology |
| • Emergency Medicine | • Pulmonology |
| • Endocrinology | • Rheumatology |
| • Gastroenterology | |

driven collaborative learning techniques. This was a multilevel plan to improve performance, not only of individual practitioners but of an entire profession, by first motivating and educating all pediatricians in the principles of CQI and then changing the standards of care by requiring quality improvement principles as part of the continuing education and certification process.

## BACKGROUND

Pediatricians and other child health care clinicians strive to ensure the health of the children and families they serve. Numerous studies, however, have shown wide and persistent variation in outcomes across providers and communities. In its report, *Crossing the Quality Chasm,* the Institute of Medicine (2001) identified problems in the system of health care delivery rather than deficiencies in individual physicians as the major impediment to quality health care for all Americans. In pediatrics, for example, where robust systems have been defined and implemented, the results have been dramatic. The Children's Oncology Group captures information on over 80% of children in the United States with cancer. Children with cancer participate in ongoing clinical trials focusing on new therapies and in studies of how to improve the delivery of existing therapies. Subsequently, the five-year survival rate of children under age 15 with acute lymphocytic leukemia was 85% in 2002 (Leukemia and Lymphoma Society 2002). This represents a more than doubling of the survival rate in the last quarter of the 20th century. However, such approaches are not widely used, leaving enormous opportunities to improve the care of children with chronic diseases. For example, the staff of the Cystic Fibrosis Foundation estimated that the average 33.5-year life of individuals with cystic fibrosis (CF) could be extend by seven years simply by applying current knowledge to every child with this condition (Schechter and Margolis 2004). Collaborative learning approaches have been developed to spread existing knowledge among practitioners. The efficacy of quality improvement approaches in a controlled setting has been demonstrated by several authors, including Margolis *et al.,* (2004) just prior to the initiation of QPSC. While clearly successful, at that point in time the use of quality improvement had been limited to specific clinical areas and/or relatively small numbers of practices. A logical priority, which was identified in 2003, was to increase impact and disseminate the learnings from previous successes by extending these quality improvement methods on a larger scale.

## COMPONENTS

The aim of QPSC is to improve the health care delivery process for children with complex medical conditions by changing the way that subspecialists practice. This change program relies on a unique process that integrates the three components outlined in Exhibit 2–2: (1) national databases/registries of key childhood illness (e.g., inflammatory bowel disease) developed and coordinated through a national data coordinating center; (2) subspecialty-wide multicenter collaborative improvement activities among pediatric sub-specialists, and (3) web-based improvement/ educational modules.

These components of this model are integrated as follows:

> National databases and a national database support center: Most conditions managed by pediatric subspecialists are not seen frequently enough to provide a single medical center with sufficient data to study or improve the treatment. Experience with children's oncology, low birth-weight infants, and cystic fibrosis have shown the value of national databases for important but relatively infrequent pediatric problems. National databases are essential for understanding variations in care and outcomes and for providing opportunities to learn from high-performing organizations. Each pediatric subspecialty identifies one or more "key" conditions, surgical procedures, or

**Exhibit 2–2**

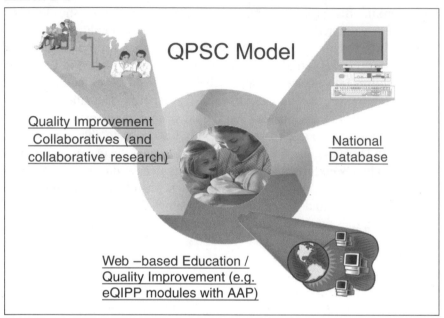

processes that are central to the specialty. After the identification of this clinical content, a practical, useful database is developed around children with that condition, procedure, or process.

National improvement collaboratives: Each subspecialty design its own collaborative improvement program around the topic selected for its database-registry. These collaborative activities help identify those process changes with the most potential and specify the sequence in which they are undertaken. Physicians have shown willingness to collect and submit performance data that is valid and complete when it is clear to them that the aim is to improve care and not to sanction "poor performers."

Education-improvement activities: A major component of the model is the use of on-line education-improvement activities as exemplified by the eQIPP program developed by the American Academy of Pediatrics. These activities enable individual subspecialists to do self-assessments of how they practice and how they can improve their quality of care for a specific disease entity. Each pediatric subspecialty develops a Web-based module alone or in conjunction with other subspecialties on subjects of broad application in the pediatric community.

## ORGANIZATIONAL STRUCTURE

An important key to success in applying CQI to a large, complex organization such as a subspecialty group is the creation of an organizational structure that motivates learning and improvement. Structures and procedures must be implemented to empower individuals and teams to take responsibility for change and continuous improvement with an outcome focus. Leadership is necessary at multiple levels; in medical care, physician leadership is crucial for the design of change, for developing incentives and opportunities, and for assembling resources. The QPSC seeks to foster that leadership by involving each subspecialty in the design and planning process. Also critical is the creation of a virtual partnership of complementary organizations to lead the process over time; these groups provide an infrastructure that guides each subspecialty through the improvement process and serves as an administrative and data coordination base for the program.

A flexible governance structure is defined by a program charter and managed by a QPSC (leadership) council that includes representatives of each of the partner organizations. The organizational structure of QPSC includes the following organizations:

- The American Board of Pediatrics (ABP): Located in Chapel Hill, NC, this organization was discussed earlier.
- The American Academy of Pediatrics (AAP): It supports the efforts of some 60,000 member health professionals on behalf of the health, well-being, and safety of infants, children, adolescents, and young adults. Members include pediatricians, pediatric medical subspecialists, and pediatric surgical specialists. Most board-certified pediatricians are members of AAP. The Academy's on-line system, Education in Quality Improvement for Pediatric Practices (eQIPP), is used to disseminate knowledge and assist subspecialty pediatricians in implementing practice improvements, as well as enabling them to meet recertification requirements.
- The UNC School of Public Health (UNC-SPH): This organization contributes expertise in epidemiology, health behavior, biostatistics,

child health at the population level, and public health leadership to QSPC. The school has operated an internet-based data collection system to support collaborative improvement activities and has developed software applications designed to support thousands of simultaneous users. The UNC SPH Instructional and Information Systems (IIS) group provides the information technology, software development, and database management systems required for this program. The Public Health Leadership Program's role is to contribute expertise on large scale organizational design, project management, and continuous improvement.

- The North Carolina Center for Children's Health Care Improvement (NC-CHI), located in the UNC School of Medicine has as its mission elimination of gaps in care for children and adolescents. It is the national program office for QPSC. This center has worked on practice-based improvement since 1992 and supported over 20 collaborative improvement programs over five years prior to the start of QPSC. Its primary role is to provide expertise and guidance in implementing collaborative improvement activities. Its Data Coordinating Center provides large-scale data management and statistical support, in conjunction with the IIS group at the UNC School of Public Health.

## Implementation Teams

Management of the implementation process involves a team-based matrix program management structure for each improvement project. The teams interact directly with each subspecialty group and cut across each of the partner organizations to insure optimal knowledge sharing and efficiency. The implementation teams for the initiation of QPSC were:

1. Collaborative learning and improvement
2. Educational module development and implementation
3. Data management and statistics
4. Software systems development and support
5. Research

Each of these teams is represented on the overall coordination team headed by a program director. The QPSC Council and the implementation teams are supported further by a set of subcommittees that coordinate design, governance, and fund-raising activities. An advisory board provides guidance and insure input from all constituencies, including patients and their families.

## Collaborative Improvement

The key CQI component of QPSC is the application of Deming's "System of Profound Knowledge" (1986). Each improvement effort within a subspecialty is framed within a generic model for managing improvement (Langley *et al.* 1996) asking "What are we trying to accomplish?"; "What changes can we make that will result in improvement?"; and "How will we know that a change is an improvement?" This approach provides a framework, at a large scale, for the use of Shewhart (PDSA) cycles to determine how to implement improvements in care within the network of collaborating provider centers. Successful changes or "best practices" are identified, summarized by the subspecialty leadership structure, and hopefully deployed across the collaborative network. Exhibit 2–3 describes the QPSC application of this system to support sub-specialty societies and physicians including the assignment of functions and feedback loops that allow for system improvement. The system is partitioned into leadership processes such as planning, service activities for subspecialty societies such as collaborative learning, and program support processes. The leadership role of the QPSC council is also clearly identified. The overall aim of this system is to improve the health of children by improving the quality of pediatric subspecialty care.

## Previous Examples

Just prior to the initiation of QPSC, the Cystic Fibrosis Foundation sponsored a very successful application of the quality improvement processes that were to be adopted on a larger scale in QPSC. The Cystic Fibrosis Collaborative made a number of between-center comparisons and found centers with life expectancies as much as 50% above the national average. The collaborative noted the potential to improve children's health outcomes by improving nutritional counseling and reducing children's exposure to tobacco smoke, thereby improving lung function. Most pediatric specialists were comfortable with the nutrition intervention, but were less knowledgeable and experienced in getting parents to stop smoking. The team went to work on improvements in both areas and preliminary analyses indicated positive results (Schechter and Margolis 2004).

**Exhibit 2–3**   QPSC System

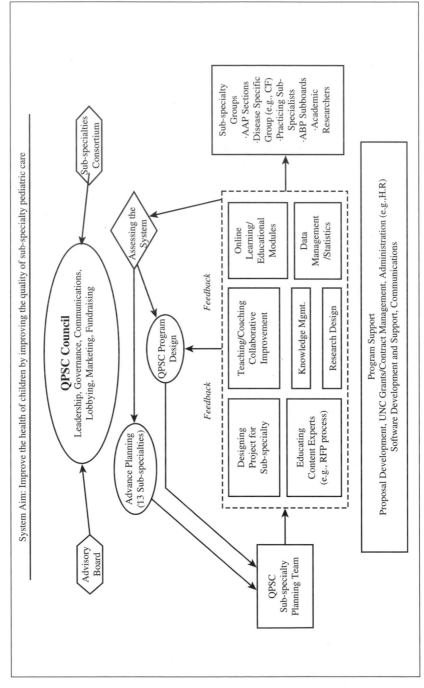

System Aim: Improve the health of children by improving the quality of sub-specialty pediatric care

## AN INCREMENTAL APPROACH

A traditional CQI transitional model of incremental change was adopted by QPSC. This meant working with one subspecialty as a "pilot group"; and through continuous learning, building on the experience gained there, expand to all 13 pediatric subspecialties. The improvement targets for each subspecialty were to include measures such as:

- Measurable improvement in children's health
- Percentage of subspecialists contributing data to the national registry
- Percentage of subspecialists participating in the national collaborative
- Percentage of subspecialists successfully completing eQIPP programs
- Number of independent, self-sustaining efforts

### The NASPGHAN Pilot

The North American Society for Pediatric Gastroenterology, Hepatology and Nutrition (NASPGHAN) was selected to be the pilot subspecialty to develop, implement, and evaluate the QSPC model. Its membership includes almost all the 800 pediatric gastroenterologists in North America. NASPGHAN formed a pediatric inflammatory bowel disease (IBD) quality improvement and research network as its first initiative. This Pediatric IBD Network for Research and Improvement (PIBDNet) conducts collaborative improvement and research on the quality and safety of care delivered by member subspecialists to children with this condition.

Inflammatory bowel disease is the most common chronic and serious pediatric gastrointestinal disorder afflicting children and adolescents. Over 45,000 children and adolescents in North America suffer from IBD and more than 4,500 new cases are diagnosed annually. Yet there is a lack of evidence as to its optimal management and the safety and effectiveness of available treatments.

**Project Objectives for PIBDNet**

The project leadership defined the following objectives of this effort:

1. Engage 200 pediatric gastroenterologists in network activities within the first year.
2. Determine the extent of variation in care of children with IBD who are initiating treatment with 9-mercaptopurine/azathioprine (6-MP/AZA) or with infliximab and identify the predictors of a successful outcome of treatment.
3. Involve 10-15 GI practices in an "innovation community" that will work collaboratively to identify, test, and develop changes that can improve IBD care.
4. Spread to all NASPGHAN members care delivery strategies that will improve the quality and safety of care for children with IBD.
5. Develop an eQIPP module on nutrition to test on-line education and QI support in the context of other subspecialty improvement activities as a means of supporting ongoing dissemination of activities.
6. Measure the effectiveness of the program in terms of the following outcomes:
    a. reductions in gastrointestinal symptoms,
    b. improved growth and nutritional management of patients prior to and during treatment,
    c. increased family self-management skills, including adherence to 6MP/AZA therapy,
    d. reduction in medication side effects (e.g., steroid side effects),
    e. appropriate diagnostic evaluation prior to treatment,
    f. safe initial 6-MP/AZA administration,
    g. surveillance for adverse effects of 6-MP/AZA and infliximab, and
    h. reporting of serious adverse effects of treatment to the FDA.

**Program Development Status**

By the summer of 2004, NASPGHAN had created the PIBDNet, and approximately 40% of the NASPGHAN membership had volunteered to participate following initial e-mail solicitation. All of the individual components of the QPSC model had been implemented by the partner organizations. However, following the platform testing and pilot initiative, each of the components of the QPSC program would require further financial support to continue to scale them up to the degree necessary to reach all subspecialists and to meet ABP's aggressive timeline to implement the model in all subspecialties by 2010.

An evaluation of the NASPGHAN pilot program, including an assessment of ways to improve the efficiency of the implementation steps, is currently underway and planning has begun to expand the model to the next subspecialties. Early observations of needed program changes include:

1. Technology improvements for data collection/management systems, including the study of ways to interface with existing electronic medical record systems,
2. Further development of data quality assurance procedures to accommodate the large number practices to be included and the variety of data to be collected for each subspecialty,
3. New disease-specific eQIPP modules for each subspecialty, and
4. Management changes related to infrastructure growth.

Ongoing fund-raising was an important component that was to be managed by the QSPC Council. Costs appeared to be of the order of a million dollars for each subspecialty plus common infrastructure costs.


## CASE ANALYSIS

This case presents a very different approach to the improvement of quality in which the responsibility falls on professional societies and board certifying agencies to push the clinical quality agenda forward. At some point in the future, then, all professionals will have to show activity and results in this arena. This is quite different from the institutional roles envisioned in TQM and CQI efforts over the recent past. This will not be a rapid change, but likely will be quite controversial.


## ASSIGNMENT QUESTIONS

### Introduction

1. What should be the role of professional societies and certifying entities in promulgating the concepts of evidence-based medicine and CQI among its professional cadres?

2. How would one go about developing the business case for CQI in this setting?

## Basics

3. The data collected on cystic fibrosis clinical outcomes are considered the most complete of any disease in the country (Gawande 2004). How can the pediatric consortium and other credentialing bodies function where complete outcome data are not so available?

## Implementation

4. Contrast and compare the approaches to transformation and organizational learning in this case with that of Intermountain Health Care (Case 1) or West Florida Regional Medical Center (Case 4). Which is more likely to be effective? So why is this case so different?

## Application

5. The approach in this case would seem to benefit from some attention to the concepts of microsystems in Chapter 15. Suggest how those concepts might be worked into the ongoing efforts of these professional organizations.

## CLASS EXERCISE

- Interview leaders in your field(s) of health care and find out what they are doing to motivate change and improvement as a professional responsibility and challenge. Compare and contrast their efforts with the approach in Case 2.

# Community-Based Quality Improvement Efforts in Kingsport, Tennessee[1]

*Curtis P. McLaughlin and Kit N. Simpson*

Quality improvement has long been a community-wide concern in Kingsport, an industrial town of 52,000 in northeastern Tennessee, involving employers, the Chamber of Commerce, the school system, the community college, and both hospitals. The effort began in 1982 with Eastman Chemical Company (ECC), then a subsidiary of Eastman Kodak, the town's primary employer. Faced with stiff foreign competition in its markets, ECC adopted a program that included a customer focus, employee empowerment, statistical methods, performance management, continuous improvement, education, and management leaders training. The program received an all-out push in 1985 and by 1988 Eastman was one of the nine finalists for the Malcolm Baldrige National Quality Award. ECC won the award in 1993. Exhibit 3–1 provides a time line outlining a number of quality efforts in the community.

## QUALITY FIRST

In 1986, Eastman executives were instrumental in Chamber of Commerce sponsorship of a QUALITY FIRST training session for community leaders at Northeast State Community College (then called Tri-Cities Community College). The program was taught by two professors

---

[1]For further background and detail see McLaughlin and Simpson, 1994, McLaughlin 1995 and McLaughlin 1998.

**Exhibit 3–1**  Key Events of Community Collaboration and Quality
Improvement Efforts in Kingsport

| Year | Activity |
|------|----------|
| 1986 | QUALITY FIRST seminars begin and include hospitals |
|      | Hospitals establish internal quality improvement efforts |
| 1988 | Midwest Business Group on health selected Kingsport for demonstration site project |
|      | KAHIP founded |
|      | Eastman quality process implemented at Holston Valley Hospital |
| 1989 | First local health care utilization studies |
|      | Kingsport Tomorrow founded |
| 1990 | Visioning process for "Kingsport 2017" completed |
|      | KAHIP becomes Health Care Task Force of Kingsport Tomorrow |
|      | Kingsport IPA and Heritage HMO start quality process |
| 1993 | Heritage offers PPO product |
|      | Learning Collaborative Project (Drive Smart) started |
|      | Eastman Chemical Company wins Baldrige award |
| 1994 | Mountain State and Premier regional hospital networks formed |
|      | KAHIP Leadership Team reconstituted |
|      | Tri-Cities Health Alliance of employers formed |
| 1995 | State of Tennessee, Governor's Highway Safety Office begins to fund regional effort |
|      | Friends-In-Need Center opens |
|      | KAHIP revises mission and vision statement |
| 1996 | KAHIP undertakes and completes strategic planning process |
|      | Holston Valley and Bristol hospitals form Wellmont Health System |
|      | State mandates that regional health departments develop health status database |
|      | Eight regional law enforcement agencies participate in NETS activity |
| 1997 | Johnson City Medical Center acquires a number of Columbia HCA hospitals including Indian Path |
| 1998 | Regional health status data becomes available through the Community Database Team |
| 1999 | CHIP replaces KAHIP with a wider geographical focus. |
| 2003 | Receives "Connecting Communities for Better Health" funding |

from Jackson Community College in Michigan, where the QUALITY FIRST program was developed with assistance from the Ford Motor Company. QUALITY FIRST is a 16-week, project-focused program that emphasizes data collection and analysis, control charting, and prevention-of-error methods, all generally based on the precepts of W. Edwards Deming. The program is implemented within a company by choosing teams of four or more participants.

## COMMUNITY COMPETITION

In the early 1990s, the Tri-Cities area, involving Johnson City, TN, Kingsport, TN, Bristol, TN, and Bristol, VA was the nation's 82nd largest metropolitan statistical area (MSA), with a 1990 population of 437,147 and 480,415 in 2000. It ranked 31st out of the 281 MSAs in manufacturing earnings as a percent of total earnings in 1988. During the first quarter of 1991, when the national unemployment rate was 7.1%, Kingsport's rate was 3.8%, Johnson City's 5.6%, and Bristol TN-VA's 5.4%. The Tri-Cities area was heavily doctored, with five acute-care hospitals (one in Bristol, two in Kingsport, and two at East Tennessee State University in Johnson City). The university also includes a medical school. By mid-1991, Kingsport had 18 obstetrician-gynecologists. Hospital lengths of stay, despite managed care, were above the national average. Advertising for hospitals and doctors abounded in the press, on billboards, and in local business periodicals.

In 1991, both Holston Valley Hospital & Medical Center (HVHMC), a nonprofit community hospital, and Indian Path Medical Center, owned by Hospital Corporation of America (HCA), operated well below their licensed bed level. HVHMC was licensed for 540 beds after giving up 50 beds to help bring in a for-profit rehabilitation hospital, but operated 350 to 375 beds, having converted its wards and semi-private rooms to all-private room status. Most community-based physicians practiced at both hospitals and belonged to the Kingsport Independent Practitioners' Association (IPA), which contracted to deliver services to Heritage National Healthplan (an HMO established and owned by John Deere). Sixty-two percent of Eastman Chemical Company's employees were covered under contracts with Heritage. The rest were covered by Blue Cross-Blue Shield of Tennessee under a contract that provided a wide range of services, including some preventive care.

## COMMUNITY COOPERATION

Kingsport also became involved in a cooperative effort to improve the community's health. In 1988, the Midwest Business Group on Health, after studying health purchasing and quality assessment tools, received funding from the John A. Hartford Foundation of New York to develop three demonstration sites for community cooperation to stress teamwork and reduce variation in health. Kingsport became the first demonstration site. Someone at HCA, which itself had invested heavily in Deming-based quality management programs, suggested Kingsport and the request was finally brought to the attention of Mr. Rob Johnson, Manager of Benefits Coordination at Eastman. He coordinated the development of the Kingsport Area Health Improvement Project (KAHIP), which involved representatives of the Kingsport Area Business Council on Health Care (KABACH), HVHMC, Indian Path Medical Center, Indian Path Pavilion (psychiatric), the IPA, and Heritage.

After going through an intensive quality training session, representatives of the KAHIP members reviewed the health problems affecting Kingsport's population and finally selected the area of respiratory diseases as its focus. Four improvement projects were undertaken:

- reducing the number of readmissions for chronically-ill respiratory patients, whom the group dubbed "frequent flyers"
- developing a more effective process for transitioning respiratory patients to nursing homes
- developing a process to encourage youth to quit/not start smoking
- determining the most appropriate means of conducting third party utilization review

Three of the teams attended the QUALITY FIRST program with their tuition paid by the Midwest Business Group on Health, and each of the four worked with an individual facilitator.

In retrospect, Rob Johnson noted that the process had been frustrating. "We didn't do a good job of using our project selection criteria. The projects we selected were difficult to deal with. They were too broad or aimed at a system instead of a process. Our data system wasn't effective enough to narrow the projects down to processes." Ownership was also a problem in this type of organization. "Everybody has ownership or nobody has ownership. Because KAHIP is a community-oriented project, no one organization could claim ownership." Three of the four teams have continued to meet and the Superintendent of Schools worked to reorganize the youth and smoking team. The team working with nursing home placements had some concrete successes and the other teams continued to collect and interpret data.

The Heritage National HMO also started its own quality management program in Kingsport and at its Illinois headquarters assisted by facilitators from Eastman and HVHMC. Under the leadership of the doctors in the IPA, a team from the IPA, the HMO and the hospitals studied the resources used for postsurgical care of gall bladder removals. The team found that there were about as many processes as there were physicians and developed a standard process. The net result was to reduce the average length of stay for this procedure by two days. Dean Anderson, operations manager of Heritage, said

> Ultimately we hope to have improvement teams in doctor's offices. Potential improvement areas we've identified included pediatric office scheduling, lab work and billing processes. We want to spread the quality virus and get all physicians involved. Physicians develop different practices, but through quality we hope to combine the various procedures into one formalized process.

Dr. Paul Pearlman, then president of the IPA, commented

> As physicians, we have to be interested in promoting health care. Physicians have varied backgrounds, so everyone manages problems differently. What we're trying to do through KAHIP is find out why there are variations and how we can reduce them to make our processes better. It shouldn't make a difference which emergency room a person goes to. What's important is that they get quality care wherever they go.

One fact that encouraged Rob Johnson was the physicians' choice of a low-cost California managed care group's practices as their cost and length-of-stay benchmarks for their gall bladder study.

KAHIP also become the task force on health for the Kingsport Tomorrow project, a community-wide program to envision Kingsport in the 21st century. Rob Johnson observed that

> We're reassessing teams, pouring over new data systems and targeting physicians' offices for facilitators. If we can't zero in on the problems with our present projects, then we'll discontinue them. There are a lot of resources yet to be tapped. We feel we

haven't accomplished a great deal, but others looking at Kingsport and KAHIP from the outside see what we're doing here and are amazed. While it's natural for us in Kingsport to cooperate, it is not in other communities.

Community cooperation was the style in Kingsport. Eastman and the other employers wanted a happy, attractive community to appeal skilled personnel for their expanding businesses. On the other hand, if health care costs could be cut, ECC could and did act unilaterally. Eastman had made a study of medical admissions for low back pain and had severely restricted payments for that service. The number of admissions and their length soon dropped sharply, especially the admissions by primary care physicians. Eastman was aware that it could achieve the lowest health care costs by selecting a subset of physicians in the town and forming a closed-panel HMO, but Rob Johnson did not want anything that confrontational yet. "That just is not Eastman's style." Furthermore, he felt that it was best to work with the total system rather than minimizing Eastman's share, since cost-shifting one way or another ended up saddling employers with the costs of uncompensated care throughout the community.

## National Center for Quality

Another cooperative venture building on the QUALITY FIRST program was the National Center for Quality. This nonprofit corporation, formed by the three chambers of commerce in 1988, is dedicated to promoting a national interest in quality and productivity improvement. It has established a core set of courses for organizations to call on. In June of 1989, Jim Wallin, Community Programs Coordinator for Eastman, was loaned to the Center as its Interim director. In January 1990, the board approved handing over the operation to Northeast State Technical Institute, and Al Thomas, Director of the QUALITY FIRST program, was asked to serve as part-time executive director of the Center.

The Center offered a number of courses:

- Seizing the Quality Initiative
- Leading the Quality Transformation
- Survey Techniques
- Quality & Performance Management for Educators
- Malcolm Baldrige National Quality Award
- Managing for Excellence in Healthcare

On August 5–6, 1991, the Center and the four area hospitals offered "A Competitive Healthcare and Quality Management Conference." The conference coordinator was Ms. Ether Luster, an assistant administrator at HVHMC. Mr. Paul Bishop, Chief Operating Officer of HVHMC, observed, "Our psychological contract with the supporters of quality management includes our making a special effort to disseminate our story." The Second Conference was held April 23–24, 1992 and included such well known presenters as Dr. Paul Batalden, Vice President of Medical Affairs for HCA, and Dr. James Roberts of the Joint Commission on Accreditation of Healthcare Organizations.

## Activities at HVHMC

Mr. Bishop, trained as a hospital administrator, was impressed with the approach and continued to send teams, more than 20 with approximately 90 participants. Documented savings at HVHMC from these team efforts included lower costs of linens, reductions in nurse turnover (costing $10,000 to $20,000 per nurse) of 6%, reductions of medication delivery lead time from the pharmacy to the nursing floors from 3 to 1¼ hours, admitting wait and processing times reduced from 30 minutes to 5.6 minutes, preadmission laboratory testing increased from 30% to 75%, and length of stay dropped one day, mostly due to the efforts of the discharge planning team.

In some ways, the QUALITY FIRST program was ideal for the Hospital. People went for training one day every other week for 16 weeks. The course was project-oriented, so people could see the effects in the work place.

### Partnerships for Excellence

Seven major projects were completed by the end of 1988, but Mr. Bishop wanted to speed up the process. So did the city manager of Kingsport. He went to Eastman Chemical, which agreed to donate the services of Mr. David J. McClaskey, a quality management coordinator, to help adapt and use his "Managing for Excellence" training course to allow HVHMC to bring quality training "in-house." David McClaskey was an examiner for the Malcolm Baldrige National Quality Award and helped develop the examiner preparation course. One assistant administrator at HVHMC, Mr. Dale Richardson, received more than 100 hours of training. Then the management team and two potential in-house facilitators—a nurse and a business manager—went through the initial 80 hours of training over about seven months. During this initial run, the participants found that about 30% of the material required modification to replace industrial illustrations with health situations. With Mr. McClaskey's cooperation, they modified the material that they now called "Partnerships for Excellence." By June 1991, the hospital was staffed with six full-time facilitators. The hospital had some 23 "natural teams" which include direct reporting relationships from the administrator through assistant administrators to department directors and to their supervisors. By June 1991, 80% of the natural teams had completed the "Partnerships for Excellence" process, with the remainder scheduled to complete the process within eight months.

The TQM program consisted of four training modules. The first 80-hour module was for natural teams (groups with common supervision). It was an introduction to Deming's 14 points, Peter's "A Passion for Customers," the Red Bead experiment, team-building exercises, listening skills, managing customer expectations, developing process measures, flow-charting, statistical thinking, and the whole QUALITY FIRST process, followed by an exercise in developing a performance management plan for the unit and planning the rollout of quality improvement in the department. There were also two modules on process teams and one on quality improvement projects averaging 40 hours each. Process and project teams were both responsible for multifunctional issues with the process teams intending to maintain their oversight of a process, while the project teams had more of an ad hoc nature.

Not all groups received the full 80 hours of training, because the program can be modularized, especially the process teams. A process team works together for an extended period of time to study an important patient care process. An example might be the "heart process" involving open heart and cardiac catheterization patients. Process teams that were started most recently required a well-trained facilitator and generated the most conflict. Mr. Bishop noted "We are still developing the process team framework. It is very hard for managers to stay out of the business of the process team long enough for them to produce results—we have found that we have had to limit participation of managers unless they are specifically assigned to the team."

When a team completed the training program, its members received certificates, called licenses (implying the need for renewal), at a celebration ceremony in front of all the managers, including first-line supervisors. Often a figure from the community and/or the hospital board was asked to hand out the certificates.

HVHMC also adopted the "Service Excellence" modules developed by the Einstein group of Philadelphia. Fifteen hundred of the hospital's 1800 employees have received this training with the rest slated to receive it by the end of 1991. Paul Bishop was genuinely pleased with the hospital and the community efforts, which were attracting national recognition. For example, he had been asked to prepare and give a presentation at the 1991 Business Week Symposium of Health Care CEOs, Rockefeller Center, NY City, June 20 to 21, 1991, which he entitled "Innovation as A Team Sport: Solutions Through Partnership." Yet when asked about issues to be worked on, he replied, "There are hundreds of them. In health care, the average time that people are satisfied with an improved service is half-an-hour. They immediately internalize the new achievement as the new standard and complain about how poor the service is." Over time, however, he felt that people were beginning to realize that the quality of care genuinely has improved.

His major concerns in 1991 beyond day-to-day implementation were:

1. how fast to change the organizational structure and the human resource infrastructure to adjust to quality management and performance management;
2. how to increase the emphasis on quality management in clinical decision-making; and
3. how to get his vision of the future of this change process across to people.

Early on, the quality assurance (QA) effort was merged with and made subordinate to the quality management program. The existing QA staff, two medical records specialists who had been doing physician utilization review, were assigned to the new head of quality management, a former nursing supervisor. They then received quality management training. The quality management department grew rapidly with the addition of the six quality management facilitators with the title of Quality Management Consultant. Their backgrounds included nursing supervision, clinical laboratory support, financial office support, quality management with the telephone company, undergraduate training in statistics, and medical records experience. The performance appraisal system had been modified some to include contributions to quality management and so had job descriptions. Yet Paul Bishop was still concerned about how fast to move away from the periodic appraisal system and move toward performance management. Some senior managers who had been successful under the old style of management and believed that "The cream rises to the top" would probably resist such a move. This didn't mean that institutionalization of the concepts of quality management wasn't pretty far along. People had internalized the concepts and terms throughout the organization. A number of physicians were quite interested in some of the projects. Some people who had complained about their supervisors' passiveness were actually saying that they saw positive changes in management, while others sometimes complained about too much time spent in meetings.

The original heart process team had not been terribly successful, because the individuals responsible for spearheading the process review had come from outside it. "We went to school on that one," one of the internal consultants said. Since then the process stewards have all come from within the process. That cuts down on barriers and defensiveness. During the past year, APM, a consulting company from New York that specializes in service line development and the team have made great strides with the heart process. The key has been in getting commitment from the physicians for improvement of the process including cost control.

*Moving on to Clinical Quality*

The hospital received its initial set of SysteMetrics/McGraw-Hill IMPAQ III reports, one of the first sets sent out, providing internal resource utilization, mortality, and complications by diagnosis, by payer, and by physician. Paul Bishop saw two major issues immediately: (1) how to adjust them for patient risk; and (2) how to transmit the information to the physicians in a way that would maintain the spirit of cooperation that existed, but still motivate review and action. HVHMC looked good on mortality and not as good on resource utilization. In some situations, Paul Bishop was not sure whether the discrepancies were due to coding errors or biases or were rooted in physician behaviors. He wanted to use this new information in a way that would enhance HVHMC's effectiveness and financial viability. On the other hand, he had been careful so far to have the quality program avoid issues that might upset physicians enough to take more of their cases to competing hospitals.

Rob Johnson at Eastman had suggested sharing the data with the IPA and letting them take ownership for the quality improvement process. "Our experiences with medical backs and gall bladders show that changes in physician practice patterns show up immediately in both hospitals. Why should Holston Valley pay all the costs of the change when Indian Path will get just as much benefit?"

This period of collaboration and cooperation in Kingsport continued through much of 1993. The combined KAHIP and IPA teams focused on additional areas of opportunity, including treatment of simple pneumonia and knee replacement surgery. The simple pneumonia protocol was fully implemented at Indian Path.

Indian Path Medical Center's administrative team also participated in the initial QUALITY FIRST training program. In 1989, they also had gone through HCA's Deming-based quality management training. (See the West Florida case in this book.) One project there had reduced outpatient registration wait time from 35 minutes to 5 minutes. However, HCA's effort was keyed to the commitment of the administration and a change of administrator in 1991 had slowed the CQI process there considerably.

## OTHER EVENTS TAKE OVER

Management changes at both hospitals in 1992 and 1993 slowed both internal and community efforts somewhat, although both hospitals continued with internal quality improvement efforts. Late in 1993, Heritage added a new product, Heritage Preferred, that moved to a more selective provider panel. For this, Heritage contracted with most of the primary care providers in the community, but only 40% to 50% of the specialists, and only one Kingsport hospital, Holston Valley. Heritage Preferred also began to purchase services regionally, for example, sending orthopedic cases to a practice in Johnson City.

Bypassed, the IPA effectively lost its place as a vehicle for community-wide process improvement. Many medical providers were angry at and suspicious of Heritage and Eastman. Provider representatives began to miss even more KAHIP meetings and, when they attended, seemed less interested in moving ahead with specific cooperative activities, especially those associated with utilization review and clinical process improvement.

Several events in 1994 further complicated Kingsport's health care marketplace. In June, Eastman Kodak announced a reorganization: Eastman Chemical would be spun off into a new corporation. This announcement came after several months of uncertainty as Eastman Kodak's management considered whether to sell Eastman Chemical or spin it off. Uncertainty mounted in the community about ownership, job security, and employee benefit structures for more than 12,000 local employees. As a result, community-based health care quality improvement virtually ceased while people waited for Kodak's decision.

The 1994 Clinton Health Plan debate, which fueled a national trend toward the formation of health care provider networks, also influenced events in the Tri-Cities area. The development of two competing networks involving all the region's hospitals also heightened the sense of competition in the medical community. The proposal to merge Health Trust and Columbia-HCA introduced still another set of uncertainties. Employers sent a strong signal to providers that they were serious about controlling health care costs. On July 1, 1994, they formed the Tri-Cities Health Alliance (TriHealth), a regional employer coalition for health care, to develop regional health care networks and offer managed care products to both large and small businesses. A full-time president and CEO was recruited from the Memphis Business Group on Health to start the organization. This further heightened the sense of competition among providers and stimulated the formation of new provider alliances and networks.

### Reconstituting KAHIP

Realizing that KAHIP wasn't working well, community leaders began discussing the nature of the organization's problems. Many team members were somewhat disgruntled, and a lack of trust was evident among the various health care providers. The IPA-related activities essentially ground to a halt, and only the smoking cessation team maintained momentum. The rapid emergence of restricted provider networks was a clear driver in the new competitive atmosphere.

The overall leadership of KAHIP had rested with a quality improvement council composed of 18 to 20 members. By late 1993, several key council members felt that this body was too big and too dominated by industry. They felt that the providers should assume more responsibility and might participate more effectively if given more of a leadership role. They discussed this among themselves and with members of the Kingsport Tomorrow board and staff. The latter group decided to reconstitute the council in early 1994. A new KAHIP Leadership Team was formed, to give health care practitioners a bigger role so as to rebuild their confidence in the process.

The KAHIP and Kingsport Tomorrow leaders talked one-on-one with many existing and potential participants in KAHIP improvement efforts, listening to their concerns, complaints, and opinions about performance gaps and potential improvements. In retrospect, they realized that this process paralleled the series of steps outlined by Perlman and Takacs

(1990) based on the stages-of-grief model outlined by Kubler-Ross. They listened to the anger of those who felt betrayed, dealt with their depression, and helped them release old expectations and accept change as a long-run reality. Perlman and Takacs refer to the final stage as "re-emergence," where new roles and identities are established and the organization redefines its mission, objectives, and goals. KAHIP developed the leadership team concept because a different, more carefully orchestrated process was needed to produce collaboration in the new competitive climate. They studied the mission and vision statements of KAHIP and revised them to meet the new realities.

"In 1995, I wouldn't have given a plugged nickel for the future of KAHIP," said one long-term member of the KAHIP's leadership team. "Today we are really beginning to see the fruits of our efforts." By late 1995, only three improvement teams were functioning and participants seemed to be focusing as much on what issues to avoid as on what new areas to address. However, the leadership team kept meeting and talking and hoping that people would emerge from their responses to the losses occasioned by managed care. They kept looking for new openings. The leadership team presented a simplified, revised mission statement in September 1995 and a new vision statement. This mission statement stated that the KAHIP mission was "to facilitate and develop cooperative health care processes that improve the health of the health status of the people of the community." The new vision statement is reproduced below. The significant vision statement changes are identified. Those items struck through were removed from the earlier mission statement. The added parts are in italics.

## KAHIP Vision

Kingsport is a ~~"national best"~~ benchmark for Health Status and Health Care

## ~~Satisfied~~ Residents/Patients

- Health care is available to all residents.
- Residents are made aware of lifestyle factors affecting their health and are taking responsibility for leading healthier lifestyles.
- ~~Residents perceive health care as high quality and good financial value.~~

## Competitive Businesses

- Superior value of health care (high quality outcomes at optimal costs) *helps* attract and retain businesses, and assists them in maintaining their competitive positions.
- *Employees are made aware of factors affecting their health and are taking responsibility for leading healthier lifestyles.*

## Effective Providers

- ~~Kingsport area health care providers are integrated into a coordinated network, which fosters cooperation and provides for continuity of patient care.~~
- ~~Integrated provider network uses continuous quality improvement (CQI) techniques to continuously improve health care processes.~~
- ~~Quality of care draws increasing patient market share to Kingsport providers to promote economies of scale.~~
- A community data system provides facts and data to serve as ~~the foundation~~ a resource for improving health care in Kingsport ~~and verifying the resultant level of excellence.~~
- *Quality, costs and scope of services attract patients to Kingsport providers.*

## Getting Outside Help

Kingsport was one of the nine U.S. and Canadian cities selected to participate in a community-wide health improvement learning project jointly sponsored by GOAL/QPC (Methuen, MA) and the Institute of Healthcare Improvement (Boston). At a 1995 meeting of project participants, members of the leadership team heard a presentation at a conference in Boston by John O'Brien, CEO of Cambridge City Hospital and Cambridge City Health Commissioner, on the process used for planning community health improvement in that city. They decided to try the approach Mr. O'Brien described in an effort to create the opening for community involvement that they were looking for.

In January 1996, KAHIP undertook a new visioning process starting with a weekend workshop for community leaders facilitated by Mr.

O'Brien. Using the process initiated during the workshop, the KAHIP and other community leaders produced a new strategic plan for 1998.

Several principles were affirmed during this process, namely:

1. continued dialogue;
2. emphasis on collaboration;
3. action where collaboration is feasible;
4. avoiding duplication of efforts;
5. emphasis on prevention;
6. broadening provider and community participation; and
7. encouraging regional collaboration where practical.

In early 1998, ten community improvement teams were functioning, six chartered by KAHIP. Planning for a similar community-wide visioning effort was underway in 1998 in Bristol, TN-VA, and local and state government financial support had been generated for specific local and regional health improvement efforts. The leadership team had been expanded to provide representation of city government, pharmacy and public mental health providers; the county public health department; more health insurance and managed care organizations; and the local YMCA. These leadership committee changes reflected the greater emphasis on prevention and wellness, on regionalization, and on wider community participation.

**Other Events**

As always, events in the community and region affected Greater Kingsport's environment for collaboration. Holston Valley Medical Center merged with Bristol Regional Medical Center to form Wellmont Health System. As its name implies, this system has developed a strong focus on wellness systems. The other hospital, Indian Path Medical Center and three small hospitals in the Johnson City area were owned by Columbia HCA, and were subject to the ups and downs of that organization. Tri-Cities Health Alliance (TriHealth), formed in 1994, had been staffed, and represented over 70 employers with some 25,000 employees. These events together with the introduction and survival of TennCare, Tennessee's managed care plan for the Medicaid eligible and uninsured, tended to make both employers and providers pay more attention to regional issues.

## Mature Projects

The three mature projects continued to expand in scope and through institutionalization in the community or both. Team membership was broadened and activities strengthened.

### Drive Smart Project

This collaborative learning project, concerned with reducing preventable injuries and death among youth from motor vehicle crashes continued to go forward. The objective of these projects had been to determine if applying continuous quality improvement techniques in a collaborative fashion in a community could help bring about significant positive change. The Kingsport team, working in tandem with a team from Twin Falls, Idaho, decided to focus on reducing "preventable" injuries to children and adolescents resulting from motor vehicle accidents. Led by Jeanette Blazier of KAHIP, the team included the Sullivan County Sheriff and representatives from private and public health providers, industry, community and parent groups, and the schools.

Assembled in 1993, this team followed the Plan-Do-Check-Act (PDCA) model. The team reviewed national data that revealed that traffic accidents are the number one preventable cause of death of children and adolescents. The data showed that this age group had four times the accident rate and twice the motor vehicle death rate of the general population and that 18% of young drivers had a crash during their first year of driving. The team collected data from the local sheriff's office on juvenile traffic accidents by school, for the five high schools in the county for the years 1991 to 1993. A Pareto chart revealed that 2 of the 11 categories, "improper driving" and "failure to yield," accounted for 54% of the 974 reported crashes. Drinking was blamed in only 6% of the cases. Further investigation showed that, while all high school students received classroom instruction, only 40% to 50% received on-road training due to lack of certified instructors and that this percentage was heading downward. It also became clear that drivers' education classes were unstandardized, underfunded, and understaffed. The use of simulation as a more cost-effective alternative was not possible due to insufficient funds.

Team members conducted benchmarking efforts and identified model curricula used elsewhere as well as state-of-the-art driving simulators. Focus groups were held with parents, students, educators, and community leaders to determine the nature of the problem and the appropriateness of the objectives selected. The team developed a cause-and-effect diagram and decided to improve the quality and reduce the variability among high school drivers' education programs locally and to increase the coverage of on-road training. This included raising funds for additional summer driving-education programs.

The team selected a "best practice," standardized drivers' education program modeled on Washington State's "Traffic Safety Education Guide." This was implemented as a pilot program in one local high school in late 1995. By 1998, the number of driving instructors in the four county high schools had been increased from two to six, the first eight-position DORON Precision Systems driving simulation system had been installed and used at Dobyns-Bennett High School in Kingsport, and the whole effort became the initial component of OUR SAFE COMMUNITY project, an ongoing project coordinated by Kingsport Tomorrow and partially funded by the State of Tennessee, Governor's Highway Safety Office. This support of $98,000 for the 1998 to 1999 fiscal year included funding for regional planning of four community efforts in northeast Tennessee.

Drive Smart also received voluntary funding from the community in the amount of $90,000 from donors and from volunteers selling programs at events held at the Bristol Motor Speedway. This helped support the purchase of more simulators as well as youth activities to increase awareness of the need for safe driving.

The other, newer component of OUR SAFE COMMUNITIES was local and regional participation in the Network of Employers for Traffic Safety (NETS), a public private partnership dedicated to reducing the deaths and injuries in the workforce. This effort included public service announcements and events and newspaper ads and billboards, as well as employer activities. In December 1997, the regional effort, the Quad-Cities Safe Community Coalition, and eight local law enforcement agencies combined to sponsor and publicize National Drunk and Drugged Driving Prevention Month. The NETS team was chartered by KAHIP.

One objective of "Drive Smart" was to demonstrate the effectiveness of the "best practice" driver-training curriculum and restructure driver training as taught in the local school systems. Individuals and groups gradually realized the applicability of this to other populations. Rehab professionals at a local hospital were using the simulator equipment with patients. Kingsport City employees were involved in a driver retraining program and the FIFTY-FIVE ALIVE program also utilized it.

*Friends-In-Needs Health Center, Inc. Project*

The initial proposal for this team was brought to Kingsport Tomorrow by the community's church groups. The objective was to provide primary health care for the uninsured, underserved working poor. This team headed by a local surgeon, included representatives from community churches, hospitals, physicians, dentists, pharmacists, the Junior League, family counseling agencies, businesses, and industry.

The team established a new community health center which officially opened July 19, 1995. An executive director was hired, a building rented and a medical director appointed. Staffing was by volunteer health providers in the community with the support of lay volunteers from various area churches.

This team's effort did not involve much use of the CQI process since those involved were already motivated and active. The KAHIP management team felt that the introduction of a new approach might slow the existing momentum.

This outpatient medical and dental clinic for the working poor registered its 1000th unduplicated patient in December 1997. It provided services, mostly from volunteer professionals and students and residents at several health profession education programs at East Tennessee State University, on a sliding fee scale, starting at 20% of fees. About half paid 20% to 30% of fees. This program has been heavily subsidized by the Holston Valley Medical Center which has provided direct financial support, indirect and in-kind support and sees about ¼ to ⅓ of the patients in its outpatient specialty clinics. Holston Valley has in turn been able to shut down its indigent care teaching clinic. Friends-In-Need has also become an associate member of the United Way of Greater Kingsport and received a $25,000 Inter-Faith Agency Grant from the Robert Wood Johnson Foundation.

While the support of the community, the health care professionals, and the churches has been strong, utilization has been below expectations. There are an estimated 6,000 to 8,000 eligible patients living or working in the clinic's service area. However, the clinic has not had resources to advertise and is unsure why it has been able to reach only 1,000 during its first two years of full operation. However, the community continued to support the effort through the churches and the program became an independent community resource.

*Youth Tobacco Prevention Project*

This project team has continued to function continuously throughout the period of turmoil in the health system. New people were brought on board from time to time to keep the process rolling. It continues to reach a wide audience with the Doctors Ought to Care (DOC) group involving at least five volunteer physicians presenting to hundreds of students in the 5th grade in 14 elementary schools, 8th grade science classes, and high school health classes. The program also interacts with the Red Ribbon drug awareness program and includes representatives of the cancer, lung, and heart societies. Now that the program has been operating long enough to see some of the same students in the elementary, middle, and high school grades, questionnaires are being developed to measure the longitudinal impact of the DOC effort.

## New Teams

In addition to NETS, four other teams were operating in Kingsport by 2000.

*Kingsport Community Alliance Linking Enforcement, Responsibility and Treatment (ALERT)*

Sponsored by Kingsport Tomorrow, Kingsport Community ALERT was a coalition of agencies, organizations and individuals working together to reduce the impact of substance abuse in the region. It is part of the Sullivan County Alliance for a Drug-Free Tennessee. Its activities were aimed at promoting awareness, linking existing programs into a more comprehensive effort, supporting and expanding programs, focusing financial and human resources to target areas of highest need, and advocating for drug-free attitudes at all levels of the community. The steering team included representatives of the treatment centers, law enforcement, parks and recreation, the schools, the housing authority, and Kingsport Tomorrow. Agreements of cooperation were signed with most of these organizations as well as the courts, the district attorney's office, First Night Kingsport, and a number of youth organizations.

*Family YMCA*

This team was a joint one lead by Wellmont and the Kingsport YMCA to develop and expand wellness services in the community. Both organizations had facilities and programs, but they focused on a joint venture to build a new community facility focused on wellness and fitness for the whole family.

*Community Database Team*

One of KAHIP's objectives for a number of years has been to develop a database focused on community health status information. In 1995 and 1996, KAHIP was working with faculty at East Tennessee State University Medical Center to develop such a database. In 1997, the state of Tennessee mandated that each regional public health entity conduct county/region health assessments and develop appropriate tracking mechanisms. In keeping with its policy of not duplicating efforts, the KAHIP effort gave way to the effort being mounted by the Sullivan County Health Department. KAHIP has continued to participate and cooperate with that effort through a newly formed Sullivan County Health Council. The data collected by this team was made available to the community during 1999.

*Immunization*

This was an effort of the Sullivan County Health Department to increase immunization rates and a pilot project supported by the state of Tennessee. A member of the KAHIP leadership team serves as a liaison with this project. The pilot has been successful in that 85% to 90% of the children in Sullivan County were immunized. It was not cost-effective to do what would be required to immunize the remaining 10% to 15%. KAHIP continued to monitor the process.

**The 1999 Situation**

The KAHIP leadership team continued to meet from 7:00 AM to 8:30 AM on the first Wednesday of each month. Most project teams continued to be successful and were expanding including the efforts against tobacco use and driving accidents. More employers were sending employees for safe driving training. The Safe Communities effort had spawned a Safe Children Coalition.

The one area where the team was less than satisfied was in the community wellness and personal fitness arena. The individuals spearheading that effort had been unable to devote adequate time to it and the team was looking for new leadership. There was an increasing realization that this effort was a key effort in preventing later health care costs.

There were also some major policy issues that would be coming up soon. Ms. Jeannette Blazier had retired as the Executive Director of Kingsport Tomorrow and this provided the opportunity to rethink whether or not KAHIP should continue to be part of Kingsport Tomorrow or become an independent entity. Ms. Blazier was still concerned about the issues, but had a new role as mayor of Kingsport.

Deere and Eastman management, together with others, had decided that the costs in Kingsport, which were the lowest of any region in the state, had been driven close to their reasonable floor. Therefore, the direction for further efforts should be in improving the quality of care. In September 1999 Tri-Health, the HMO, and key employers invited Dr. Mark Chassin to give a series of presentations on health quality of care for KAHIP and other local groups. The board of the Midwest Business Group on Health, which was meeting in Kingsport as the guest of board member Rob Johnson from Eastman, was also invited to attend.

The KAHIP leadership team also continued to study the data assembled by the health department on the health of the community. They hoped to identify the areas of health need where new initiatives could be mounted effectively. Note that not all of the areas of concern in the 1998 strategic plan had yet been addressed. Access to behavioral health care and the value aspects of health care including health care quality and cost were still in the plan, but not operationalized. That is not at all surprising given the sensitivities reported earlier (McLaughlin 1995).

## KAHIP Ends

Meanwhile, Kingsport Tomorrow moved ahead with its Vision 2017 process. One concern was that the regionalization of health care services and payer organizations went well beyond the city and Sullivan County.

In 2000, KAHIP was reorganized into the Community Health Improvement Partnership (CHIP) with much broader regional representation. However, it still operated under the umbrella of Kingsport Tomorrow. CHIP's new vision is to "facilitate and develop cooperative processes that improve the health status of our community and region." The rest of CHIP's vision statement virtually reproduces the KAHIP version (McLaughlin and Simpson 1994).

Friends-in-Need Health Center was spun off and so was the Drive Smart/TN Association of Highway Safety Leaders which became part of the TN Governor's Highway Safety Office. Kingsport Community ALERT increased public involvement and established Greater Kingsport's Promise: Alliance for Youth.

The new CHIP leadership team identified three priority health issues for Northeast TN and Southwest VA:

- Cardiovascular disease under a new Heart Care Partners team.
- Tobacco control, so the Youth Tobacco Prevention project became the Nicotine-Free Mountain Empire Team
- Lack of physical activity, supported by the revised Active Community Team

A Care Data Exchange team was formed to improve outcomes for patients through evidence-base practices and exchange of regional health information among health providers. The Care Data Exchange team developed a pilot proposal and in 2003 received funding from the "Connecting Communities for Better Health" program funded in cooperation with eHealth Initiative and HRSA.

Kingsport Tomorrow has also provided links on its Web site to local organizations dealing with teen pregnancy, peer education, eating disorders, and suicide prevention. Check out www.kingsporttomorrow.org and browse the site. Be sure to click on the icons for projects, as well as opening the sections on events and Vision2017. What seems to be the latest trend in KAHIP/CHIP's progression?

## Lessons Learned

In the rapidly changing and uncertain health care environment, it is the role of leadership of any community collaboration effort to stand tall and maintain communication, avoid taking sides, and look for the possible amid the anger and mistrust that change can generate. When competition is intense in the community, keeping people communicating may become a legitimate end in itself. If those affected are going to reemerge from their anger and grief, leaders need to provide alternative modes of community collaboration.There were a number of useful learnings ffrom KAHIP, which include:

- As the community deals with its anger and distrust, it is the role of leadership to look for possible areas of synergy that can encourage more collaboration on broader community and on regional bases.
- In a community with widespread knowledge of continuous improvement philosophy and techniques, it makes sense to encourage other agencies to take the initiative and the credit and not worry about whether or not a specific process is adopted.
- The structure of the leadership team must reflect the areas where people are ready to move. In 1994 to 1995, the focus was on addressing the felt need for providers for more representation. In 1996 to 1999, the focus was on more representation of community-based and governmental organizations that have specific interests and even mandates that can contribute toward health collaboration and improvement. By 2000 to 2004, the focus of CHIP seemed more clinical.
- Team composition must be flexible to reflect both local and regional markets and activities. The appropriate definition of the relevant region will vary with the issue being addressed and will change over time with shifting areas of concern and realignments of markets and interest.
- The role of the public health system for assessment, policy assessment, and assurance and for collaboration in an era of reduced government and managed care (Halverson *et al.* 1998b) cannot be ignored and can be encouraged. Similarly, the roles of other government entities such as law enforcement, parks and recreation, and schools can be included as the planning process is institutionalized in the community.
- Focusing on positive outcomes with one population segment, such as youth, can lead to interactions with other segments, as in the Safe Driver program which now interacts with similar concerns from NETS and FIFTY-FIVE ALIVE.

- Continuous improvement principles need to be continually applied to the collaborative process. For example, all KAHIP team meetings have added an initial, five-minute learning activity in which one member is assigned to present some new information for the benefit of the team member.

## CASE ANALYSIS

This is an early and highly regarded application of TQM techniques directly from industry. One interesting aspect of the case is that it clearly shows the role of the dominant employer in the community, Eastman Kodak and its successor, Eastman Chemical. It represents a long-term community-based implementation of TQM supported by the business community of Kingsport. Unfortunately, it did not begin with the felt need of the community's health care professionals for change. Therefore, as the relationships between employers, providers, and payers changed, so did the nature of the KAHIP effort. However, the concepts of CQI were firmly rooted in the community and its various organizations. However, there were many ups and downs as the relationships among the actors and the interests of the community shifted over time.

## ASSIGNMENT QUESTIONS

### Introduction

1. What were the strategic reasons behind the decisions of the two hospitals and the city to invest heavily in TQM?
2. What messages were sent by having the KAHIP effort embedded in the Kingsport Chamber of Commerce?

### Basics

3. What were the strengths and weaknesses of the TQM program as it was implemented here?
4. What was the role of local industry and community resources in this effort? How was consumer satisfaction represented in this process?
5. Why did this program seem to attract so much national attention?

## Implementation

6. What seemed to be the involvement of the Sullivan County Department of Health in the early stages of this effort?
7. How would one go about introducing a parallel activity to KAHIP in your community?
8. Given the current status of the community-based effort, how successful would you consider it to be?

## Application

9. What functions of a local health department seem to have devolved on KAHIP, at least in the early stages of the community effort?
10. There is no chapter in the book on community-based health improvement efforts. What would you want to see included in such a chapter after reading and discussing the case?

## CLASS EXERCISE

Investigate the current status of KAHIP, CHIP, and any successor organizations in Kingsport, TN, using the Internet. Are there parallel efforts in your communities? If not, why not? If so, compare and contrast those efforts with those of the Kingsport community. Do not forget to include the local health department in the exercise.

The authors wish to acknowledge the extensive cooperation of two members of the KAHIP leadership team: Jeanette D. Blazier, Executive Director of Kingsport Tomorrow, Inc., and James S. Herbert, Jr., Senior Employee Benefits Manager, Eastman Chemical Company. Both cooperated extensively through interviews and reviewed earlier drafts of this effort. The authors also wish to thank the American College of Healthcare Executives, the Kenan-Flagler Business School of the University of North Carolina at Chapel Hill and the Physician Executive MBA Program of the College of Business Administration, University of Tennessee Knoxville who at various times have supported this research.

# West Florida Regional Medical Center

*Curtis P. McLaughlin*

West Florida Regional Medical Center (WFRMC) is a Hospital Corporation of America (HCA)-owned and operated, for-profit hospital complex on the north side of Pensacola, Florida. Licensed for 547 beds, it operated approximately 325 beds in December 1991 plus the 89-bed psychiatric Pavilion and the 58-bed Rehabilitation Institute of West Florida. The 11-story office building of the Medical Center Clinic, P.A., was attached to the hospital facility, and a new cancer center was under construction.

The 130 doctors practicing at the Medical Center Clinic and its satellite clinics admitted mostly to WFRMC, whereas most of the other doctors in this city of 150,000 practiced at both Sacred Heart and Baptist Hospitals downtown. Competition for patients was intense, and in 1992 as many as 90% to 95% of patients in the hospital would be admitted subject to discounted prices, mostly Medicare for the elderly, CHAMPUS for military dependents, and Blue Cross/Blue Shield of Florida for the employed and their dependents.

The continuous quality improvement (CQI) effort had had some real successes over the previous four years, especially in the areas where package prices for services were required. All of the management team had been trained in quality improvement techniques according to HCA's Deming-based approach, and some 25 task forces were operating. The experiment with departmental self-assessments, using the Baldrige Award criteria and an instrument developed by HCA headquarters, had spurred department heads to become further involved and begin to apply quality improvement techniques within their own work units. Yet John Kausch, the Center's CEO, and his senior leadership sensed some loss of interest among some managers, whereas others who had not bought into the idea at first were now enthusiasts.

## THE HCA CQI PROCESS

John Kausch had been in the first group of HCA CEOs trained in CQI techniques in 1987 by Paul Batalden, M.D., Corporate Vice President for Medical Care. John had become a member of the steering committee for HCA's overall quality effort. The HCA approach was dependent on the active and continued participation of top local management and on the Plan-Do-Check-Act (PDCA) cycle of Deming. Exhibit 4–1 shows that process as presented to company employees. Dr. Batalden told the case writer that he did not work with a hospital administrator until he was convinced that that individual was fully committed to the concept and was ready to lead the process at his or her own institution—a responsibility that included being the one to teach the Quality 101 course on site to his or her own managers. John Kausch also took members of his management team to visit other quality exemplars, such as Florida Power and Light and local plants of Westinghouse and Monsanto.

In 1991, John Kausch became actively involved in the Total Quality Council of the Pensacola Area Chamber of Commerce (PATQC), when a group of Pensacola area leaders in business, government, military, education, and health care began meeting informally to share ideas in productivity and quality improvement. From this informal group emerged the PATQC under the sponsorship of the Chamber of Commerce. The vision of PATQC was "helping the Pensacola area develop into a total quality community by promoting productivity and quality in all area organizations, public and private, and by promoting economic development through aiding existing business and attracting new business development." The primary employer in Pensacola, the U.S. Navy, was using the total quality management (TQM) approach extensively, was quite satisfied with the results, and supported the Chamber of Commerce program. In fact, the first 1992 one-day seminar presented by Mr. George F. Butts, consultant and retired Chrysler Vice President for Quality and Productivity, was held at the Naval Air Station's Mustin Beach Officer's Club. Celanese Corporation, a Monsanto division, and the largest nongovernmental employer in the area, also supported PATQC.

The CQI staffing at WFRMC was quite small, in keeping with HCA practice. The only program employee was Ms. Bette Gulsby, M.Ed., Director of Quality Improvement Resources, who served as staff and "coach" to Mr. Kausch and as a member of the quality improvement council. Exhibits 4–2 and 4–3 show the organization of the council and

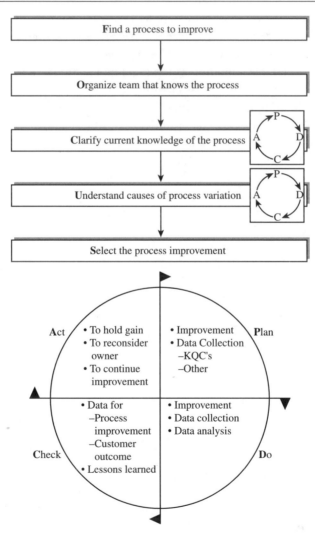

**Exhibit 4–1**  HCA's FOCUS–PDCA Cycle. Source: Hospital Corporation of America, Nashville, Tennessee, ©1988, 1989. Not for further reproduction.

the staffing for Quality Improvement Program (QIP) support. The "mentor" was provided by headquarters staff, and in the case of WFRMC was Dr. Batalden himself. The planning process had been careful and detailed. Exhibit 4–4 shows excerpts from the planning processes used in the early years of the program.

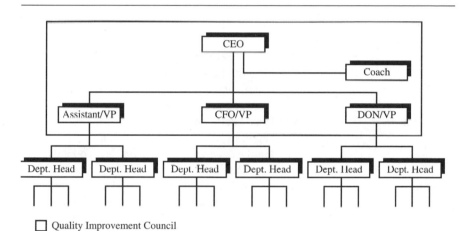

☐ Quality Improvement Council

**Exhibit 4–2** Organization Chart with Quality Improvement Council.

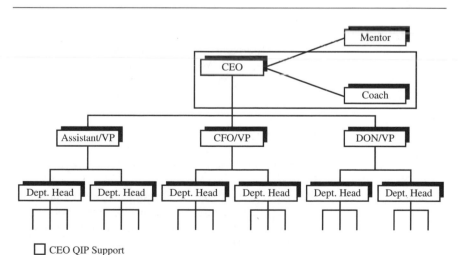

☐ CEO QIP Support

**Exhibit 4–3** Organization Chart with CEO QIP Support Mentor.

**Exhibit 4–4**  Planning Chronology for CQI

| | |
|---|---|
| **Initiation Plan—3 to 6 months, starting May 25, 1988** | |
| May 25: | Develop initial working definition of quality for WFRMC. |
| May 25: | Define the purpose of the Quality Improvement Council and set schedule for 2–4 PM every Tuesday and Thursday. |
| May 25: | Integrate Health Quality Trends (HQT) into continuous improvement cycle and hold initial review. |
| June 2: | Start several multifunctional teams with their core from those completing the Leadership Workshop with topics selected by the Quality Improvement Council using surveys, experience, and group techniques. |
| June 2: | Department Heads complete "CEO assessment" to identify customers and expectations, determine training needs, and identify department opportunities. To be discussed with assistant administrators on June 15. |
| June 16: | Present to QIC the Task Force report on elements and recommendations on organizational elements to guide and monitor QIP. |
| June 20: | Division meetings to gain consensus on Department plans and set priorities. QIC reviews and consolidates on June 21. Final assignments to Department Heads on June 22. |
| June 27: | Draft initial Statement of Purpose for WFRMC and present to QIC. |
| June 29–July 1: | Conduct first Facilitator's Training Workshop for 16. |
| July 1: | Task Force reports on additional QIP education and training requirements for:<br>• Team training and team members' handbook<br>• Head nurses<br>• Employee orientation (new and current)<br>• Integration of community resources (colleges and industry)<br>• Use of HCA network resources for Medical Staff, Board of Trustees |
| July 19: | Task Force report on communications program to support awareness, education, and feedback from employees, vendors, medical staff, local business, colleges and universities, and HCA. |
| August 1: | Complete the organization of the Quality Improvement Council. |

*continues*

**Exhibit 4–4**  continued

**Quality Improvement Implementation Plan to June 30, 1989**

| | |
|---|---|
| Fall: | Pilot and evaluate "Patient Comment Card System." |
| Oct. 21: | QIC input to draft policies—guidelines regarding forming teams, quality responsibility, and guidelines for multifunctional teams. Brainstorm at Oct. 27 meeting, have revisions for Nov. 10 meeting, and distribute to employees by November 15. |
| Oct. 27: | Review proposals for communicating QIP to employees to heighten awareness and understanding, communicate on HCA and WFRMC commitments; key definitions, policies, guidelines; HQT; QIP; teams and improvements to date; responsibility and opportunities for individual employees; initiate ASAP. |
| Nov. 15: | Prepare statements on "On further consideration of HCA's Quality Guidelines;" discuss with department heads, hospital staff, employee orientation; use to identify barriers to QI and opportunities for QI. Develop specific action plan and discuss with QIC. |
| Dec. 1: | Identify and evaluate community sources for QI assistance—statistical and operational—including colleges, companies, and the Navy. Make recommendations. |
| Early Dec.: | Conduct Quality 102 course for remaining Dept. Heads. Conduct Quality 101 course for head nurses and several new Dept. Heads. |
| Jan. 1, 1989: | Develop and implement a suggestion program consistent with our HCA Quality Guidelines, providing quick and easy way to become involved in making suggestions/identifying situations needing improvement, providing quick feedback and recognition; and interfacing with identifying opportunities for QIP. |

**QIP Implementation Plan, July 1989–June 1990**

| | |
|---|---|
| Aug. 1: | Survey Department Heads to identify priorities for additional education and training. |
| Sept. 14–15: | Conduct a management workshop to sharpen and practice QI methods. To include practice methods; to increase management/staff confidence, comfort; to develop a model for departmental implementation; to develop process assessment/QIP implementation tool; to start Quality Team Review. |

*continues*

**Exhibit 4–4** continued

| | |
|---|---|
| September: | Develop a standardized team orientation program to cover QI tools and group process rules. |
| Fall: | Expand use of HQTs and integrate into Health Quality Improvement Process (HQIP)—improve communication of results and integration of quality improvement action plans. Psychiatric Pavilion to evaluate and implement HQT recommendations from "Patient Comment Card System"—evaluate and pilot. |
| October: | Incorporate QIP implementation into existing management/communication structure. Establish division "steering committee functions" to guide and facilitate departmental implementation. Identify QI project for each Department Head/Assistant Administrator. Establish regular Quality Reviews into Department Manager meetings. |
| December: | Evaluate effectiveness of existing policies, guidelines, and practices for sanctioning, supporting, and guiding QI teams. Include Opportunity Form/Cross Functional Team Sanctioning; Team leader and Facilitator responsibilities; Team progress monitoring/guiding; Standardized team presentation format (storyboard). Demonstrate measurable improvement through Baxter QI team. |
| Monthly: | Monitor and improve the suggestion program. |
| January: | Pilot the Clinical Process Improvement methodology. |
| All year: | In all communications, written and verbal, maintain constant message regarding WFRMC commitment to HQIP; report successes of teams and suggestions; and continue to educate about principles and practices of HQIP strategy. |
| January: | Successfully demonstrate measurable improvement from focused QIP in one department (Medical Records). |
| Spring: | Expand use of HQTs and integrate into HQIP.<br>• Pilot HQT in Rehab Center.<br>• Evaluate and implement Physicians' HQT.<br>• Pilot Ambulatory Care HQT. |
| Summer: | Expand use of HQTs and integrate into HQIP.<br>• Human Resources—Pilot HQT.<br>• Payers—Pilot HQT. |

WFRMC has been one of several HCA hospitals to work with a self-assessment tool for department heads. Exhibit 4–5 shows the cover letter sent to all department heads. Exhibit 4–6 shows the Scoring Matrix for Self-Assessment. Exhibit 4–7 shows the Scoring Guidelines, and Exhibit 4–8 displays the five assessment categories used.

**Exhibit 4–5**   Departmental Quality Improvement Assessment

In an effort to continue to monitor and implement elements of improvement and innovation within our organization, it will become more and more necessary to find methods which will describe our level of QI implementation.

The assessment or review of a quality initiative is only as good as the thought processes which have been triggered during the actual assessment. Last year (1990) the Quality Improvement Council prepared for and participated in a quality review. This exercise was extremely beneficial to the overall understanding of what was being done and the results that have been accomplished utilizing various quality techniques and tools.

The Departmental Implementation of QI has been somewhat varied throughout the organization and although the variation is certainly within the range of acceptability, it is the intent of the QIC to better understand each department's implementation road map and furthermore to provide advice/coaching on the next steps for each department.

Attached please find a scoring matrix for self-assessment. This matrix is followed by five category ratings (to be completed by each department head). The use of this type of tool reinforces the self-evaluation which is consistent with continuous improvement and meeting the vision of West Florida Regional Medical Center.

Please read and review the attachment describing the scoring instructions and then score your department category standings, relative to the approach, deployment, and effects. This information will be forwarded to Bette Gulsby by April 19, 1991, and following a preliminary assessment by the QIC, an appointment will be scheduled for your departmental review.

The review will be conducted by John Kausch and Bette Gulsby, along with your administrative director. Please take the time to review the attachments and begin your self-assessment scoring. You will be notified of the date and time of your review.

This information will be utilized for preparing for the next Department Head retreat, scheduled for May 29 and 30, 1991 at the Perdido Beach Hilton.

**Exhibit 4–6**   A Scoring Matrix for Self-Assessment

| APPROACH | DEPLOYMENT (Implementation) | EFFECTS (Results) |
|---|---|---|
| • HQIP design includes all eight dimensions* <br> • Integration across dimensions of HQIP and areas of operation | • Breadth of implementation (areas or functions) <br> • Depth of implementation (awareness, knowledge, understanding, and applications) | • Quality of measurable results |

*The eight dimensions of HQIP are: leadership constancy, employee mindedness, customer mindedness, process focused, statistical thinking, PDCA driven, innovativeness, and regulatory proactiveness.

| | | | |
|---|---|---|---|
| 100% | • World-class approach: sound, systematic, effective HQIP based, continuously evaluated, refined, and improved. <br> • Total interaction across all functions. <br> • Repeated cycles of innovation/improvement. | • Fully in all areas and functions. <br> • Ingrained in the culture. | • Exceptional, world-class, superior to all competition in all areas. <br> • Sustained (3 to 5 years), clearly caused by the approach. |
| 80% | • Well developed and tested, HQIP based. <br> • Excellent integration. | • In almost all areas and functions. <br> • Evident in the culture of all groups. | • Excellent, sustained in all areas with improving competitive advantage. <br> • Much evidence that they are caused by the approach. |
| 60% | • Well planned, documented, sound, systematic. HQIP based, all aspects addressed. <br> • Good integration | • In most areas and functions. <br> • Evident in the culture of most groups. | • Solid, with positive trends in most areas. <br> • Some evidence that they are caused by the approach. |
| 40% | • Beginning of sound, systematic, HQIP based; not all aspects addressed. <br> • Fair integration | • Begun in many areas and functions. <br> • Evident in the culture of some groups. | • Some success in major areas. <br> • Not much evidence that they are caused by the approach. |
| 20% | • Beginning of HQIP awareness. <br> • No integration across functions. | • Beginning in some areas and functions. <br> • Not part of the culture. | • Few or no results. <br> • Little or no evidence that any results are caused by the approach. |
| 0% | | | |

**Exhibit 4–7** Departmental Quality Improvement Assessment Scoring Guidelines

In order to determine your department's score in each of the five categories, please review the Scoring Matrix for self-assessment. The operational definitions for Approach, Deployment, and Effects are listed in the small boxes on the top of the scoring matrix. Each criteria is divided into percentage of progress–implementation (i.e., 0% to 100%). For example, you may determine that your departmental score on category 3.0 (QI Practice) is:

| APPROACH | DEPLOYMENT | EFFECTS |
|:---:|:---:|:---:|
| 20% | 20% | 20% |

    This means that your departmental approach has fair integration of QIP practice, your departmental deployment is evident in the culture of some of your groups, and your departmental effects are not actually evidence that they are caused by the approach.

    Please remember that this is a self-assessment and only you know your departmental progress. This assessment is not a tool to generate documentation. However, if you would like to bring any particular document(s) to your review, please do so. This is only meant to provide a forum for you to showcase your progress and receive recognition and feedback on such.

    Remember, review each of the self-assessment criteria of approach, deployment, and effects and become familiar with the levels or percentages described. You have three scores for each Departmental QI Assessment Category (categories 1.0–5.0)

## FOUR EXAMPLES OF TEAMS

### IV Documentation

The nursing department originated the IV Documentation Team in September 1990 after receiving documentation from the pharmacy department that over a 58-day period there had been $16,800 in lost charges related to the administration of intravenous (IV) solutions. Pharmacy attributed the loss to the nursing staff's record keeping. This was the first time that the nursing department was aware of a problem or that the pharmacy department had been tracking this variable. There were other lost charges, not yet quantified, due to recording errors in the oral administration of pharmaceuticals as well.

The team formed to look at this problem found that there were some 15 possible reasons why the errors occurred, but that the primary one was that documentation of the administration of the IV solution was not entered into the medication administration record (MAR). The MAR was kept at the patient bedside, and each time that a medication was administered the nurse was to enter documentation into this record.

The team had to come to understand some terms as they went along. The way that Pharmacy kept its books, anything that was sent to the floors but not billed within 48 to 72 hours was considered a "lost charge." If an inquiry was sent to the floor about the material and what happened and a correction was made, the entry was classified as "revenue recovered." Thus the core issue was not so much one of lost revenue as one of unnecessary rework in pharmacy and on the nursing floors.

The team developed Pareto charts showing the reasons for the documentation errors. The most common ones were procedural—for example, "patient moved to the operating room," or "patient already discharged." Following the HCA model, these procedural problems were dealt with one at a time to correct the accounting for unused materials. The next step in the usual procedure was to develop a run chart to show what was happening over time to the lost charges on IVs. Here the team determined that the best quality indicator would be the ratio of lost charges to total charges issued. At this point pharmacy management realized that it lacked the denominator figure and that its lack of computerization led to the lack of that information. Therefore, the task force was inactive for three months while Pharmacy implemented a computer system that could provide the denominator.

Ms. Debbie Koenig, Assistant Director of Nursing, who was responsible for the team, said that the next step would be to look at situations where the MAR was not at the patient bedside but perhaps at the nursing station so that a nurse could not make the entry at the appropriate time. This was an especially bothersome rework problem because of nurses working various shifts and because occasionally an agency nurse had been on duty and was not available to consult when pharmacy asked why documentation was not present for an IV dose of medication.

**Exhibit 4–8** Departmental QI Assessment Categories

---

### 1.0 DEPARTMENTAL QI FRAMEWORK DEVELOPMENT

The QI Framework Development category examines how the departmental quality values have been developed, how they are applied to projects in a consistent manner, and how adoption of the values throughout the department is assessed and reinforced.
Examples of areas to address:

- Department Mission
- Departmental Quality Definition
- Departmental Employee Performance Feedback Review
- Departmental QI Plan
- QI Methods

| APPROACH | DEPLOYMENT | EFFECTS |
|----------|------------|---------|
| _____% | _____% | _____% |

### 2.0 CUSTOMER KNOWLEDGE DEVELOPMENT

The Customer Knowledge Deployment category examines how the departmental leadership has involved and utilized various facets of customer-mindedness to guide the quality effort.
Examples of areas to address:

- HQT Family of Measures (patient, employee, etc.)
- Departmental Customer Identification
- Identification of Customer Needs and Expectations
- Customer Feedback/Data Review

| APPROACH | DEPLOYMENT | EFFECTS |
|----------|------------|---------|
| _____% | _____% | _____% |

### 3.0 QUALITY IMPROVEMENT PRACTICE

The Quality Improvement Practice category examines the effectiveness of the department's efforts to develop and realize the full potential of the work force, including management, and the methods to maintain an environment conducive to full participation, quality leadership, and personal and organizational growth.
Examples of areas to address:

- Process Improvement Practice
- Meeting Skills
- QI Storyboards

*continues*

**Exhibit 4–8** continued

- QI in Daily Work Life (individual use of QI tools, i.e., flow chart, run chart, Pareto chart)
- Practice Quality Management Guidelines
- Departmental Data Review
- Plans To Incorporate QI in Daily Clinical Operations
- Identification of Key Physician Leaders

| APPROACH | DEPLOYMENT | EFFECTS |
|----------|------------|---------|
| _____% | _____% | _____% |

**4.0   QUALITY AWARENESS BUILDING**

The Quality Awareness Building category examines how the department decides what quality education and training is needed by employees and how it utilizes the knowledge and skills acquired. It also examines what has been done to communicate QI to the department and how QI is addressed in departmental staff meetings.

Examples of areas to address:

- JIT Training
- Employee Orientation
- Creating Employee Awareness
- Communication of QI Results

| APPROACH | DEPLOYMENT | EFFECTS |
|----------|------------|---------|
| _____% | _____% | _____% |

**5.0   QA/QI LINKAGE**

The QA/QI Linkage category examines how the department has connected QA data and information to the QI process improvement strategy. Also examined is the utilization of QI data-gathering and decision-making tools to document and analyze data. (How the department relates the ongoing QA activities to QI process improvement activities.)

Examples of areas to address:

- QA Process Identification
- FOCUS-PDCA Process Improvement
- Regulatory/Accreditation Connection (Joint Commission)

| APPROACH | DEPLOYMENT | EFFECTS |
|----------|------------|---------|
| _____% | _____% | _____% |

## Universal Charting

There was evidence that a number of ancillary services results, "loose reports," were not getting into the patients' medical records in a timely fashion. This was irritating to physicians and could result in delays in the patient's discharge, which under DRGs [diagnosis-related groups] meant higher costs without higher reimbursement. One employee filed a suggestion that a single system be developed to avoid people running over other people on the floor doing the "charting." A CQI team was developed and led by Ms. Debbie Wroten, medical records director. The 12-member team included supervisors and directors from the laboratory, the pulmonary lab, the EKG lab, medical records, radiology, and nursing. They developed the following "Opportunity Statement":

> At present six departments are utilizing nine full-time equivalents 92 hours per week for charting separate ancillary reports. Rework is created in the form of repulling of inhouse patient records creating an ever-increasing demand of chart accessibility. All parties affected by this process are frustrated because the current process increases the opportunity for lost documentation, chart unavailability, increased traffic on units creating congestion, prolonged charting times, and provides for untimely availability of clinical reports for patient care. Therefore, an opportunity exists to improve the current charting practice for all departments involved to allow for the efficiency, timeliness, and accuracy of charting loose reports.

The team met, assessed, and flow-charted the current charting processes of the five departments involved. Key variables were defined as follows:

- Charting timeliness—number of charting times per day, consistency of charting, and reports not charted per charting round.
- Report availability—indicated by the number of telephone calls per department asking for reports not yet charted.
- Chart availability—chart is accessible at the nurses' station without interruption.
- Resource utilization—manhours and number of hours per day of charting.

Each department was asked to use a common "charting log" track for several weeks of the number of records charted, who did the charting, when it was done, the preparation time, the number of reports charted, the number of reports not charted (missed), and the personnel hours consumed in charting. The results are shown in Exhibit 4–9.

These data gave the team considerable insight into the nature of the problem. Not every department was picking up the materials every day. Two people could cover the whole hospital in three-quarters of an hour each or one person in 1.5 hours. The clinical chemistry laboratory, medical records, and radiology were making two trips per day, whereas other departments were only able to chart every other day and failed to chart over the weekends.

The processes used by all the groups were similar. The printed or typed reports had to be sorted by floors, given room numbers if missing, taken to the floors, and inserted into patient charts. If the chart was not available, they had to be held until the next round. A further problem identified was that when the clerical person assigned to these rounds was not available, a technical person, who was paid considerably more and was often in short supply, had to be sent to do the job.

A smaller team of supervisors who actually knew and owned the charting efforts in the larger departments (medical records, radiology, and clinical chemistry) was set up to design and assess the pilot experiment. The overall team meetings were used only to brief the department heads to gain their feedback and support. A pilot experiment was run in which these three departments took turns doing the runs for each other. The results were favorable. The pilot increased timeliness and chart availability by charting four times per day on weekdays and three times per day on

**Exhibit 4–9** Charting Log

| Department | Mean Records | | Mean Hours | | |
| | Per Day | Range | Per Day | Range | Comments |
|---|---|---|---|---|---|
| Medical Records | 77.3 | 20–40 | 1.6 | 0.6–2.5 | Daily |
| Pulmonary Lab | 50.3 | 37–55 | 1.0 | 0.7–1.5 | MWF |
| Clinical Lab | 244.7 | 163–305 | 3.2 | 1.9–5.4 | Daily |
| EKG Lab | 40.2 | 35–48 | 0.8 | 0.1–1.0 | Weekdays |
| Microbiology | 106.9 | 3–197 | 1.4 | 0.1–2.2 | Daily |
| Radiology | 87.1 | 6–163 | 1.5 | 0.1–2.9 | Daily |

weekends. Report availability was improved, and there were fewer phone calls. Nursing staff, physicians, and participating departments specifically asked for the process to be continued. The hours of labor dropped from 92 weekly to less than 45, using less highly paid labor.

Therefore, the team decided that the issues were important enough that they should consider setting up a separate Universal Charting Team to meet the needs of the entire hospital. However, an unanticipated hospital census decline made impractical the possibility of requesting additional staffing, etc. Consequently, the group reevaluated the possibility of continuing the arrangement developed for the pilot using the charting hours of the smaller departments on a volume basis. It was discovered that this had the effect of freeing the professional staff of the smaller departments from charting activities and a very minimal allocation of hours floated to the larger departments. It also increased the availability of charters in the larger departments for other activities.

The payroll department was then asked to develop a system for allocating the hours that floated from one department to another. That proved cumbersome, so the group decided to allocate charting hours on the basis of each department's volume. "In the event that one or more departments experiences a significant increase/decrease in charting needs, the group will reconvene and the hourly allocation will be adjusted."

The resulting schedule has the lab making rounds at 6:00 AM and 9:00 AM and radiology at 4:00 PM and 9:30 PM Monday through Friday, and Medical Records at 6:00 AM, 1:00 PM, and 8:00 PM on Saturday and Sunday. Continuing statistics were kept on the process, which is shown in Exhibit 4–10. The system continued to work effectively.

## Labor, Delivery, Recovery, Postpartum (LDRP) Nursing

Competition for young families needing maternity services had become quite intense in Pensacola. WFRMC Obstetrical (OB) Services offered very traditional services in 1989 in three separate units—labor and delivery, nursery, and postpartum—and operated considerably below capacity.

A consultant was hired to evaluate the potential growth of obstetrical services, the value of current services offered by WFRMC, customers' desires, competitors' services, and opportunities for improvement. Focus group interviews with young couples (past and potential customers) indicated that they wanted safe medical care in a warm, homelike setting with

**Exhibit 4–10** Universal Charting Team FOCUS–PDCA Outline

**F**

**Opportunity Statement:**
At present, six departments are utilizing 9 full-time equivalents 92 hours a week for charting separate ancillary reports. Rework is created in the form of repulling of inhouse patient records creating an ever-increasing demand of chart accessibility. All parties affected by this process are frustrated because the current process increases the opportunity for lost documentation, chart unavailability, increased traffic on units creating congestion, prolonged charting times, and provides for untimely availability of clinical reports for patient care.
Therefore, an opportunity exists to improve the current charting practice for all departments involved to allow for the efficiency, timeliness, and accuracy of charting loose reports.

**O**

Team members include:
Debbie Wroten, Medical Records Director—Leader
Bernie Grappe, Marketing Director—Facilitator
Joan Simmons, Laboratory Director
Mary Gunter, Laboratory Patient Services Coordinator
Al Clarke, Pulmonary Services Director
Carol Riley, Pulmonary Services Assistant Director
Marlene Rodrigues, EKG Supervisor
Patti Travis, EKG
Debra Wright, Medical Records Transcription Supervisor
Mike West, Radiology Director
Lori Mikesell, Radiology Transcription Supervisor
Debbie Fernandez, Head Nurse

**C**

Assessed and flow charted current charting practices of departments.
Clarified and defined key quality characteristics of the charting process:

Charting Timeliness—number of charting times per day, consistency of charting, and reports not charted per charting round.
Report Availability—indicated by the number of telephone calls per department asking for reports not yet charted.
Chart Availability—chart is accessible at nurses' station for charting without interruption.
Resource Utilization—manhours and number of hours per day of charting.

**U**

Gathered data on departments charting volumes and time spent on charting.

---

| Department: | | | | | | | |
|---|---|---|---|---|---|---|---|
| | | | *Charting Log* | | | | |
| *Date* | *Charting Tech vs. Clk.* | *Prep Time* | *# Reports Charted* | *# Reports Not Charted* | *Charting Time (amt)* | *Hour of Day* | *Comment* |
| | | | | | | | |
| | | | | | | | |
| | | | | | | | |
| | | | | | | | |
| | | | | | | | |
| | | | | | | | |
| | | | | | | | |
| | | | | | | | |
| | | | | | | | |
| | | | | | | | |
| | | | | | | | |
| | | | | | | | |

*continues*

**Exhibit 4–10** continued

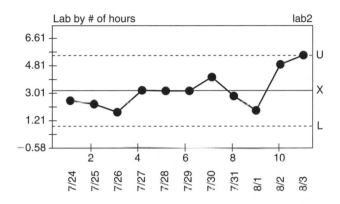

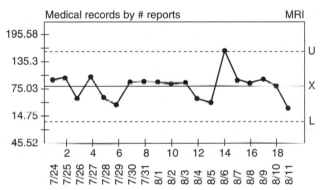

**S**
**P**

Data gained through the pilot indicated that significant gains were available through the effort to justify proceeding with the development of a Universal Charting Team.

The team developed a flow chart of the charting process using a universal charting team rather than previous arrangements. In order to pilot the improvement, the group decided to set up a UCT using current charters from the three major charting departments-medical records, laboratory, and radiology. The team also developed written instructions for both the charters and participating departments. A subgroup of the team actually conducted a one-day pilot before beginning extensive education to ensure that the UCT would work as planned and to be sure that the charters from each of the large departments were well versed on possible situations that might occur during the pilot.

**D**

Piloted proposed Universal Charting Team using current charting personnel from radiology, laboratory, and medical records to chart for all departments.

**C**

Pilot results were positive and indicated that the UCT concept offered significant advantages over the previous charting arrangements. Results were:

*continues*

**Exhibit 4–10** continued

> Timeliness/Chart Availability—Pilot reduced daily charting to four scheduled charting times daily for all departments. Smaller departments did not chart daily prior to pilot. The charting team also reduced the number of occasions that charters from different departments were on the nursing unit needing the same chart.
>
> Report Availability—Telephone calls were reduced and nursing staff, physicians, and participating departments specifically asked for UCT following the pilot.
>
> Resource Utilization—Number of manhours spent charting and preparing to chart was reduced from 92 hours weekly to less than 45 hours. The improvement also allowed the use of less expensive staff for charting.

The group reached consensus that the easiest configuration for the UCT would be to set up a separate UCT that would serve the needs of the entire hospital. This was to be proposed to administration by the team as the conclusion of their efforts. However, an unanticipated hospital census decline made impractical the possibility of requesting additional staffing, etc. Consequently, the group reevaluated the possibility of continuing the arrangement developed for the pilot using the charting hours to the smaller departments on a volume basis. It was discovered that this had the effect of freeing the professional staff in the smaller departments from charting responsibilities while a very minimal allocation of hours floated to the larger departments, and it increased the availability of charters in the larger departments for other activities. The payroll department was then involved in order to develop the proper mechanism and procedure for floating hours.

This modification of the previous pilot was piloted for a month with continued good results. Streamlining of the hours floating process may be necessary to place less burden on the payroll department.

Since no major changes were required following the pilot, the group has elected to adopt the piloted UCT format. Allocation of charting hours is based on a monthly review of charting volumes for each department. In the event that one or more departments experiences a significant increase/decrease in charting needs, the group will reconvene and the hourly allocation will be adjusted.

**LESSONS LEARNED**

Because of the size and the makeup of the team, which included a number of department heads, it was found helpful to set up a smaller team of three supervisors who actually knew and owned the charting efforts in the major departments. This group designed and assessed the initial pilot and actually piloted the pilot before bringing departmental charters into the process. As a result, overall team meetings were used primarily to brief department heads and gain their feedback and consensus.

the least possible number of rules. Most mothers were in their thirties, planning small families with the possibility of only one child. Fathers wanted to be "actively involved" in the birth process. The message came back, "We want to be actively involved in this experience and we want to make the decisions." The consultant challenged the staff to develop their own vision for the department based on the focus group responses, customer feedback, and nationally trends.

It became clear that there was a demand for a system in which a family-centered birth experience could occur. That system needed to revolve around the customers' preferences rather than making the customers follow a rigid traditional routine. Customers wanted all aspects of a normal delivery to happen in the same room. The new service would allow the mother, father, and baby to remain together throughout the hospital stay, now as short as 24 hours. Friends and families would be allowed and encouraged to visit and participate as much as the new parents desired. The main goals were to be responsive to the customer's needs and to provide safe, quality medical care.

The hospital administration and the six obstetricians practicing there were eager to see obstetrical services grow. They were open to trying and supporting the new concept. The pediatricians accepted the changes, but without great enthusiasm. The anesthesiologists were opposed to the change. The OB supervisor and two of the three nursing head nurses were also opposed to any change. They wanted to continue operations in the traditional manner. When the hospital decided to adopt the new LDRP concept, it was clear that patients and families liked it but that the nursing staff, especially management, did not. The OB nursing supervisor retired, one head nurse resigned, one was terminated, and the third opted to move from her management position to a staff nurse role. Ms. Cynthia Ayres, R.N., Administrative Director, responsible for the psychiatric and cardiovascular services, was assigned to implement the LDRP transition until nursing management could be replaced.

One of the issues involved in the transition was clarification of the charge structure. Previously each unit charged separately for services and supplies. Now that the care was provided in a single central area, the old charge structure was unnecessarily complex. Duplication of charges was occurring, and some charges were being missed because no one was assuming responsibility.

Ms. Ayres decided to use the CQI process to develop a new charge process and to evaluate the costs and resource consumption of the service. Ms. Ayres had not been a strong supporter of the CQI process when it was first introduced into the organization. She had felt that the process was too slow and rigid, and that data collection was difficult and cumbersome. Several teams were organized and assigned to look at specific areas of the LDRP process.

To reach a simplified charge process, as well as a competitive price, all aspects of the process had to be analyzed. Meetings were held with the nursing and medical staff. Management of OB patient and physician preferences in terms of supplies and practices were analyzed. A number of consensus conferences were held to discuss observed variations. For example, each of the six obstetricians specified a different analgesic for pain control. All of these drugs appeared effective for pain control, but their cost per dose ranged from $10 to $75. The physicians agreed that the $10 product was acceptable since the outcome was the same.

Another standard practice was sending placentas to the pathology laboratory for analysis after every normal delivery. This involved labor time, lab charges, and a pathologist's fee for review. The total procedure cost $196. When questioned about the practice, the current medical staff did not feel it was necessary medically nor the current practice nationally, but felt that they were just following the rules. Upon investigation, the team found that an incident involving a placenta had occurred 15 years ago that had led the service chief (since retired) to order all placentas sent to the lab. The obstetricians developed criteria for when it was medically necessary for the lab review of a placenta. This new rule decreased the number of reviews by 95%, resulting in cost savings to the hospital and to patients.

The team reviewed all OB charges for a one-year period. They found that in 80% of the normal deliveries, 14 items were consistently used. The other items were due to variations in physician preferences. The teams and the physicians met and agreed which items were the basic requirements for a normal delivery. These items became the basic charges for package pricing.

The team met weekly for at least one hour for over a year. Some meetings went as long as five hours. Initially, there was a great deal of resistance and defensiveness. Everyone wanted to focus on issues that did not affect himself or herself. The physicians objected that they were being forced to practice "cookbook medicine" and that the real problem was "the hospital's big markup." Hospital staff continued to provide data on actual hospital charges, resource consumption, and practice patterns. The hospital personnel continued to emphasize repeatedly that the physicians were responsible for determining care. The hospital's concern was to be consistent and to decrease variation.

Another CQI team, the Documentation Team, was responsible for reviewing forms utilized previously by the three separate units. The total number of forms used had been 30. The nursing staff was documenting vital signs an average of five times each time care was provided. Through review of policies, standards, documentation, and care standards, the number of forms was reduced to 20. Nurses were now required to enter each care item only one time. The amount of time spent by nurses on documentation was reduced 50%, as was the cost of forms. Data entry errors were also reduced.

The excess costs that were removed were not all physician-related. Many had to do with administrative and nursing policies. Many were due to old, comfortable, traditional ways of doing things. When asked why a practice was followed, the typical response was, "I don't know; that's just the way we've always done it." The OB staff became comfortable with the use of CQI. They recognized that, although it requires time and effort, it does produce measurable results. The OB staff continued to review their practices and operations to identify opportunities to streamline services and decrease variation.

**Pharmacy and Therapeutics Team**

In late 1987, a CQI team was formed jointly between the hospital's Pharmacy and Therapeutics (P&T) Committee and the pharmacy leadership. The first topic of concern was the rapidly rising costs of inpatient drugs, especially antibiotics, which were then costing the hospital about $1.3 million per year. The team decided to study the process by which antibiotics were selected and began by asking physicians how they selected antibiotics for treatment. Most of the time physicians ordered a culture of the organism believed to be causing the infection from the microbiology lab. A microbiology lab report came back identifying the organism and the antibiotics to which it was sensitive and those to which it was resistant. Some physicians reported that they would look down the list until they came to an antibiotic to which the organism was sensitive and order that. That list was in alphabetical order. A study of antibiotic utilization showed a high correlation between use and alphabetical position, confirming the anecdotal reports. Therefore the team recommended to the P&T committee that the form be changed to list the antibiotics in order of increasing cost per average daily dose. The doses used would be based on current local prescribing patterns rather than recommended dosages. The P&T committee, which included attending physicians, approved the change and reported it in their annual report to the medical staff. Exhibit 4–11 shows what happened to the utilization of "expensive" antibiotics

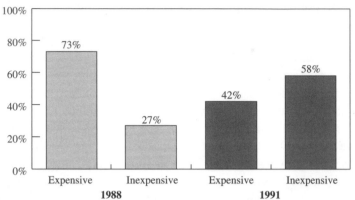

**Exhibit 4–11** Antibiotic Utilization Ratio, Expensive: Inexpensive Doses Dispensed (expensive ≈ $10.00 per dose)

(more than $10 per dose) from 1988 to 1991. These costs were not adjusted at all for inflation in drug prices during this period. The estimated annual saving was $200,000.

Given this success, the team went on in 1989 to deal with the problem of the length of treatment using antibiotics. Inpatients did not get a prescription for ten days' supply. Their IM and IV antibiotics were continued until the physician stopped the order. If a physician went away for the weekend and the patient improved, colleagues were very reluctant to alter the medication until he or she returned. The team wrestled with how to encourage the appropriate ending of the course of treatment without hassling the physicians or risking undue legal liability problems. They settled on a sticker that was placed in the chart at the end of three days stating that the treatment had gone on for three days at that point and that an ending date should be specified if possible. The hospital newsletter and the P&T committee annual report noted that the physician could avoid this notice by specifying a termination date at the time of prescribing. This program seemed to be effective. Antibiotic costs again dropped, and there were no apparent quality problems introduced as measured by length of stay or by adverse events associated with the new system.

In 1990 the team began an aggressive Drug Usage Evaluation (DUE) program, hiring an assistant director of pharmacy clinical services to administer it. The position had to be rigorously cost-justified. DUE involved a review of cases to determine whether the selection and scheduling of powerful drugs matched the clinical picture presented. For example, if the physician prescribed one of three types of antibiotics known to represent a risk of kidney damage in 3% to 5% of cases, the DUE administrator ordered lab tests to study serum creatinine levels and warn the physician if they rose, indicating kidney involvement. There was a sharp decline in the adverse effects due to the use of these drugs. This program was expanded further to incorporate looking at other critical lab values and relating them to pharmacy activities beyond antibiotics, for example, use of IV solutions and potassium levels. By 1991, the unadjusted antibiotic costs for roughly the same number of admissions had dropped to less than $900,000.

## LOOKING AHEAD

One of the things that had concerned John Kausch during 1991 was the fact that implementation had varied from department to department. Although he had written in his annual CQI report that the variation had certainly been within the range of acceptability, he was still concerned about how much variation in implementation was appropriate. If maintaining enthusiasm was a concern, forcing people to conform too tightly might become a demotivator for some staff. This issue and the four mentioned at the beginning of this case study should all be addressed in the coming year.

## CASE ANALYSIS

This is a hospital with a large group of physicians closely tied to it, both economically and geographically. It is also operating in an area of intense competition and tight cost controls. The fact that 90% to 95% of the hospital's compensation is case-based (DRGs) and not procedure-based has a profound impact on management motivation. Intense support for the CQI implementation was provided by Dr. Batalden and his staff at HCA corporate headquarters.

## ASSIGNMENT QUESTIONS

### Introduction

1. What were the strategic reasons behind West Florida Regional Medical Center's (WFRMC's) decision to invest heavily in TQM?
2. How did the program undertaken at WFRMC reflect this strategic impetus?

### Basics

3. What were the strengths and weaknesses of the TQM program as it was implemented here?
4. What were the influences of corporate headquarters in this effort?
5. What effort has been made to measure the impact of the program on the hospital, especially in terms of supporting its strategic directions?

### Implementation

6. What effort has been made to use TQM to support tactical programs within the hospital?
7. What should John Kausch do next in dealing with continuous improvement?

### Application

8. If West Florida Regional Medical Center was to introduce an internal medicine residency program, how should the concepts of microsystems be incorporated into its current quality efforts?

## CLASS EXERCISE

Visit a large local health delivery institution. Document how they are motivating participation in continuous improvement by various types of clinical and administrative staff. Compare and contrast their approach with the HCA approach outlined in the West Florida case.

# CASE 5

# Rex Healthcare and Service Line Teams

*Curtis P. McLaughlin and Linda C. Jordan*

Rex Healthcare is a private, nonprofit organization founded in 1894 by Raleigh N.C. tanner, John Rex. It provides a wide range of services to the research triangle area. The main Rex campus is a 62-acre site in west Raleigh convenient to I-40 and I-440. This campus includes the 394-bed Rex Hospital, the 140-bed Rex Convalescent Center, and the Rex Cancer Center. Patients utilizing the Rex Heart Center also have access to the Rex Wellness Centers in Raleigh and Cary. Rex Home Services serves patients in seven counties through approximately 100,000 home health visits a year. Exhibit 5–1 shows the various centers and campuses of Rex Healthcare.

ReXMeD is a physician-hospital organization (PHO) formed in late 1995. By April 1998, ReXMeD had credentialed 45 primary care physicians and over 200 specialty physicians, all of whom were stockholders together with the hospital in this for-profit limited liability company. The Rex primary care network included over 50 board-certified primary care physicians, physician assistants, and nurse practitioners in 12 practices in Raleigh, Cary, Garner, and Wake Forest. Over 800 total physicians were members of the Rex medical staff. Rex has a long history of innovation, having been a North Carolina pioneer in a number of radiological techniques, hospital management training, the comprehensive cancer center, and employee childcare. The introduction of clinical care service lines in 1996 was a continuation of that history of innovation.

**Exhibit 5–1** Special Centers and Services of Rex Healthcare

In Raleigh:
- Rex Hospital
- Rex Cancer Center
- Rex Convalescent Center
- Rex Same Day Surgery Center
- Rex Wellness Center
- Rex Family Birth Center
- Rex Emergency Department Fast Track Services
- Rex Heart Center
- Rex Breast Care Center
- Rex Primary Care (multiple sites)
- ReXMeD (PHO)
- Healthnet Information and Resource Center
- Rex Senior Health Center (downtown)
- Rex Business Health Services (occupational medicine)
- RexAware (employee assistance program)
- Rex Emergency Response Team
- Rex Urgent Care Centers

In Cary and Apex
- Rex Healthcare of Cary (primary care)
- Rex Wellness Center
- Rex Urgent Care Center
- Rex Convalescent Care Center (107 beds)

In Garner
- Rex Healthcare of Garner-Garner Family Physicians

In Wake Forest
- Rex Healthcare of Wake Forest (primary care)

Regionally
- Rex HomeHealth Services

## QUALITY AT REX

Rex Hospital has an excellent reputation for quality. A 1995 consumer survey conducted by the Endresen Research Group of Seattle, Washington identified Rex as the preferred hospital in Wake County. It received

National Research Corporation's 1996 and 1997 Quality Leaders awards. This Lincoln, Nebraska-based research organization conducted surveys of 165,000 households in 100 metropolitan areas nationwide with about 2,500 hospitals. Rex was selected as one of the best 119 nationwide based on questions about overall preference, quality of care, best physicians and nurses, best image and reputation, best community health programs, and most personalized care. Rex has consistently earned the Gallup survey's premier rating in several patient categories as well as "Likelihood to Recommend and Likelihood to Choose Again," placing it in the top 20 percent of Gallup hospitals nationwide. In 1997, Rex was honored by *Working Woman Magazine* as one of the "Best 100" workplaces for working women. It has also earned the North Carolina Governor's Award for Excellence for its Workplace Wellness Program.

The hospital's mission–vision statement read as follows:

> Rex is a patient-centered healthcare delivery system in working partnership with the medical staff. We are a healthcare leader, designing innovative and flexible solutions that achieve superior patient outcomes and customer satisfaction. Through the integration of clinical, financial, and administrative systems, we are cost effective and deliver a continuum of care that meets the dynamic health needs of our community. We are committed to creating a culture that continually improves services, sustains a high quality team-oriented work environment, and provides for all of our community healthcare for life.

## COMPETITION IN THE RESEARCH TRIANGLE

The research triangle area has a population of approximately 1.2 million, about half of whom live in Wake County. It is generally considered to be over-doctored with the University of North Carolina and Duke University medical schools in adjacent Orange and Durham counties. Wake County and the easterly counties of Johnson, Franklin, and Harnett have a combined population of three-quarters of a million. The market population was growing rapidly, was youthful, and had very low unemployment. There were three substantial hospitals in Wake County—Wake Medical Center, historically the county hospital; Raleigh Community Hospital, formerly Columbia-owned, but purchased in 1998 by Duke

Medical Center; and Rex. Wake Medical had a slightly higher share of market than Rex did, but Rex was dominant in ambulatory surgery, women and children's services and oncology. Rex's payer mix was good with the highest percentage of commercial and managed care patients. The Wake County market in 1997 was:

| | |
|---|---|
| HMO | 43% |
| Commercial–Other | 33% |
| Medicare | 8% |
| Medicaid | 5% |
| Uninsured | 10% |

Physician practices were consolidating with MedPartners and FPA Medical Management having practices in the county, with WakeMed having started an medical service organization (MSO) and Rex a physician-hospital organization (PHO) while both Duke and Carolina were developing independent practice associations (IPAs) in the area. In 1997, Wake County hospital discharges per 1,000 dipped below 100 and hospital days per 1,000 below 500.

## HISTORY OF QUALITY AND PERFORMANCE IMPROVEMENT EFFORTS AT REX

Exhibit 5–2 provides a chronological list of quality events at Rex. Early efforts to implement clinical pathways were not as successful as hoped, because the software was used for documentation rather than for variance identification, but were again being encouraged and the overall infrastructure to support this effort was being restructured.

### Structure for Governance and Implementation

The leaders at Rex established a Joint Conference Committee (JCC) to oversee performance improvement activities. It included representatives from the board of trustees, medical staff executive committee, and Rex Healthcare executive staff. Its purpose was to direct the selection of organizational measures for important processes, prioritize and reprioritize these measurement activities, and establish performance objectives for

**Exhibit 5–2** Chronological Events at Rex Healthcare

| Date | Event |
|------|-------|
| 1894 | Rex Hospital founded in Raleigh, NC |
| Before 1995 | Installs Trendstar cost reporting system |
| 1995 | Rex named preferred hospital in Wake County by Endreson Research Group survey |
| | Case Management and Performance Improvement–Risk Management Departments created (October) |
| | ReXMeD PHO formed (November) |
| 1996 | Case Management Services implemented (January) |
| | Master Performance Improvement Plan developed (February) |
| | Service Line Teams implemented (March) |
| | Performance Improvement Committee replaces Hospital Quality Assurance Committee (August) |
| | Mediqual Atlas data collection starts |
| | Starts using Gallup survey of customer satisfaction |
| | Starts using Health Management Council Clinical Benchmark cost data |
| | HCIA hospital discharge benchmarking data set introduced |
| | Named as one of "Best 100" workplaces for working women by Working Mother's Magazine |
| 1997 | Arthur Andersen report suggests organizational structure for performance improvement with matrix of functional teams and service line teams |
| | Received National Research Corp.'s Quality Leader Award |
| | Earned State of North Carolina Governor's Award for Excellence for its Workplace Wellness Program |
| | MedPartners acquires Cardinal and Piedmont IPA bringing its Raleigh membership to about 500 physicians |
| 1998 | Duke University Medical Center announces purchase of Raleigh Community Hospital from Columbia–HCA |

them. It received regular reports from the Performance Improvement Committee (PIC) concerning process improvements and outcomes. This organizational relationship is outlined in Exhibit 5–3.

The Performance Improvement Committee was an interdisciplinary medical review committee reporting to both the medical staff executive committee and the JCC. Its functions were to oversee organizational compliance with the performance improvement plan adopted by the leadership;

**Exhibit 5–3**  Performance Improvement Reporting Structure

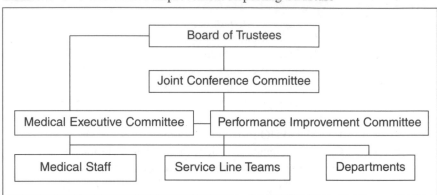

identify and recommend priorities and priority changes to the JCC; receive and review regular reports from all of the service line teams, committees, and departments; identify opportunities to improve performance; and recommend and establish "action teams" where indicated. Priorities were based on their potential to enhance patient care, achieve corporate goals, improve the financial strength of the organization, and/or improve quality of work life for employees and physicians.

## Introduction of Service Lines

Service lines grouped inpatients according to similar diagnosis-related groups (DRGs) so that the care team could better meet the patients' needs. Ten services lines were developed. They were:

1. Oncology
2. Neuroscience
3. Orthopedics
4. Cardiovascular
5. Medicine
6. General Surgery
7. Women and Children
8. Pulmonary–Nephrology
9. Emergency Services
10. Primary Care Division

The objective of the service line team was to promote accountability for the care of its population across the continuum of care. Representation on the teams was multidisciplinary and was determined by the particular needs of the population served. Each team had a physician team leader and a nursing team coordinator. The service line team members assessed data on an ongoing basis to identify opportunities for improvement and promote achievable patient outcomes and satisfaction. Each team's charge also included cost-effective utilization of resources, identification of the need for clinical pathways, and minimization of risks where feasible. It compared internal performance over time, compared Rex's performance with similar facilities, and compared performance to other sources such as practice guidelines as appropriate. It initiated intensive assessments by establishing action teams when variations in performance occurred or when opportunities to improve were identified.

The objective of an action team was to provide intensive assessment, analysis, and recommendations for improvement. The expected outputs were recommendations, an implementation plan, and a measurement plan. Rex adopted the FOCUS-PDCA methodology of process improvement. It was included in the leadership development core training program offered to all employees. Education included the use of performance improvement tools, analysis of data, and leading and facilitating teams. New employee orientation included an introductory session on this process improvement methodology.

## 1995–1996 Reorganization

The reorganization into service line teams highlighted the need to change the way that the staff services that support quality improvement were organized. Rex Hospital had traditional and separate departments of utilization review—quality assurance, social work, and continuous service improvement (also responsible for pathway development). Pathway implementation had not been as successful as hoped except for orthopedics. To prepare for an environment of more risk-based reimbursement and to counter reduced margins, these departments were intensified, re-engineered, and integrated to have greater impact on clinical and financial outcomes without adversely affecting existing high quality levels.

In October 1995, two new departments were created—case management and performance improvement–risk management. Case management combined utilization review–quality assurance and social work and added a pre-entry case management function. Within three months, the new case management model with concern for clinical, financial, and quality improvement was implemented in the inpatient setting. Nurse case managers and medical social workers were assigned to each of the eight inpatient core specialties and became core members of the service line teams. By 1998, the Case Management Program included the following:

- Pre-entry coordination
- Screening and referral
- Assessment
- Problem identification
- Care planning
- Utilization management
- DRG analysis
- Variance management
- Discharge planning
- Psychosocial intervention
- Crisis management

At the same time, the performance improvement–risk management (PI–RM) department was established to support the organization's quality assurance, quality improvement, outcomes management, risk management, and clinical pathway development. It coordinated, analyzed, and reported improvement data. Wherever possible, measurement activities were incorporated into processes and performed and reviewed concurrently by caregivers. The PI–RM department coordinated systems for the collection of specific data (Atlas, RiskKey) and worked directly with other departments to acquire other data (Trendstar, Gallup, National Nosocomial Infection Survey). These data were compiled and initial analysis performed. Comparison was made to historical experience, reference databases, accreditation guidelines, and practice guidelines. These data and analyses were then presented to service line teams, departments, and committees on a routine basis. Exhibit 5–4 lists the measures regularly collected or acquired. Quality control issues were reported to the Performance Improvement Committee on a "report-by-exception" basis. Regular Performance Improvement Service Line Reports were issued as well. An example is shown in Exhibit 5–5.

**Exhibit 5–4** Reporting Systems Used for Performance Improvement

Atlas
Variance Reports
Clinical Path Variance Reports
Infection Control Surveillance
Comments
Improvement Initiatives
JCAHO Indicator Monitors
Gallup Satisfaction Results
Department Specific Monitoring Reports
MMI Clinical Indicators
HCIA comparative hospital discharge summary data
Trendstar internal cost reports
Sentinel Events
Quality Control in the Organization– = or > 30 cases up to 5% sample
    quarterly
• preoperative and postoperative diagnosis discrepancies
• adverse drug reactions
• confirmed transfusion reactions
• adverse anesthesia events
• appropriateness of admissions and hospital stays
• patient satisfaction
• staff views regarding performance and improvement operations
• autopsy results
• restraints
• risk management activities
• quality control activities for clinical labs, diagnostic radiology, dietetic,
    nuclear medicine, radiation oncology, medication administration equip-
    ment, pharmacy equipment used to prepare medications
Additional measures identified and prioritized by Joint Conference
    Committee:
• patient care functions
• organization functions
• high risk, high volume, high cost, problem-prone procedures–processes.

The key coordination mechanism for performance improvement continued to be the PIC. It fulfilled a wide variety of roles and its agenda
became extensive and complex. For example, the calendar for the
September 1998 meeting called for third quarter Gallup results, the quarterly Infection Control report, review of quarterly HCIA data, and quarterly

**Exhibit 5–5**   Example of Service Line Report

PERFORMANCE IMPROVEMENT SERVICE LINE REPORT
WOMEN AND CHILDREN DATE _____

| GLOBAL INDICATORS | BENCHMARK | Q1 | Q2 | Q3 | Q4 |
|---|---|---|---|---|---|
| 1.  C/S | ** 20% | | | | |
| 2.  APGAR <4 @ 5" | ** 18 | | | | |
| 3.  Meconium aspiration | ** 13 | | | | |
| 4.  NB w/ cerebral hemorrhage | ** 1 | | | | |
| 5.  Pts ≥ 24 wks. gestation who do not receive baseline monitoring | ** 5 | | | | |
| 6.  Use of Pit w/o fetal monitoring | ** 11 | | | | |
| 7.  C/S for fetal ind not started w/in 30" | ** 8 | | | | |
| 8.  Neonates delivered in a Level I or II facility @ < 34 wks. & tr. to NICU | ** 29 | | | | |
| 9.  Neonates deliv. >34 wks.& tr to NICU | ** 130 | | | | |
| 10.  Maternal deaths | ** 0 | | | | |
| 11.  Neonatal deaths | | | | | |
| ≥ 34 wks. | | | | | |
| < 34 wks. & </= 500 gms. | ** 10 | | | | |
| 12.  Neonatal temp <35 C in first 4 hours of life | ** 5 | | | | |
| 13.  Pneumothorax after neonatal resuscitation using ppv | ** 1 | | | | |
| 14.  Neonates w/intubation prior to use of ppv | ** 42 | | | | |

** Based on MMI

| Gallup Survey Results | | | | |
|---|---|---|---|---|
| Service Line Overall | | | | |
| Rex Overall | 3.59 | 3.56 | 3.55 | N.A. |
| **Resource Management** | | | | |
| Cost per Case | | | | |
| Cost Index | | | | |

informational presentations from the cardiovascular, medical, and surgical service line teams and from the Rex Convalescent Center team. In addition, it included a quarterly report on risk management issues, medical staff review of clinical pathway team recommendations, and review of other procedural changes. Also, it would consider additional items that might come up such as sentinel event reports, adverse drug reaction re-

**Exhibit 5–6** Quarterly Schedule of PIC Presentations

| October 1998 | November 1998 | December 1998 |
|---|---|---|
| Safety | Procedure Review | Gallup customer satisfaction survey |
| Pharmacy & Therapeutics Committee | Pulmonary Service Line Team | Infection Control |
| Risk Management | Orthopedics Service Line Team | Cardiovascular Service Line Team |
| Oncology Service Line Team | Women and Children's Service Line Team | Medicine Service Line Team |
| Neuroscience Service Line Team | Nursing Performance Improvement Team | Surgery Service Line Team |
| Rex Home Services | | |
| Emergency Department Service Line Team | | |
| Blood Utilization Committee | | |
| Cancer Committee | | |

ports, and accreditation concerns. At other meetings, the PIC reviewed plans and performance of the performance improvement–risk management department and reports required by the hospital's liability insurance carrier; analyzed safety issues, pathway utilization, and variance reports; reviewed proposals for new action teams; approved forms for reporting; and reviewed Atlas Mediqual, Trendstar, and other benchmarking systems. Exhibit 5–6 shows the schedule of reviews planned for each of the monthly PIC meetings during the fourth quarter of 1998.

**Future Plans**

By mid-1998, the assessment of the services showed that service line team leadership was in place with adequate staff support and functioning with clear targets. The next step was to begin to involve the service line teams (SLTs) in the 1999 budget process to allow service line savings to track back to the bottom line. In 1999, the hospital would try to develop an affordable team reward system that could be implemented in 2000. This would have to be coordinated with the development of job description changes reflecting the new organizational structure and supported through a new communication plan to explain the changes to all the Rex community. Beyond that, the leadership saw the need to increase medical staff involvement in SLTs and action teams, to move the program beyond acute care, and balance the focus on outcomes, satisfaction, and cost effectiveness. They also saw needs to develop mechanisms and/or incentives for following protocols, to streamline the approval process of SLT actions, and to streamline and clarify data sources and processes for decision-making.

## CASE ANALYSIS

This case illustrates the organizational complexities introduced by the need for outcomes measurement as well as process enhancement. This hospital was much further along than most at this point in time, but it still had a number of issues to deal with in the future, such as the roles of administration, of the performance and measurement committee, and of the medical staff in this transition period and in the long run.

## ASSIGNMENT QUESTIONS

### Introduction

1. Evaluate the mission statement of Rex Hospital.
2. How does the competitive environment of the Triangle influence the situation here?

### Basics

3. How has the historical development of quality systems at Rex Hospital affected the evolution of its quality improvement effort?

4. Evaluate the performance improvement reporting structure as outlined in Exhibit 5–3.

5. Evaluate the makeup of the service line team and explain its impact on the quality improvement effort.

## Implementation

6. What do you think of the 1995–1996 reorganization creating the two new departments: case management and performance improvement-risk management?

7. What recommendations do you have about the reporting systems used for performance improvement (Exhibits 5–3 and 5–4)?

8. What further recommendations do you have to the individuals responsible for clinical quality improvement at Rex Hospital?

## Application

9. Rex Hospital has since been acquired by the University of North Carolina Health Care System (www.unchealthcare.org). How would you modify its quality improvement programs to enhance their potential contribution to teaching CQI to health professionals in training?

## CLASS EXERCISE

Visit a large local health care institution and find out how they are currently measuring and reporting on quality. Is their system outcomes oriented? Does it report by product line or some other way? What information is reported to various levels of management, with what frequency, with what links to corporate strategy, with what impacts on quality of care and on profitability?

# Dr. Johnson, Network Medical Director

*William Q. Judge and Curtis P. McLaughlin[1]*

Charles A. Johnson, D.O., M.B.A., reviewed his six months of experience as a network medical director for the Southeast region of Vigilant–Xtra Mile Healthcare located in Atlanta, Georgia. He was one of two physicians responsible for developing and managing the professional medical network of providers and hospitals serving this market, which included the states of Alabama, Georgia, and Mississippi. His duties involved recruiting providers, negotiating contracts, promoting the company's disease management approaches, credentialing physicians, maintaining National Committee for Quality Assurance (NCQA) accreditation, reviewing cost and quality data as well as provider report cards, arranging education efforts for outliers, and controlling the unit cost side of the firm's medical loss ratio in that market.

Dr. Johnson had a full plate of responsibilities that were new to him and his organization. Furthermore, he had limited staff to which to delegate duties and there were overlapping responsibilities with two other medical directors in his office that needed to be coordinated carefully. Despite these challenges, he felt fortunate to have a supportive and

---

[1]This case was prepared by Professor William Q. Judge, College of Business Administration, University of Tennessee Knoxville and Professor Curtis P. McLaughlin for use at both universities as a basis for class discussion rather than to illustrate the effective or ineffective handling of an administrative matter. All rights reserved. Not to be reproduced without permission.

powerful boss and he was convinced that Vigilant–Xtra Mile Health-care was the wave of the future. His immediate challenge was funda-mentally a matter of time management. Although Dr. Johnson was highly organized, he felt he was constantly "putting out unexpected fires" and these urgent projects tended to push out longer-term strate-gic issues. For example, in the last month, his schedule had been con-sumed by several unexpected activities including: (1) supervising a database cleanup; (2) addressing open enrollment administrative glitches in January; (3) being available for audits of the Medicare pro-gram by HCFA and the state of Georgia; (4) preparing for a mock NCQA audit; and (5) dealing with supervisory and human relations is-sues within his unit. These issues tended to get in the way of refining his network of providers and overseeing quality, but they had to be ad-dressed. Dr. Johnson hoped that with time things would settle down.

## PERSONAL BACKGROUND

When Charles Johnson graduated in 1970 from Baldwin-Wallace College in Berea, Ohio with a B.S. in zoology and philosophy, he went to work as a pharmaceutical salesman in Ohio and Western Pennsylvania. He was suc-cessful there, but he wanted direct patient contact, so he decided to pursue a medical degree. In 1973, he entered the Midwestern University–Chicago College of Osteopathic Medicine. Graduating in 1977, he interned at Hospital Corporation of America (HCA) Northlake Hospital in Tucker, Georgia. In 1979, he founded the East Cobb Family Practice in Marietta, Georgia and joined the staff of the Archway Hospital. He became board certified by the American Board of Osteopathic Family Practitioners and a fellow of the American Academy of Family Practice in 1986 and a diplomat of the American Board of Medical Management in 1997.

In the late 1980s, Dr. Johnson and his partner differed markedly over the importance of managed care. His partner did not want to participate, while he was convinced it was the wave of the future. When he witnessed the loss of 20% of his patients after Lockheed Marietta moved all of its employees to managed care, he was convinced that he needed to change his practice. He had been participating in management workshops pro-vided by the American College of Physician Executives (ACPE) and decided to enter Emory University's weekend executive MBA program. He found this to be a valuable learning experience, particularly his thesis project which involved a study of methods of evaluation for small medical practices. When he graduated in June 1991, he installed a total quality management effort in his family practice and asked his partner to leave within 90 days. After his partner left, Dr. Johnson increased the volume of the practice 83% within 12 months while accepting managed care patients and adding a new partner, two physician assistants, and a nurse practitioner.

Dr. Johnson tried to start a group practice without walls in conjunction with other providers, but it failed within six months due to lack of capital and physician management skills and involvement. Then in late 1994, he received four offers to sell his practice. One of the offers came from an organization that was connected to the hospital where he practiced. Ultimately, he decided to sell his practice to this organization and become involved in the management of the resulting organization. Thus, he became one of the founding members and Chief of Family Medicine for Dominion Northwest Physician's Group, a group with 180 physicians and 60 locations and affiliations with 13 hospitals in the greater Atlanta region. There he spent half of his time in management and half the other in patient care delivery.

The job with Dominion Northwest was a useful transition for him. He negotiated contracts for the physicians and was involved in developing methods for equitably dividing capitated payment among the specialists and primary care physicians. He was on the contracting committee of the Dominion Physician–Hospital Organization (PHO) and the Physician's Group, and on the strategic planning and the informatics committees as well as the physicians' advisory board. He learned more about working in large organizations with hours spent in committee meetings and dealing with larger bureaucracies. With time, however, he became convinced that this organization did not have sufficient physician involvement in decision making to satisfy him in the long run, but he kept on learning about medical management and leadership.

Then an executive recruiter called him about the job at Vigilant–Xtra Mile HealthCare (Vigilant–XMHC). Dr. Johnson felt he had nothing to lose in looking at it, especially since it was in Atlanta. He concluded that it was the type of job that would allow him to make a difference at a higher level. Vigilant–XMHC was looking for a physician with management skills, with a good reputation and credentials, and one well-connected to the local network. Dr. Johnson had been very active in the Georgia Academy of Family Practice, was on the board of directors of Blue Ridge Area Health Education Center (AHEC) and of a couple of managed care plans, in addition to his involvement with administrative duties within Dominion.

In 1994, Governor Zell Miller appointed Dr. Johnson to the nine-member Georgia Joint Board of General Practice that oversaw the allocation of $50,000,000 in state residency and training funds. Dr. Johnson worked with the other members to formulate state policy on funding of graduate medical education and to redesign all state funding mechanisms for medical education. He was currently secretary-treasurer of the board. He has also served as a preceptor for Emory University and the West Virginia College of Osteopathic Medicine and on the 6th District (Newt Gingrich's former district) Medicare Advisory Board Task Force on Alternative Plans for Medicare. In short, his connections and experience were ideal for the job.

The job carried with it a salary comparable to a good primary care practitioner income with major upside potential in the long run. There were very good benefits and he was part of the regional management team. Fortunately, Dominion-Northwest allowed Dr. Johnson to opt out of the remaining two years of his employment contract and he joined Vigilant–XMHC in August 1997.

His counterpart, Chris Donovan, M.D., was a native of the West Indies who had previous experience as a medical director with Domina in Charlotte, NC. He was also new to the organization as he joined Vigilant–Xtra Mile HealthCare about the same time as Dr. Johnson did. Drs. Johnson and Donovan had a good working relationship. Their responsibilities were basically the same, except for different parts of the market.

## CORPORATE BACKGROUND

Vigilant and Xtra Mile Healthcare merged in April 1996, bringing together two quite different firms. Vigilant was a traditional full-line insurance company founded in 1899 with 48 highly decentralized HMO operations and a rather conservative business outlook. It was headquartered in Boston. In contrast, Xtra Mile Healthcare was founded in Wheeling, West Virginia in 1978. It was a highly centralized and entrepreneurial company developed and managed by physicians. For example, Vigilant had 50 different claims processing centers, while XMHC had only one. In addition to structural differences, their growth strategies were also quite different. Vigilant had been buying primary care practices, while Xtra Mile HealthCare did not buy any practices.

The resulting merger was a giant company with revenues in excess of $17 billion, more than half of which was in health care products. It divided the nation into six regions that are depicted in Exhibit 6–1. In 1998, Vigilant–Xtra Mile Healthcare provided health care services to 23 million Americans in 50 states through networks involving 300,000 physicians and 3,000 hospitals. Roughly one insured American in 12 was covered for health care by the resulting organization.

The merged company developed a number of strategies aimed at capitalizing on its extensive asset base and unique array of competencies. First and foremost, it would offer a full line of health care insurance products (e.g., indemnity, preferred provider organization [PPO], point-of-service [POS], HMO, senior HMO) on a national basis to offer "one-stop shopping" to nationally-based organizations. The firm would not purchase medical practices or facilities, but would maintain an open panel of physicians and nonexclusive contracts with hospitals and ancillary providers. Its basic HMO contracting model called for primary care physicians (PCPs) to serve as gatekeepers on quality based-capitation, with special-

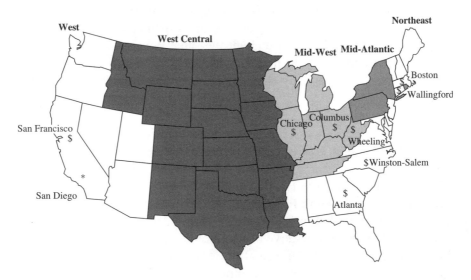

**Exhibit 6–1** Six Regions of Vigilant–Xtra Mile HealthCare.

ists paid on a discounted fee-for-service or capitated basis and hospitals paid at a negotiated rate by the case or per diem.

By 1997, Vigilant–XMHC had an approved HMO in 23 states and the District of Columbia covering 73% of the population and had applications pending in the rest. Each physician recruited to the network was expected to service all Vigilant–XMHC health care products under one contract. This consistent national presence and full range of health care products allowed the company to approach large national employers on a highly competitive basis. The fact that they could also supply disability insurance, group life insurance, retirement plans, 401Ks, dental insurance, and variety of other products to the same benefits managers nationwide was considered a strong competitive advantage. The company is a leading provider of Medicare managed care services and could also service the company's retirees.

The two companies had been highly profitable in 1995 and 1996. However, profit margins narrowed and medical loss ratios rose sharply in 1997. The stock had dropped sharply from 1996 levels. The economies in operations and from scale that had been expected took much longer to achieve. Dr. Johnson talked about the loss of human capital during the reorganization that cost it dearly. According to Dr. Johnson,

> In our efforts to re-engineer the organization, a lot of administrative help was eliminated. In so doing, we let go of a lot of Ms. Smiths. You know, Ms. Smith was the one in the local office who knew that Dr. Jones never checked box 30 on the HCFA 1500 form, but checked it for him rather than sending it back to his office.

The resulting delays and other glitches with new offices and employees slowed down claims processing and overstated initial earnings, with costs catching up later. However, the new organization was now getting more integrated and claims processing was functioning better in 1998. The new Vigilant–Xtra Mile HealthCare organization was partially decentralized into six regions. The Southeast region consisted of four markets stretching from Mississippi to Florida to Maryland.

## Organizational Structure

The overall corporate headquarters was located with Vigilant in Boston, while the health care operations were headquartered at XMHC in

Wheeling. The six regional offices reported to the Wheeling corporate offices. There were three medical director hierarchies in the company. Network medical directors, of which Dr. Johnson was one, reported to the general manager for each market who in turn reported to the regional manager. Patient management medical directors were involved with utilization management, preauthorizations, length-of-stay reviews, case management development, retrospective reviews, and disease management enrollment. They came under the regional medical director who reported directly to the core team at Wheeling. Finally, there was also a regional quality medical director who reported to quality management staff in Boston. A detailed comparison of these three types of medical directors is listed in Exhibit 6–2.

Dr. Johnson supervised a team of eight individuals—two provider relations managers who in turn led five professional service coordinators, and an administrative assistant shared with Dr. Donovan. The professional service coordinators were the ones out on the firing line with the providers. There were numerous dotted line relationships among the various medical directors. In fact, when he was hired, Dr. Johnson had only dotted line relationships and no direct reports, so he recommended a reorganization in which he took on budgetary and supervisory responsibility for a portion of the provider services staff. He also made a determined effort to be seen as a contributor to the management team of the market and the region. For example, he hosted a weekend strategic planning session for the regional management team at his summer home at Lake Lanier.

This meant considerable added workload due to supervision, performance review, objective setting, and process improvement. He typically worked from 7:00 AM to 6:00 PM two days a week, and 9:00 AM to 6:00 PM the other three, and then usually had a couple of dinner meetings each week. Weekend activities such as a strategic planning retreat or a mock NCQA site visit exercise might tie up one weekend a month. Typically, he responded to about 60 internal e-mail messages a day and a large number of telephone calls. A two-month review of his calendar showed that he spent on average four hours a day in meetings about 60% in the office and 40% outside. When he took the job, he was told to expect to be traveling four days a week. However, this market's business was very heavily concentrated in Georgia and in Atlanta in particular.

**Exhibit 6–2** Excerpts from the Job Descriptions of Medical Directors at Vigilant–Xtra Mile HealthCare

| Job Characteristics | Patient Management Director & Quality Management Director | Network Medical Director |
|---|---|---|
| Fundamental Role | Develop and manage a health services organization focused on reducing medical cost and improving clinical outcomes, member satisfaction, and provider satisfaction | Develop and manage a health services organization focused on reducing medical cost and improving clinical outcomes, member satisfaction, and provider satisfaction |
| Central Activities | Implement utilization and quality management programs through timely policy interpretation and local application | Provide strategic and operational direction for the delivery of performance based medical management |
| | Manage budget | Manage budget and risk drivers |
| | Provide marketing support through sales presentations, site visits and support for requests for proposals | Analyze and report business performance data to customers and colleagues |
| | Render medical necessity determinations | Handle Vigilant funds as if they were his/her own |
| | Chair committees in accordance with market and contractual needs | Participate in internal and external health industry development efforts |
| | Participate in national, regional, local work groups as required | Participate in management of local profit and loss |
| | Serve as liaison between field organization, home office, and governmental agencies | Serve as liaison with regulatory and accrediting agencies and other business units within the company |
| | Develop local medical review and coverage policies | Develop and maintain strong provider relationships |
| Leadership | Maintains a customer driven passion for excellence and commitment to action and change | Maintains a customer driven passion for excellence and commitment to action and change |
| Direction Setting | Ability to make timely and high quality decisions as well as implement them | Ability to make timely and high quality decisions as well as implement them |
| Selection | Hire, develop and reward staff to effectively support the company's strategy | Hire, develop and reward staff to effectively support the company's strategy |
| Communication | Excellent verbal and written skills as well as negotiation and conflict resolution skills | Excellent verbal and written skills as well as negotiation and conflict resolution skills |
| Business Knowledge | In-depth knowledge of managed care, financial, business processes, and strategies and objectives | In-depth knowledge of managed care, financial, business processes, and strategies and objectives |
| | Job specific technical knowledge | Job specific technical knowledge |
| Other Requirements | Board certification is highly desired; State License must be active & unencumbered | Board certification is optional |
| | Demonstrated commitment to professional development (e.g., CME, conferences) | Demonstrated commitment to professional development (e.g., seminars) |

## Management of Quality

In 1990, XM Data Driven, Inc. (XMDD) was established as a XMHC quality measurement subsidiary. With over 280 employees, it had access to a data warehouse of claims information from hospitalization, outpatient visits, pharmacy claims, and laboratory reports of 15 million enrollees. It was a pioneering and innovative unit with Xtra Mile Healthcare, developing clinical algorithms, identifying and risk-stratifying seriously ill members for disease management interventions, providing risk-adjusted performance reporting systems, maintaining a disease registry for members with any of more than 65 chronic illnesses, and working with participating academic medical centers to conduct applied research. A fuller description of XMDD is provided in Exhibit 6–3. An example of the type of report cards that they provide to management and to providers is shown in Exhibit 6–4.

**Exhibit 6–3** XMDD Description

---

The XMDD's Health Services Research Program is the dedicated research and development unit of Vigilant–Xtra Mile HealthCare™. Physicians, Ph.D.–level researchers, methodologists, nurses, statisticians, programmers, medical coders, and other experienced professionals make up this unit. Staff conduct applied research and develop methodologies that measure and improve the quality and efficiency of health care services for Vigilant-Xtra Mile HealthCare's membership. One of the main goals of the Health Services Research Program is to evaluate the outcomes and cost-effectiveness of managed care programs.

The XMDD Health Services Research Program has access to an abundance of health-related data on more than 14 million insured members throughout the United States, and routinely analyzes both primary and secondary data for hundreds of practical applications. Research conducted by this unit is designed to benefit four primary customers which include: (1) individual members, (2) providers, (3) plan sponsors, and (4) the Vigilant–Xtra Mile HealthCare system.

When working with external organizations on collaborative research, XMDD staff provide methodological, data acquisition, and technical support, and assist with the grant application process as well.

**Examples of XMDD Health Services Research:**

- Health Profiling—Using a number of different data sets, clinical logic has been created to identify individuals with any of 65 chronic diseases. Each

---

*continues*

**Exhibit 6–3** continued

individual's disease-specific health status can be categorized and used in a number of applications. For instance, an individual's health profile is used as a predictor in risk–stratification models to determine who should be entered into disease management programs. Health status is also used as a risk adjuster in physician performance compensation models. Furthermore, these profiles are used to calculate employer group disease-specific prevalence rates, which help employers determine the best benefits package to purchase from Vigilant–Xtra Mile HealthCare.

• Risk-Stratification Modeling—XMDD has created empirically driven risk-stratification models designed to identify individuals who are at high risk for certain types of disease-specific acute exacerbations. These multivariate predictive models use previous utilization patterns to assign chronically ill individuals into one of five risk strata. After extensive cross-validation, these models are used to determine appropriate disease management resources that are consistent with the health needs of each category of individuals.

• Clinical Outcomes Studies and Program Evaluation—Both pilot and long-standing managed care programs are evaluated to determine their impact on members' health status. A number of different econometric, epidemiological and statistical quasi-experimental models have been employed to evaluate these programs while controlling for important confounding variables.

• Severity-Adjusted Performance Measurement—Severity-adjusted performance measurement models have been developed for hospitals, specialists, and primary care providers. These multivariate statistical models are used to provide feedback to providers and institutions about their performance relative to others in their field. Additionally, performance measurement information is used to determine a portion of each provider's reimbursement. By accounting for differences in patient mix by factoring in characteristics such as age, gender, and comorbidities, the playing field is leveled between providers, and performance results are more valid.

• Health System Research—A number of research projects are under way to further investigate the health system overall. Cost-effectiveness and practice pattern variation studies, for example, have been undertaken to more fully understand costs and utilization of the country's health system. Additionally, the impact of different insurance arrangements on utilization and health status are being studied. Results from these studies will help Vigilant–Xtra Mile HealthCare better understand how to resource high-quality health services

**Exhibit 6–4** Sample XMDD Report Card for Asthma

Practice Type: Family Practice Region: XX  
Office Address: 1 Street, Anytown, PA 19074  
Number of our current insureds identified with asthma: 232  

Office Number: XX  
Reporting Period: 10/1/94–9/30/95

| | Office | XMHC Average |
|---|---|---|
| **PREVALENCE MEASURES** | | |
| 1. Estimated overall prevalence of asthma | 4.5% | 4.0% |
| 2. Estimated overall prevalence of asthma age 0–9 | 9.0% | 7.9% |
| 3. Estimated overall prevalence of asthma age 10–19 | 7.2% | 6.8% |
| 4. Estimated overall prevalence of asthma age 20–39 | 5.7% | 4.0% |
| 5. Estimated overall prevalence of asthma age 40+ | 2.5% | 2.8% |
| **ASTHMA TREATMENT PATTERNS** | | |
| 6. Asthmatics on prescription drugs for asthma | 65.8% | 66.4% |
| 7. Asthmatics receiving sympathomimetics | 58.3% | 58.3% |
| 8. Asthmatics receiving theophylline | 6.4% | 11.0% |
| 9. Asthmatics receiving only theophylline | 0.0% | 0.7% |
| 10. Asthmatics receiving cromolyn | 8.0% | 8.7% |
| 11. Asthmatics receiving inhaled steroids | 21.4% | 18.8% |
| 12. Average annual number of beta agonist prescriptions for asthmatics receiving any beta agonist | 4.29 | 3.72 |
| 13. Asthmatics on beta agonists receiving 2 or more prescriptions in one month | 18.3% | 17.9% |
| 14. Asthmatics receiving one or more course of oral steroids | 17.1% | 18.3% |
| **ACCESS MEASURES** | | |
| 15. Asthmatics seeing the PCP at least once | 92.5% | 86.9% |
| 16. Average number of annual PCP visits per asthmatic | 5.74 | 4.69 |
| 17. Asthmatics seeing a pulmonologist | 8.8% | 4.69 |
| 18. Asthmatics seeing an allergist | 14.5% | 11.7% |
| **PROCESS MEASURES** | | |
| 19. Asthmatics with an outpatient chest x-ray | 8.4% | 8.9% |
| 20. Asthmatics age 8+ receiving pulmonary function tests | 8.3% | 10.1% |
| 21. Asthmatics receiving allergy testing | 3.1% | 10.1% |
| 22. Asthmatics receiving allergy immunotherapy | 7.5% | 8.0% |
| 23. Asthmatics using a home nebulizer | 2.2% | 2.4% |
| 24. Asthmatics with at least one antibiotic prescription | 63.1% | 71.3% |
| 25. Asthmatics on theophylline who have at least one theophylline level drawn | 10.0% | 71.3% |
| 26. Average annual number of theophylline levels in asthmatics on theophylline | 0.10 | 0.29 |
| 27. Asthmatics receiving at least one home care visit | 3.5% | 0.29 |
| **OUTCOME MEASURES** | | |
| **ASTHMA RELATED CONDITIONS** | | |
| 28. Emergency room visits specifically for asthma/1000 asthmatics/year | 57 | 86 |
| 29. Total admissions (acute) specifically for asthma/1000 asthmatics/year | 44 | 40 |
| 30. Total inpatient days (acute) specifically for asthma/1000 asthmatics/year | 44 | 40 |
| **ALL CONDITIONS FOR ASTHMATIC MEMBERS** | | |
| 31. Total emergency room visits for all conditions/1000 asthmatics/year | 154 | 242 |
| 32. Total admissions (acute) for all conditions/1000 asthmatics per year | 128 | 149 |
| 33. Total inpatient days (acute) for all conditions/1000 asthmatics/year | 493 | 572 |
| **SATISFACTION MEASURES**\*\* | | |
| 34. Overall satisfaction with medical care at the PCP office of asthmatic members | 100.0% | 95.9% |
| 35. Satisfaction with the ability to make appointments for illnesses | 95.4% | 92.1% |
| 36. Satisfaction with the response to an emergency call within 30 minutes | 98.6% | 93.0% |

\* Adjusted for age, sex, plan type, office type and pharmacy severity level  
NA: Not Available or Not Applicable  
\*\*Percentage of respondents with Good, Very Good, or Excellent

Vigilant–Xtra Mile HealthCare believed that ultimately the market would be defined by quality. This was so important to Vigilant–XMHC that the company had established a unique quality-driven compensation system for primary care physicians. The incentives in this system are balanced to attempt to avoid both over and under utilization. Each practice receives a capitation payment which is adjusted for the age and gender of the covered population. This payment is further adjusted by a quality factor that is revised every six months. The example below in Exhibit 6–5 illustrates how the quality factor is determined.

Offices that failed to make a score of at least 2% received a 10% reduction in capitation payments during the subsequent six months. Those that maintained a score of at least 2% received an increase in their semimonthly capitation payments equal to the percentage score. Thus, the ABC practice would have received a 14.55% increment in its capitation payments.

Each practice also received a six-month Quality-Factored Distribution based on its three utilization components (hospital, specialist, and ER) year-to-date which was adjusted by the Quality Review and Comprehensive Care Components (in the example above 4.25% + 8.50% = 12.75%). If the practice had achieved a combined Quality Review and Utilization Component Score of at least 4% (4.25% + 1.80% = 6.05%), it was eligible for an Office Status Payment of 5%, if it had remained open for XMHC enrollment throughout the period or if it had accepted current patients as XMHC members throughout that period.

The large employers that the company sought out tended to insist on NCQA certification. Therefore, one of Dr. Johnson's main performance objectives was to have the network meet the NCQA requirement of meeting its own written quality standards. He spent much time and effort making sure that the network conformed to NCQA requirements such as having a certain percentage of members within 15 minutes travel time of a primary care provider in the network and working with practices to help them achieve NCQA's Health Plan Employer Data and Information Set (HEDIS) standards for their patients. Another standard was that of keeping provider turnover below 5% per year.

The costs of achieving these standards can be substantial. In six months, the region had gone through an NCQA audit exercise, a Georgia exercise for Medicare and a federal exercise for Medicare. Then there were the operational costs of maintaining standards. For example, NCQA standards required recredentialing each network physician every two years. With over 7,000 physicians in their network in Georgia, that was a

**Exhibit 6–5** Sample Quality Factor Calculation

Based on the quality of care, comprehensive service, and utilization, the ABC Practice earned the following quality factor which is multiplied by their sex- and age-adjusted base capitation payment for the previous two weeks:

**Quality Review Components:**

| | |
|---|---|
| a. Member Surveys (compared to others in HMO, range: −0.75 to + 3.0) | 2.00% |
| b. Focused Medical Chart Reviews (2/yr., comparative, −0.75 to + 3.0) | 0.75% |
| c. Member Transfer Rates (comparative, −0.75 to + 1.5) | 0.50% |
| d. Philosophy of Managed Care (cooperation and participation with XMHC quality programs (subjective, −0.75 to + 3.0) | 1.00% |
| **Quality Review Subtotal** | **4.25%** |

**Comprehensive Care Components:**

| | |
|---|---|
| a. Membership Size (members/doctor or practice, e.g.: range = 0, 1% at 100/doctor, 1.5% at 200/doctor, 2% at 300/doctor) | 1.00% |
| b. Schedule Office Hours (range = 0, 0.5% for 50–59, 1.0% for 60–69, and 1.5% for > 70 hours/week) | 0.50% |
| c. Available Office Procedures (e.g., flexible sigmoidoscopy = 1.0%) max. = 3%) | 1.00% |
| d. Program Education (completing XMHC educational courses (e.g., Current Concepts in Cancer = 0.5%,) max. sum = 2%) | 0.50% |
| e. Internal Practice Coverage (1% if coverage is by practice for continuity) | 1.00% |
| f. Catastrophic Care (practice has greater than the HMO type average total costs for catastrophic cases (e.g., > $20,000 = 1.5%) | 1.50% |
| g. Patient Management (1% if practice supports and participates in XMHC patient management and directs hospital care of own patients) | 1.00% |
| h. Practice Growth (XMHC membership growth (e.g., > 10% = 1.0%) | 1.00% |
| i. Computer Links to XMHC (transmits encounter and referral data electronically = 1.0%) | 1.00% |
| **Comprehensive Care Subtotal** | **8.50%** |

*continues*

**Exhibit 6–5** continued

| Utilization Components: | |
|---|---|
| a. Hospital Utilization at the average bracket (range $= -0.8$ to $+1.8\%$) | 0.80% |
| b. Specialist Utilization one bracket greater than average ($-0.8$ to $+1.8\%$) | 0.40% |
| c. Emergency Room Utilization one bracket less than average ($-0.8$ to $+1.4\%$) | 0.60% |
| **Utilization Subtotal** | **1.8%** |
| **TOTAL QUALITY FACTOR =** | **14.55%** |

substantial workload, the cost of which made Dr. Johnson consider strategies for narrowing the network where possible. HMOs in Georgia were licensed county by county by the state. As geographic coverage was expanded, the number of physicians to be credentialed expanded. He found himself having to trade off greater choice for his patients with the costs of providing the larger provider network in the served areas as well as allocating scarce resources between served areas and new target market areas.

One decision that Dr. Johnson had to make was how much time to spend requesting and reviewing report cards on the physicians in the network. XMDD could generate an almost infinite number of reports like the one in Exhibit 6–4. They could also generate statistical reports identifying outlier individuals and practices. Much of the data on over or underutilization was of more concern to the regional medical director responsible for patient management, but that medical loss ratio was part of his performance evaluation also.

## DR. JOHNSON'S OBSERVATIONS ABOUT THE JOB

Dr. Johnson had been in the job only 6 months when this case was written. So far, he was quite happy with the job and with its potential. He observed that Dominion-Northwest had been a useful transition for him to enable him to see the comparative advantages of various types of health care organizations and to get used to working in a large organization. He was no longer seeing patients, but he was comfortable with that fact.

He had already "seen enough patients to fill Fulton County Stadium three times" and no longer found practice much of a challenge. He often compared the practice of medicine to flying an airplane: "When you need a skilled pilot, that individual is important and one's skills are critical during the unique takeoff and landing periods. However, in between takeoffs and landings, most of the system is on autopilot and that gets old over time. The same is true of medicine."

There were always the fires to fight and there were always special projects related to process improvement. For example, the company had just gone through a major database cleanup of its provider records. Many physicians had changed their affiliations due to mergers and acquisitions and thus their tax ID numbers, but had not informed their payers. A wrong provider ID number on a claim could hold up payment and distort the company's data on activities and costs. That had been a major effort for his group.

He observed that most physicians would not be comfortable with the length of time that it took to get things done in a large organization. They, like he, were used to dealing with and reaching closure on a presenting problem every fifteen minutes. Recruiting a substantial group practice into the network might take as much as a year with a meeting every month to establish a trusting relationship and to work out the details of the contract.

Medical directors also had to be comfortable working as part of a management team, to influence others where possible, but take orders when necessary. They would have to know when to keep quiet and when to speak up. For example, in the disease management arena, the core management at Wheeling would often decide which disease management programs were "network impactable" and he would have to make them work. He noted that he still had more to learn about the politics of large organizations and about the insurance industry in general, about group selection, underwriting, claims management, contracting, and marketing. He certainly felt that he had a better idea of what groups such as independent practice associations (IPAs) could or could not do effectively. Having seen the information system investment that Vigilant–Xtra Mile Health Care had to support membership enrollment, claims processing, disease management and utilization review, he saw no way that much smaller, physician-led organizations could compete. On the other hand, he felt that insurance organizations knew relatively little about managing practices or running hospitals and were better off not trying to integrate them.

Dr. Johnson was aware of the high turnover rate among medical directors in the industry. In his own words: "The health care environment is in turmoil and one needs a mentor, someone looking out for him, if one is to survive. One has to be careful to avoid the lose-lose situations that many medical directors had gotten into." By way of example, he cited medical directors of Medicaid managed care organizations when the Georgia state legislature decreed a 20% cut in funding, or those whose jobs were eliminated during mergers. He knew a local medical director working for MedPartners who was let go when the merger with Phycor was announced. Now that that merger did not go through, they were recruiting a replacement.

He noted that most physicians are not at all prepared for the practices of large organizations. He had heard them speak quite heatedly about the experience of a terminated medical director at another HMO who was given 20 minutes under observation to clean out her desk, escorted to the door with a security person on each side, and asked to hand over her keys at the door. After a few months in a data-driven organization, he fully understood why. Why give anyone a chance to download proprietary information onto a computer disk or destroy a data set? However, no practicing physician would ever expect to be mortified that way.

Dr. Johnson also felt that most physicians would have difficulty with having to clear so many decisions with the legal department or with public relations. Yet, while there were policies and procedures governing most everything, he did not feel that they would constrain his team from setting aggressive goals, developing plans to compete in the markets that they chose, and implementing them quickly and efficiently. However, most physicians would have trouble at first being resource constrained in what could be accomplished. When he was in practice, if he felt the practice would benefit from a piece of equipment, he bought it. It meant a loss in the profits distributed at the end of the month, but there was still enough. But when he wanted a additional employee to serve as a practice management coordinator, a highly skilled professional services consultant to go into network practices and help them solve billing or cost problems, he had to work hard to justify that position and show how it would contribute to meeting financial targets.

## The Future

Dr. Johnson saw the provider community consolidating, which would give them more power in the negotiations with payer networks. He felt that payers would have to learn how to do a better job of partnering with the providers so that in sharing the risks they would both succeed. Thus far, providers had a very poor track record in profiting by taking on risk and he felt that one of his jobs in the future would be in helping them succeed.

He also saw many opportunities for expanding the network. There were many areas of Georgia, Mississippi, and Alabama that did not have rationalized provider networks. He recognized a need to tell the managed care story more effectively given the current hostility in the profession and in the media which was being echoed politically in Georgia and Washington, DC. He also saw the need to become more effective in negotiating good contracts, closely observing quality and utilization, and providing communities access to the good providers. There were many opportunities, many issues, and many unknowns to be faced.

## CASE ANALYSIS

This case is about the roles of medical directors in the quality efforts of large HMO companies and insurers. In this case, the primary focus is on gatekeeper contracts rather than PPO contracts. Dr. Johnson is just one of three types of medical directors in the firm, each reporting to a different level of the organization. The reader can use case data to review the apparent criteria used by the company in recruiting its market medical directors individually and as a team. There is also considerable information about the company's databases and their methods of motivating quality performance among participating primary care physicians.

## ASSIGNMENT QUESTIONS

### Introduction

1. Review Dr. Johnson's job history. What experiences contributed to his becoming a job applicant that was attractive to Xtra Mile? How relevant are these to his current position and to his future career?

2. Review the set of job descriptions. What seems to be the salient differences between the three types of medical directors at this firm? What does that tell you about what Xtra Mile really expects out of each medical director? Is that consistent with their other quality measurement and control systems evident in the case?

3. What do you believe Dr. Johnson's career depends on? If you were in charge, what practical and operational evaluative measures would you use?

## Basics

4. Dr. Johnson observes that he expects to make a bigger difference at Xtra Mile than he could have at the local integrating hospital system? Why do you think he believes that? How realistic do you think he was being about this? Why?

5. What does this case tell you about the advantages of scale that a large provider can bring to bear on the measurement of health care processes and outcomes? Can a small IPA ever overcome that?

6. What do you think of the "quality" incentive system outlined in the final exhibit of the case? What behaviors does it seem designed to motivate? How much do you think it will actually impact on the PCP practices? How would you go about motivating them?

## Implementation

7. What advice can you offer Dr. Johnson about doing his job better in the future? Are you satisfied with his time allocation, or do you recommend some changes of strategy or tactics?

8. Would you be interested in this job? What is attractive about it? What is not attractive about it? What have you learned from it that you want to take with you in your attitudes toward any potential job search?

## Application

9. The other payer-oriented cases are Cases 7 and 8. Compare and contrast the approach at Xtra Mile with the governmental ones in the other two cases? How and why are all three so different?

## CLASS EXERCISE

Find out what a specific health care insurer is doing to improve quality. Is that organization making use of the data that it has in house? Is it using other consortia or available data bases to enhance clinical performance? What is behind the selection of that specific approach? How likely are other payers to use their accumulated data to enhance clinical quality?

# CASE 7

# North Carolina Science to Service Project

*Beth Melcher and Christina Rausch*

The Science to Service Project (NCS2S) was established to support the commitment of North Carolina Division of Mental Health, Development Disabilities, and Substance Abuse Services (MH/DD/SAS) to implement evidence-based practices in North Carolina. The project was initiated in June 2003 when Beth Melcher, PhD, was hired as project director. It was funded with a $100,000 grant from the Substance Abuse and Mental Health Services Administration's (SAMHSA) Center for Mental Health Services (CMHS) and the National Institute for Mental Health (NIMH). This grant was part of Round 1 of their State Implementation of Evidence-Based Practices–Bridging Science and Service Grant Program.

The goals of the project, outlined in Exhibit 7–1, were ambitious. Notification of the grant award was received in August 2003 requiring a slight adjustment of some timelines. Over the course of the year, the project was to educate providers, consumers, families, and administrators about evidence-based mental health practices (EBPs), evaluate current service implementation, and, with input from a broad consortium of stakeholders, develop a comprehensive statewide implementation agenda that would guide policy decisions and state plan revisions. The recommendations of that study and its agenda were completed in July 2004. Now NCS2S staff was concerned about the willingness of the state, the payers, the providers, and the politicians to implement that agenda.

**Exhibit 7–1** Initial Goals of Grant 1 R24 MHO68779–01

**Goal: Improve service delivery by integrating the results of science-based research into service delivery by:**
   a. Educating treatment providers, and consumers and their families about new evidence-based practices (EBPs) and
   b. Helping researchers and policy makers gain a better understanding of how clinicians can better access and use research

**Objective 1: To expand and strengthen the integration of a statewide network of community-based consumers and family members, advocates, MH providers, researchers, educators, and policy makers:**

1. Identify key stakeholders (e.g., consumers and family members, advocates, providers, researchers, educators, and policymakers) representing geographic regions of the State to be on the Steering Committee (July 15, 2003)
2. Establish a working committee to develop the science to service agenda (July 31, 2003)
3. Conduct a track on EBPs at regional and state meetings of the major MH consumer and family organizations in NC (August 31, 2003)
4. Establish a conference planning committee to oversee the planning and implementation of a statewide conference (July 31, 2003)
5. Establish a research committee to evaluate the implementation of EBPs in public sector settings (July 31, 2003)

**Objective 2: To oversee the development of a statewide science to service agenda:**

1. Identify the needs of the targeted stakeholders (e.g. consumers and their families, administrators, program managers, and treatment providers) (December 31, 2003)
2. Identify existing experts and other resources in MH research in the State (December 31, 2003)
3. Develop priorities for implementation of identified EBPs in local management entities (LMEs) (Incorporated into final agenda 5/04)
4. Design an implementation plan that addresses training needs, financing mechanisms, and programmatic and policy issues. (May 31, 2004)

*continues*

**Exhibit 7–1** continued

---

**Objective 3: To convene a conference that will present information on the implementation of evidence-based practice (EBP) strategies.**

1. Develop a conference agenda with input from consumers and family members, advocates, providers, researchers, educators, and policymakers (August 31, 2003)
2. Identify EBPs (e.g. Implementation Resource Kits) to be showcased at the conference (August 31, 2003)
3. Identify national experts to present on EBPs, with local clinicians, consumers and their families, to discuss implementation issues in NC (September 30, 2003)
4. Conduct the conference in November 2003

**Objective 4: To conduct a pilot knowledge adoption study, which will provide information to improve mental health service delivery in the State of North Carolina**

1. Develop a pilot study on the implementation of the ACT (Assertive Community Treatment) teams, with input from providers, researchers, educators, policymakers, advocates, consumers and family members (December 31, 2003)
2. Conduct an evaluation of knowledge adoption (e.g. fidelity of implementation and data collection, barriers to implementation (June 30, 2004)

---

## HISTORICAL BACKGROUND

The 1998 Schizophrenia Patient Outcomes Research Team (PORT) study, supported by the federal government, found that fewer than half of the patients studied had received care that met treatment standards. The 1999 Surgeon General's Report on Mental Health concluded that "a wide variety of community-based services are of proven value for even the most severe mental illnesses" yet they are not being "translated into community settings." As new drugs reduced the degree of severity in many mentally ill patients, the system had to respond with newly identified practices that focused on the delivery of recovery-oriented services in the community, including psychosocial support, employment training, housing, and education, to adults with serious mental illness and children having serious mental disturbances.

The comprehensive system reviews and evidence-based practice implementation activities at the federal level support the 2003 President's New Freedom Commission on Mental Health report, *Achieving the Promise: Transforming Mental Health Care in America.* While the Commission found that recovery from mental illness is now a real possibility, "for too many Americans with mental illnesses, the mental health services and supports they need remain fragmented, disconnected and often inadequate." The Commission declared that the goal of a mental health system was recovery and laid out six major goals for a transformed system. These are:

1. Americans understand that mental health is essential to overall health
2. Mental health care is consumer- and family-driven
3. Disparities in mental health services are eliminated
4. Early mental health screening, assessment, and referral to services are common practice
5. Excellent mental health care is delivered and research is accelerated
6. Technology is used to access mental health care and information

As a result of the report, federal agencies began evaluating programs, working together collaboratively, and realigning policies and resources to support the report's recommendations. In response to the increased attention to the lag between science and service, the SAMHSA and the Robert Wood Johnson Foundation initiated the national Implementing Evidence-Based Practices Project to reduce the amount of time for effective treatments to be incorporated into the mental health system. The project identified the first cluster of six evidence-based practices and developed implementation resource kits ("toolkits") to support implementation activities. The first six practices are Assertive Community Treatment (ACT), Supported Employment, Medication Management Approaches in Psychiatry, Illness Management and Recovery, Family Psychoeducation, and Integrated Dual Disorder Treatment.

## THE NORTH CAROLINA SITUATION

North Carolina's once proud mental health system had begun to lag behind other states. In the interim, the state avoided many of the mistakes made by other states, but by the mid-1990s, its systems were in serious disarray. Its four state mental hospitals operated independently from the community mental health system and the community system was organized along the quasi-autonomous area community mental health center model of the 1970s. In the 1980s the state had assumed the dominant role of funding these centers based on federal block grants but with limited accountability to local or state governments. The signs and symptoms of the systems problems included:

- The state's "Carolina Initiative" managed Medicaid mental health care waiver had been cancelled
- Problems at the state's mental hospitals, especially Dorothea Dix in Raleigh, had threatened their Medicare and Medicaid certification
- The State Auditor's 2000 Report, *Study of the State Psychiatric Hospitals and the Area Mental Health* Programs indicated that the hospitals were completely outdated and outmoded and should be replaced.
- The state's community treatment programs usually failed to meet what were likely to become future programmatic requirements and were badly lacking in what the federal government referred to as evidence-based practices for the severely and persistently mentally ill

The 2000 State Auditor's report called for the state to:

- Define specific target populations requiring specialized services that matched the needs of the targeted groups
- Require the development of new community-based capacities
- Change the funding mechanisms (i.e., coordination with Medicaid; establishment of "bridge" funding to support reorganization of services)
- Develop a statewide training plan to support the development of these new capacities

## NORTH CAROLINA'S RESPONSE

In 2001, the North Carolina General Assembly adopted comprehensive legislation to reform the public mental health, developmental disabilities, and substance abuse service (MH/DD/SAS) system. This action was taken in response to public demands for improved services, better access, and more accountability. The General Assembly had commissioned several studies to guide their efforts, including the 1998 *Efficiency Study of the State Psychiatric Hospitals* and the 2000 State Auditor's report. The legislation passed by the General Assembly in 2001 incorporated many of the recommendations from the state auditor's report, including the identification of target populations and promotion of services based on "best practices" for those populations. To implement the legislation, the state was required to develop a detailed state plan, including specific standards or outcomes for specific populations and service requirements based on best practice standards. This plan was to be revised yearly to reflect new developments and feedback from families, consumers, citizens, and other stakeholders. State Plan 2001 began to layout the structure of how target populations would be defined and what evidence would be reviewed to determine "best practice" for these populations. State Plan 2002 established the values and philosophical foundation for how these services would be provided (i.e., person-centered, recovery-oriented, systems of support) and the broad categories of what would be included in the array of services and supports (e.g. housing, transportation, work, crisis response). By 2003, the state plan presented a structure of how services should be offered and coordinated. It also articulated the specific practices it considered "best," both evidence-based and emerging best practices.

The 2001 legislation and subsequent plans also called for the "divestiture" of the local area mental health units' service activities and making area mental health programs directly accountable to county commissioners. The idea had been to reduce the number of area organizations involved and consolidate them into regional local management entities (LMEs) that would contract with willing providers to deliver the services and then assume the oversight functions that many considered to have been in conflict with their past service delivery roles. Some saw this as a transition from a quasi-governmental agency to an HMO-type structure which would gradually move from current mixture of budget-based state appropriations and Medicaid and Medicare fee-for-service funding to a capitation system for funding similar to that of Washington State and other states. The adoption of "evidence-based practices" that for many meant moving from office-based therapy and case management to active treatment in the community and divestiture, which were entangled in many people's minds as the NCS2S Project surveys confirmed.

## PROJECT STARTUP

The project was not housed in the MH/DD/SAS headquarters in Raleigh, NC, but in the Governor's Institute on Alcohol and Substance Abuse in Research Triangle Park, NC about 15 miles away. Dr. Melcher was recruited three-quarters time from her position as legislative advocate for the North Carolina affiliate of the National Alliance for the Mentally Ill. She had been ten years with NAMI North Carolina, five of them as its Executive Director. Christina Rausch, MSW, joined the project in September 2003 as a planning researcher. She was employed by the Governor's Institute and assigned to work full-time on the Science to Service Project.

The activities of the grant were established and guided by the North Carolina Science to Service Consortium. Its individual members represented a range of stakeholder groups including families, consumers, policy makers, researchers, agency administrators, and providers. This group was responsible for developing the conference agenda, overseeing the needs assessment surveys completed during the grant, and crafting the Science to Service Agenda report. Duke University, UNC Chapel Hill, NAMI North Carolina, the North Carolina Mental Health Consumers' Organization, and associations of both providers and area MH/DD/SA programs were some of the groups represented. Both UNC School of Social Work and Sheps Center for Health Services Research (affiliated with UNC) conducted the research studies that were part of this grant's activities. This resulted in a comprehensive, detailed agenda report on the needs and challenges of the state. However, since this planning document was crafted outside of state government departments, generating commitment and "ownership" by state agencies to provide leadership to implement its recommendations had been challenging. In addition, the departure in the middle of the grant period of the head of MH/DD/SAS, who had recently come from and then returned to Michigan, and strongly supported organizational and treatment practice changes, posed a unique challenge.

## PROJECT ACTIVITIES

### Raising Awareness

Over the course of the year, the NC Science to Service Project collaborated with nearly every major stakeholder group in the state to develop and offer EBP workshops at state meetings, including: NC Psychiatric Association, Mental Health Association of North Carolina, NC Psychological Association, NAMI North Carolina, North Carolina Mental Health Consumers' Organization, NC Community Support Providers Council, NC Council of Community Programs (the Association of Area Programs becoming LMEs), and National Association of Social Workers-North Carolina. These efforts reached over 1,000 individual attendees. In addition, presentations on EBPs were offered through the Area Health Education Centers (AHEC) on four occasions in different regions of the state. In an effort to expand participation and greater knowledge of EBPs, the NC Science to Service Project worked in collaboration with the AHEC and the NC Council of Community Programs to offer "toolkit" workshops consisting of half-day overviews of each evidence-based practice. Presentations were produced on CDROM for wider distribution.

During the grant period, the project developed a comprehensive Web site to provide information on EBPs including essential elements, fidelity scales, frequently asked questions, and links to other sites. Various national organizations and other states implementing EBPs were contacted. They outlined for NCS2S some of the barriers they had faced, possible solutions, and implementation strategies. Some of these organizations were: NASMHPD, Ohio SAMI CCOE, West Institute, Dartmouth PRC, Indiana ACT Center, and the departments of mental health in a wide range of states (many involved as original pilot sites in the federal implementing EBP project). Finally, the NC Council of Community Programs played a major role in partnership, hosting the project's November conference, publishing articles in its newsletter, and incorporating EBPs and the Science to Service project in other activities throughout the year (such as its Spring Policy Forum).

### Needs Assessments

A needs assessment among stakeholders was conducted by researchers at UNC School of Social Work with input and guidance from

the Consortium Research Committee. It focused on families and consumers, administrators, and front-line providers. A review of local planning documents also was completed to determine plans for development
of EBPs. A series of focus groups with families and with consumers
identified what they knew about EBPs in adult mental health services,
what EBPs were being received, perceived barriers to the provision of
EBPs, opinions about EBPs, and what were seen as important services
in adult mental health.

The needs assessment provided the state with a comprehensive baseline
of awareness of EBPs and perceived barriers and needs as the state began
implementation efforts. The assessment provided guidance to the consortium in the development of implementation strategies and priorities.

## Knowledge Assessments

Telephone surveys were conducted with administrators and program
managers to determine:

- Staff and administrator knowledge about EBPs
- Organization needs for support, training, and/or education on EBPs
- Possible incentives for implementation of EBPs in their programs
- Possible barriers to implementing EBPs in their programs
- Challenges to sustainability and fidelity for EBPs in their programs
- Methods regarding the selection and evaluation of the provider net-
  work with regard to EBPs
- EBP services for non-English speaking consumers

Front-line providers responded to a written survey to measure
providers' views and knowledge around adult mental health EBPs.
Specifically, surveys asked about providers' familiarity with each of the
EBPs, their agency's level of provision of each EBP, their need for training in EBPs and preference in training modality, and their views on challenges to EBP implementation, fidelity, and sustainability. In addition,
providers were asked about the needs of non-English speaking consumers in their community. The review of the local planning documents
revealed little reference to EBPs or incorporation of EBPs into service
planning activities.

During the needs assessments conducted with consumers, family members, providers, and local management entity administrators, it became clear that there were major problems with the definition of "evidence-based practices" and with which practices would qualify. Providers and administrators believed they were providing services using best practices, although they were not clear on the evidence-based specific models. Most importantly, the state had not clarified which practices it recognized as evidence-based, leading to confusion in the assessments and among providers and administrators in the system. The Science to Service Project agenda affirmed the six evidence-based practices recognized by SAMHSA/Dartmouth as "evidence-based," and encouraged the state to send out a policy memo documenting the state's definition. In addition, the agenda document recommended a structure for continuously defining which practices were evidence-based on a state level.

**Priority Setting**

The Science to Service agenda document was developed by the consortium's three committees focused on the broad areas of awareness, workforce development, and system infrastructure. Its implementation plan identified priorities for implementation of identified EBPs, beginning with ACT and Supported Employment. These priorities were identified by a committee of the consortium and, based on the expressed desire of consumers and families, identified funding mechanisms and comprehensive training opportunities. An extensive review of the literature was conducted, information about North Carolina experience and the impact of reform efforts was considered, and the expertise of consortium members was utilized. The plan was completed in May and received public comment until June 15th. The plan identified three major goals:

- Goal 1: Stakeholder interest and demand for effective evidence-based services are increased
- Goal 2: Clinicians and clinical supervisors have the knowledge and skills necessary to deliver evidence-based services
- Goal 3: Mechanisms are established at the state and local level to support and maintain effective services

Detailed objectives and strategies were offered for each goal to provide North Carolina with a comprehensive strategic plan to support implementation of evidence-based practices. The final plan (agenda) was presented to the Director of the Division of MH/DD/SAS on August 2, 2004. It was also made available at www.ncs2s.org. A brochure was developed to raise awareness of EBPs and the Science to Service agenda report.

A database was developed with information about what research was being conducted within the state on mental health. Conversations regarding the use of this information were initiated but there was relatively little demand for it. Most interest was directed toward how to translate replicated research into practice. Recommendations on a process to promote this implementation were incorporated into the Science to Service agenda.

**Awareness Objective**

The development of the Science to Service agenda brought together a range of stakeholder experts to work on a joint project and to learn and have greater appreciation of the challenges facing various constituencies in implementation efforts. This effort benefited greatly from the experience of other states participating in the EBP pilot projects. The integration of research and academic interests into the consortium discussion was especially useful. This has resulted in ongoing discussions regarding future research opportunities on EBP implementation activities. The experience suggested, however, that making those research opportunities a reality will require state level guidance, encouragement, and incentives. The agenda proposed a mechanism to accomplish that. Although the project started out as a "top-down" effort, through the consortium membership and the efforts to develop the plan and raise awareness, a group of "champions" for evidence-based practices has begun to develop that will continue to promote implementation efforts in the state.

**Conference Objective**

The Conference Committee, comprised of a broad range of stakeholder representatives from the Science to Service Consortium, decided in July to collaborate with the North Carolina Council of Community Programs statewide conference in November in order to attract the largest and broadest possible audience. Nearly 150 individuals attended the two-day EBP track representing providers, families, consumers, administrators, and policy makers. Robert Drake, MD, PhD, of the New Hampshire-Dartmouth Psychiatric Research Center presented on overview of evidence-based practices, the national evidence-based practices project, and the development of the "toolkits." Molly Finnerty, MD, presented on New York's experience implementing evidence-based practices. The ACT and Integrated Dual Disorders Treatment toolkits were highlighted in workshops presented by Marvin Swartz, MD, of Duke University and Patrick Boyle, Director of Training, from the IDDT Center of Excellence in Ohio. After each presenter, a panel of local clinicians, consumers, and family members responded to the information presented and led a facilitated discussion with the audience.

### Adoption Research Objective

The originally proposed pilot study was to examine clinician adoption and use of ACT teams, looking specifically at one established site and at one newly established site. It was anticipated that 21 Area Programs/LMEs would have ACT teams in place by January 2003. The goal was to develop an understanding of ACT implementation issues in North Carolina and to develop a framework for evaluating the subsequent roll out of ACT teams to the other areas of the state. To gather the data necessary to answer these questions a program evaluation was to be developed built upon the previous technical assistance efforts in North Carolina.

The Research Committee of the North Carolina Science to Service Consortium was established and met in August and September. The committee was very supportive of the goals of evaluating adoption and use of ACT and gaining an understanding of implementation issues. Practical reality forced the committee to revisit the goal of developing a framework to evaluate rollout of ACT. In fact, due to accelerating reform efforts in North Carolina and the expectation that ACT services be provided in all communities, identified ACT Teams in North Carolina exceeded 40 in the fall of 2003, double the anticipated 21 stated in the grant. In fact, "rollout" already had occurred. Very little information was available about these teams and even less about their fidelity to ACT principles. Committee members felt it was imperative to expand the scope of the study and to survey all ACT teams in North Carolina to establish a baseline of functioning and to assist in determining training needs. Consequently, members felt it would be far more useful to survey all teams on elements of the Dartmouth Assertive Community Treatment Scale (DACTS) instead of doing a complete DACTS assessment on only two teams. Committee members also were interested in assessing the impact of various training and technical assistance efforts on implementation and fidelity of those teams that had received such assistance.

As a result of these discussions, Joe Morrissey, PhD, and Piper Meyer, PhD, at the Cecil G. Sheps Center for Health Services Research at the University of North Carolina, developed a series of telephone surveys. The "Operational Status of ACT Teams" survey provided extensive qualitative data on the team and its operations as well as probing training needs and perceived challenges and barriers. The "Operational Status Fidelity Scoring Form" was more directly tied to elements of the DACTS and this information was entered into a database for analysis. The final survey instrument was the "ACT Team Checklist" which had three versions, one for those teams that had received state-supported technical assistance from a consultant, one for teams that received state-supported training in Madison, Wisconsin, and one for teams that received no state-supported assistance to get a sense of training value, needs, and barriers.

A final element of the proposed ACT Team study was a record review. Research committee members determined that, given the limited resources available, resources would be better used conducting the modified study. Investigator Joe Morrissey wrote,

> . . . The message from this research is loud and clear—well functioning ACTTs prevent hospitalization. So there's no real reason for us to replicate it in NC. What we are doing in the pilot will yield much more valuable information about the state's current capacity and needs for ACTTs, information that can be used to build future efforts to enhance the evidence-base of current practice."

In addition, two focus groups were conducted by the UNC School of Social Work to assess consumer satisfaction and perceptions of Assertive Community Treatment. Overall, consumers were very satisfied with ACT services but identified the need to enhance vocational supports.

The ACT Team survey offered the first systematic assessment of ACT Teams in the state and a measure of the fidelity of these teams to the ACT model. It found that compared to National Fidelity Standards, NC ACT Teams:

- Had smaller staffs
- Had smaller case loads
- Used less psychiatrist time
- Had fewer multidisciplinary staff members.

This seemed to be due in part to the rural nature of many of the counties involved.

The recommendations of that study were that the state:

- Develop a training and support network for ACT team leaders
- Provide training on measuring fidelity to the practice model and incorporate fidelity measures into clinical supervision
- Educate leaders about alternative services for rural communities
- Provide ongoing ACT training for new ACT Teams and new staff

## GENERAL ISSUES AND OBSERVATIONS

The final grant report noted that implementation of evidence-based practices often focused on raising awareness of these practices and supporting the workforce to change practice. This planning effort emphasized the necessity, and the complexity, of building state and local infrastructure to support not only the implementation of EBPs, but the sustainability of these practices. There is limited experience from other states or national guidance in this area. The bulk of the North Carolina implementation plan focused on the difficult task of building this infrastructure.

Implementation of evidence-based practices in North Carolina had been made more complex by the comprehensive system reform efforts that were reconfiguring the institutions historically responsible for providing mental health services. While this offered the opportunity to align care in more effective ways, many policy and program leaders, providers, and consumers felt overwhelmed by the magnitude of change. A major leadership challenge was the promotion of evidence-based practices as an integral part of reform rather than an additional undertaking or an initiative competing for already limited resources.

## STAFF CONCLUSIONS

When queried by the federal grantors about their candid observations and lessons learned, the staff reported as follows:

- Do not minimize the need for and the time it takes to raise awareness and create buy-in of major constituency groups, especially providers. Identify "champions" within these constituency groups early on and support them to carry the message.
- Simply having researchers and community providers work together on a project or grant does not result in more collaborative research efforts. They may understand each other better and develop positive personal relationships, but the conduct of research and the transfer of research to practice will require more planning and structural support. There is relatively little funding for research and increasingly available funding is from federal sources through state agencies. State agencies need to establish a collaborative structure of various stakeholders to develop research priorities and provide coordinated support of these efforts.
- Strong, consistent, visible state leadership is essential to send a message of support to the broad constituency, but especially to state bureaucracy. Retraining of state agency staff is essential as these individuals often are directly responsible for the development of policy and support structures that will sustain implementation efforts.
- Having a consistent, clear message about exactly what the state's expectations are regarding evidence-based practices is crucial. The state must define what they mean by the term "evidence-based practice," which specific practices qualify, and what essential elements of that practice are critical. Otherwise, everyone believes they are doing evidence-based practices.
- State-level policies and systems need to be in alignment with EBPs if a state wants to take EBPs statewide. These include data systems that can track which EBP services people receive and their outcomes. It also includes a state level quality improvement process that includes evidence-based practices as a major role. (Portions of the agenda report dealing with administrative infrastructure supports covering quality improvement are reproduced in Exhibit 7–2.)

- Workshops that presented compelling research on the effectiveness of six evidence-based practices did not lead to implementation, nor did it necessarily encourage all persons to support EBPs. Administrators and practitioners need compelling reasons to implement beyond the strength of the research. In addition, consumers questioned the recovery base of the six EBPs and the need for randomized controlled trials (rather than qualitative studies) to prove "evidence."
- Actual implementation occurs in the communities and will be successful when there is strong leadership that supports collaboration among consumers, families, providers, and local government leaders.
- Families and consumers play a critical advocacy role in promoting implementation of EBPs in their communities. They are unlikely to advocate for practices they do not feel ownership of, and presentations by the Science to Service Project alone do not create ownership.

*Text continues on p. 600*

**Exhibit 7–2** Excerpts from Agenda Report of NC Science to Service Project
July 2004

---

**Strategy 3.4: The State is encouraged to develop a strong quality improvement process and capacity to support model fidelity to evidence-based practices.**

- The State is encouraged to hire or contract for expertise to examine its data system and evaluate state system and provider LME performance to determine if the desired outcomes are being achieved (i.e. helping consumers gain competitive employment, reduce psychiatric hospitalizations). It is recommended that reports developed by the State be regularly posted and easily accessible to the public on the web.
- The State is encouraged to support the development of technical assistance to LMEs and providers to advance quality improvement systems that foster continuous learning and improvement and involve a collaborative process between providers and LMEs.
- The State must identify quality improvement domains and consumer outcomes, gather data, and provide timely and useful feedback to LMEs and the public.
- It is recommended that the State ensure that utilization management protocols reflect and are consistent with the outcomes and recom-

---

*continues*

**Exhibit 7–2** continued

> mended amount of treatment in the evidence-based practice toolkits. This will require breaking this information out for the EBPs embedded in the Community Support and Community Support Team definitions, such as Family Psychoeducation, Wellness Management and Recovery, and Integrated Dual Disorder Treatment.
> - With regard to EBPs, it is recommended that the State and LME quality improvement processes initially focus on the domains of:
>   - access to evidence-based practices as measured by:
>     - the number of EBP programs available in counties and in the state
>     - eligible consumers on waiting lists for EBP services
>     - eligible consumers denied access to EBP services due to unavailability;
>   - process as measured by fidelity to the EBP model; and
>   - consumer outcomes affected by EBP services.
> - In addition to these quantitative data, it is recommended that qualitative data be gathered from consumers, LMEs, and providers regarding barriers to implementation. This data should be used to inform State and local QI processes.
> - The contract between the State and the LMEs is encouraged to require the use of fidelity scales when one is available and have an independent entity complete that assessment. It is recommended that the State develop an independent process involving experienced EBP fidelity scale evaluators, perhaps through the Council of Community Programs accreditation process, to administer fidelity scales to programs providing evidence-based practices. It is recommended that results of this evaluation should be provided to the LME, program administrator, clinical supervisor, and to the LME and provider QI committees. Programs are encouraged to develop a plan for continuous improvement and submit these to the LME.
> - The State Consumer and Family Advisory Committee (CFAC) should have input into which outcomes the Division monitors for quality, and should receive regular quality improvement reports from the Division.
>
> **Strategy 3.5: LMEs must be responsible for developing EBP programs that adhere to model fidelity in their provider community and improve consumer outcomes.**
> - As soon as it is feasible, LME and program staff should receive training about fidelity scales and appropriate ways to use these measures to improve quality. LMEs should begin to actively monitor fidelity to

*continues*

**Exhibit 7–2** continued

> evidence-based practices and work collaboratively with programs to
> improve model fidelity.
> - It is recommended that LMEs track consumer outcome data to deter-
>   mine the effectiveness of services. This data should be regularly re-
>   viewed and provided to the QI committee.
> - Consumers and families should be actively involved in gathering con-
>   sumer satisfaction data and it is recommended that CFACs receive
>   reports of LME QI activities and provide input to the QI committee.
> - CFACs should also be included in the selection of LME indicators of
>   quality, the analysis of information gathered, and the development
>   of strategies to improve quality.
>
> **Strategy 3.6:  Providers of EBP services are encouraged to use
> fidelity measures and outcome data to improve services through their
> internal quality improvement process.**
> - Provider organizations should receive training about fidelity scales and
>   appropriate ways to use these measures to improve quality.
> - Provider organizations should monitor fidelity and track consumer out-
>   comes data and use the information gathered within their QI system.
>   Consumers of the provider agency should be involved in this process.
>
>
> **Outcome Evaluation**
>
> *Gathering Quality Data*
>
> Establishing outcome measures and data systems to collect and ana-
> lyze those measures for quality improvement purposes is essential for
> system improvement. Many states have established comprehensive qual-
> ity systems. New York, for example, uses consumer assessment teams to
> collect qualitative information about satisfaction with services. In many
> instances, collection of outcome data is embedded into the routine
> process of service provision and coordination. For example, a case man-
> ager can gather baseline information during admission that can be
> shared throughout the system through computer networks. For ease of
> administration New York has developed short global indicator approach
> to measurement, including a 12-item quality of life assessment. At this
> time, such real-time data systems are not available to local level deci-
> sion makers in North Carolina.

*continues*

**Exhibit 7–2** continued

Historically North Carolina has used the Client Outcome Indicators (COI) tool to measure client-specific outcomes on quality of life measures over time. This measure is referenced in the proposed State/LME contract and will continue to be used to assess system outcomes. Historically, however, this measure has been controversial. Concerns have been raised about the complexity and cost of gathering data, the relevance of the items, and the timeliness and usefulness of data analysis. The proposed contract between the State and LMEs also contains the mandate to measure several consumer outcomes, including employment, housing, and recidivism.

The State is early in the process of establishing a quality management system and exactly what data it needs to collect is still under discussion. In addition, there is significant variability among local LMEs in the capacity to collect and analyze outcomes. This becomes a critical function, however, when LMEs are responsible for developing and managing a network of providers for a broad continuum of services. Outcome data should be utilized in quality improvement activities, report cards, and for monitoring of contracts.

Other states have utilized outcome measures and data that provide relevant information about the status of EBPs. For example, access to EBPs may be measured by the number of counties with each service or the number of consumers receiving an EBP. Outcomes of service can be measured by the changes in consumers' lives versus similar consumers who received another service. Kansas, for example, has been collecting consumer outcome data for over 15 years on a variety of areas important to consumers, such as vocational status. Their system requires only 20 minutes each quarter for each worker to complete their entire caseload and provides a 48 hour turnaround for reports back to the agencies. These reports are also integrated with grant development, on-site reviews, and technical assistance. The implementation resource kits created by the national Implementing Evidence-Based Practices Project also includes an outcome tool that is designed to measure those areas that the identified evidence-based practices impact

Once the data is collected, it is important that it is analyzed and provided back to those who will be able to use the information. For this reason, it may be helpful to get input from front-line clinicians, supervisors, provider agency administrators, and LMEs when developing outcome measures. One key to making the data useful will be to provide information in reports that clearly answer key questions that stakeholders have and directly send them to the appropriate group.

*continues*

**Exhibit 7–2** continued

Where the data is sent, who will do the analysis and formulate the report, who will disseminate the information and how, and who will receive the information are all key questions.

In addition, what measures (if any) should be standardized and collected statewide is an issue that should be considered. Currently, the system performance standards in the proposed Division/LME contract only requires that employment, housing, and recidivism outcomes are collected, leaving the choice of other outcomes on the local level. While this provision allows for locally relevant data collection, it does not allow the State to measure other crucial indicators of the quality of services statewide nor the impact of statewide policies and other efforts. In addition, LMEs cannot benchmark performance against other similar entities.

North Carolina has recently been recognized for promoting innovations in data collection and management. New initiatives have begun to integrate data throughout the Department of Health and Human Services and allow customizable reports through the Decision Support Information System that respond to information needs. These innovations provide great opportunities for supporting the implementation of evidence-based practices. To reach its potential, there are four major areas that the State outcome and data system will need to respond to in order to adequately measure the provision and effectiveness of evidence-based services.

1. The current inability to measure access to or effectiveness of Family Psychoeducation, Wellness Management and Recovery, and Integrated Dual Diagnosis Treatment services.
   - Currently, the state collects information about which services consumers receive from the billing system based on Medicaid service definitions. The four practices above are potentially billable under a new proposed bundled service definition, Community Support Team. Consumer outcomes are measured through the COI, which can be linked to the billing system through a unique client identifier in a unified Data Warehouse. However, because the four practices above are bundled and have no unique service definition/billing code, it is currently impossible to directly link these four practices to the outcomes they produce for specific consumers.
2. The current inability to measure the provision or effectiveness of the Medication Management EBP.
   - The State does not have a method to measure the number of consumers receiving atypical antipsychotic medications. Although

*continues*

**Exhibit 7–2** continued

> Medicaid data captures Medicaid eligible consumers, medications non-Medicaid consumers receive are not tracked. The COI does not ask a question regarding which medicine a consumer is taking.
>
> 3. The current inability to measure access to services statewide through penetration rates (as indicated by the number of consumers who are eligible for EBP services that actually receive these services).
>    - In order to determine a penetration rate, it is necessary to link information about clients who will benefit with those that actually receive the service. Currently, documentation does not survey which evidence-based practices a particular consumer will benefit from (judged by the criteria in the implementation resource kits). And as mentioned above, it is currently not possible to track the individual evidence-based practices a consumer receives within a bundled service.
>
> 4. LMEs, providers, and consumers do not currently have access to data about the effectiveness of services.
>    - While State data systems have the capability to create customizable reports, few users have access to this data. In addition, reports about the effectiveness of services are not produced and disseminated to the public. Other states have publicly published reports about the number of consumers employed in Supported Employment programs, for example, and release employment statistics per individual program to the public.
>
> **Strategy 3.7: Meaningful outcomes and helpful data systems must be identified and implemented to improve quality and inform policy and planning on the State and local level.**
>
>    - The State is encouraged to engage in a dialog with LMEs, providers, and consumers/family members regarding meaningful outcomes the State should be gathering for statewide comparison.
>    - Minimally, the State is encouraged to gather and utilize LMEs outcome measures relative to EBP for access (number of programs statewide and per county, eligible consumers on waiting lists for EBP services, and eligible consumers denied access to EBP services due to unavailability), process (model fidelity), and outcomes (recidivism, housing, employment, atypical antipsychotic use). . . .
>    - The State, in collaboration with the LMEs, is encouraged to review whether modifications to the COI instrument and process can

*continues*

**Exhibit 7–2** continued

> address concerns and improve the relevance of data. Efforts should be made to link specific outcomes to the service a particular individual receives, and effectiveness data should be available publicly.
> - LMEs and providers are encouraged to gather additional consumer outcomes to further evaluate the effectiveness of evidence-based and emerging best practices.

## FUTURE DIRECTION

The project will focus its efforts on awareness building with major constituency groups, advocacy with state agencies, supporting collaborative training and research efforts, and providing technical assistance to local programs. Specifically, the project will:

- Work closely with consumers and family members through CFACs and advocacy groups to increase awareness of and demand for evidence-based practices
- Provide consultation to Local Management Entities to create the infrastructure to support evidence-based practices
- Work with universities and community colleges to integrate content on evidence-based practices into course curricula
- Disseminate information about evidence-based practices and implementation
- Monitor the implementation of the statewide agenda and encourage adoption of the recommendations included in the report
- Continue to work closely with a new EBP training project coordinated through one of the regional AHEC centers

In addition, North Carolina has been awarded a Mental Health: Systems Transformation (CMS) grant that will be managed by the Science to Service Project. This grant will be used to assist local management entities to develop models for implementing EBPs into their infrastructure.

## CASE ANALYSIS

This case shows how the federal government agencies and mental health experts are attempting to influence the quality of care in state-controlled public mental health programs. There have been widespread differences of opinion about best practices and about the need for transformation and change in the mental health system. Various states are at very different places in this transition. Now the federal government has developed and implemented a policy aimed at transformation and change which is to finance projects like NCS2S in states that seem likely to benefit from it.

## ASSIGNMENT QUESTIONS

### Introduction

1. What factors are influencing the decision of the federal and state governments to encourage the adoption of evidence-based practices into the state's public mental health systems?
2. How does the approach to continuous quality improvement adopted here differ from that of the Medicare and Medicaid programs? Why the differences?

### Basics

3. Interpret the NCS2S strategy of a consortium and the series of presentations and meetings as a method of team building as outlined in Chapter 6.

### Implementation

4. Evaluate the NCS2S strategy as a method of managing transformation and learning in the rapidly changing public mental health system.
5. The NCS2S case says little about changing the training programs for new mental health professionals to incorporate changing definitions of evidence-based practices. Present a proposal to deal with this need.

## Application

6. Interpreting the public mental health programs of a state as a public health issue, what do the models and interpretations in Chapter 14 suggest should be the role of NCS2S or its successor programs in the future?

## CLASS EXERCISE

Follow up on the SAMHSA and NIMH Web sites to determine whether new evidence-based practices are being added to the six arrayed in the case. What kinds of pressures is the federal government applying to foster their implementation? How is your state government responding? Is it changing service definitions, certification requirements, reimbursement mechanisms, or organizational structures to keep up? Compare your state's response with that of other leading states like New York and Washington State.

# CASE 8

# Transforming Health Care: The President's Health Information Technology Plan[1]

*"By computerizing health records, we can avoid dangerous medical mistakes, reduce costs, and improve care."*
*–President George W. Bush, State of the Union Address,*
*January 20, 2004*

On April 27, 2004, the White House published *Promoting Innovation and Competitiveness: President Bush's Technology Agenda: A New Generation of American Innovation.* The report outlined a plan to ensure that most Americans have electronic health records within the next ten years. A fundamental assumption of the plan is that better health information technology is essential to a vision of a health care system that puts the needs and the values of the patient first and gives patients information they need to make clinical and economic decisions in consultation with dedicated health care professionals. This report addresses longstanding problems of preventable errors, uneven quality, and rising costs in the nation's health care system.

[1]This case was prepared by the editors with only minor editorial changes to verbatim material excerpted from the original government documents *Transforming Health Care: The President's Health Information Technology Plan* (www.whitehouse.gov/infocus/technology/economic_policy/200404/chap3) and *Health Information Technology Strategic Framework Report: Executive Summary* (www.hhs.gov/healthit/onchit/executivesummary) both accessed 12/11/04.

## THE PROBLEM: CHALLENGES TO THE U.S. HEALTH CARE SYSTEM

The U.S. health care system has a long and distinguished history of innovation. Discoveries move from the laboratory bench to the bedside, as basic research results are translated into new understanding of diseases, better diagnostic tools, and innovative treatments. At the same time, our health care system faces major challenges. Health care spending and health insurance premiums continue to rise at rates much higher than the rate of inflation. Despite spending over $1.6 trillion on health care as a Nation, there are still serious concerns about preventable errors; uneven health care quality; and poor communication among doctors, hospitals, and many other health care providers involved in the care of anyone person. The Institute of Medicine estimates that between 44,000 and 98,000 Americans die each year from medical errors. (2000) Many more die or have permanent disability because of inappropriate treatments, mistreatments, or missed treatments in ambulatory settings. Studies have found that as much as $300 billion is spent each year on health care that does not improve patient outcomes—treatment that is unnecessary, inappropriate, inefficient, or ineffective.

All these problems—high costs, uncertain value, medical errors, variable quality, administrative inefficiencies, and poor coordination—are closely connected to our failure to use health information technology as an integral part of medical care. The innovation that has made our medical care the world's best has not been applied to our health information systems. Other American industries have harnessed advanced information technologies, to the benefit of American consumers. Our air travel is safer than ever, and consumers now have ready and safe access to their financial information. Unlike these other industries, medicine still operates primarily with paper-based records. Our doctors and nurses have to manage 21st century medical technology and complex medical information with 19th century tools. America's medical professionals are the best and brightest in the world, and set the standard for the world. It is a testament to their skill that they are able to achieve high-quality care in this antiquated system. In this outdated, paper-based system:

- A patient's vital medical information is scattered across medical records kept by many different caregivers in many different locations— and all of the patient's medical information is often unavailable at the time of care. For example, patients with medical emergencies too often are seen by doctors with no access to their critical medical information, such as allergies, current treatments or medications, and prior diagnoses.

- Physicians keep information about drugs, drug interactions, managed care formularies, clinical guidelines, and recent research in memory—a difficult task given the high volume of information.
- Medical orders and prescriptions are handwritten and are too often misunderstood or not followed in accordance with the physician's instructions.
- Consumers lack access to useful, credible health information about treatment alternatives, which hospitals and physicians are best for their needs, or their own health status.
- Physicians do not always have the best information to select the best treatments for their patients, resulting in an unacceptable lag time before new scientific advances are used in patient care. They also do not have ready access to complete information about their patients, do not know how other doctors are treating their same patients, or how other health care providers around the country treat patients with the same condition. These conditions set the stage for preventable medical errors.

## THE SOLUTION—HEALTH INFORMATION TECHNOLOGY

President Bush's plan presents an ambitious goal of assuring that most Americans have electronic health records within the next ten years. Specifically:

- Within the next ten years, electronic health records will ensure that complete health care information is available for most Americans at the time and place of care, no matter where it originates. Participation by patients will be voluntary.
- These electronic health records will be designed to share information privately and securely among and between health care providers when authorized by the patient.

An underlying premise of the report is that innovations in electronic health records and the secure exchange of medical information will help transform health care in America—improving health care quality, preventing medical errors, reducing health care costs, improving administrative efficiencies, reducing paperwork, and increasing access to affordable health care.

The steps we need to take across the Nation are already underway in some places. Health information technologies—electronic medical records, computerized ordering of prescriptions and other medical tests, clinical decision support tools, and secure exchange of authorized information—improve quality, reduce medical errors, and prevent deaths. In the past three years, some communities, hospitals, clinicians, patient groups, and information technology companies have acted to improve their health information systems. These pioneering communities are taking the initiative and showing that health care can and must be modernized.

The report envisions a dramatically changed system:

- When arriving at a physician's office, new patients will not have to enter their personal information, allergies, medications, or medical history, since it will already be available.

- A parent, who previously had to carry the child's medical records and x-rays in a large box when seeing a new physician, will now keep the most important medical history on a keychain, or simply authorize the new physician to retrieve the information electronically from previous health care providers.

- Arriving at an emergency room, a senior with a chronic illness and memory difficulties can authorize her physicians to access her medical information from a recent hospitalization at another hospital—thus avoiding a potentially fatal drug interaction between the planned treatment and the patient's current medications.

- Three patients with unusual sudden-onset fever and cough that would not individually be reported, will be able to show up at separate emergency rooms, and the trend will instantly be reported to public health officials, who will alert authorities of a possible disease outbreak or bioterror attack.

## The President's Health Information Technology Plan

To achieve this ten-year goal, the plan proposes the following steps to urge coordinated public and private sector efforts that will accelerate broader adoption of health information technology.

### Adopting Health Information Standards

The completion and adoption of standards will allow medical information to be stored and shared electronically while assuring privacy and security. The necessary work is already well underway and much of it has already been completed. In the last several years, the Department of Health and Human Services (HHS) has been collaborating with the private sector and other Federal agencies to identify and endorse voluntary standards that are necessary for health information to be shared safely and securely among health care providers. Federal agencies are accelerating their use of these standards. As part of this effort, HHS has recently negotiated and licensed a comprehensive medical vocabulary and made it available to everyone in the Nation at no cost. The results of these projects include standards for:

- Transmitting X-Rays Over the Internet: Today, a patient's chest x-ray can be sent electronically from a hospital or laboratory and read by the patient's doctor in his office.
- Electronic Laboratory Results: Laboratory results can be sent electronically to the physician for immediate analysis, diagnosis, and treatment, and could be automatically entered into the patient's electronic health record if one existed. For example, a doctor could retrieve this information from his office for a hospitalized patient, assuring a prompt response and eliminating errors and duplicative testing due to lost laboratory reports.
- Electronic Prescriptions: Patients will save time because prescriptions can be sent electronically to their pharmacists. By eliminating illegible handwritten prescriptions, and because the technology automatically checks for possible allergies and harmful drug interactions with other drugs, standardized electronic prescriptions help avoid serious medical errors. The technology also can generate automatic approval from a health insurer.

*Doubling Funding to $100 Million for Demonstration Projects on Health Care Information Technology*

To build upon the progress already made in the area of health information technology standards over the last several years, the proposed FY 2005 budget includes $100 million for demonstration projects that will help test the effectiveness of health information technology and establish best practices for more widespread adoption in the health care industry.

- This increase builds on the FY 2004 budget which included $50 million, and these new resources will support more local and regional grants so that pioneering communities, physicians, and hospitals can show that health care can be transformed by adopting and implementing health information technology.

- In April 2004, more than 600 applications for funding were received for these grants, and HHS will be awarding grants this summer, following their peer-reviewed process for selecting grantees.

*Using the Federal Government to Foster the Adoption of Health Information Technology*

As one of the largest buyers of health care—in Medicare, Medicaid, the Community Health Centers program, the Federal Health Benefits program, Veterans medical care, and programs in the Department of Defense, the federal government can create incentives and opportunities for health care providers to use electronic records, much like the private sector is doing today. The President will direct these agencies to review their policies and programs and propose modifications and new actions, and forward the recommendations to him within 90 days.

*Creating a New, Sub-Cabinet Level Position of National Health Information Technology Coordinator*

In the presentation of the report, President Bush announced creation of a new sub-Cabinet level post at HHS, to provide national leadership and coordination necessary to achieve his ten-year goal. The individual will report directly to the HHS Secretary, and will be charged by the President with:

- Guiding ongoing work on health information standards and working to identify and implement the various steps needed to support and encourage health information technology in the public and private health care delivery systems.
- Coordinating partnerships between government agencies and private sector stakeholders to speed the adoption of health information technology.

## IMPLEMENTATION

The new sub-cabinet level Office of the National Coordinator for Health Information Technology (ONCHIT) was established and on May 6, 2004, Secretary Tommy G. Thompson appointed David J. Brailer, MD, PhD, to this new position. Executive Order 13335 required the National Coordinator to report within 90 days operation on the development and implementation of a strategic plan for to guide the nationwide implementation of health information technology in both the public and private sectors.

In fulfilling the requirements of this executive order. ONCHIT issued a report, the Executive Summary of which is reproduced in part below:

> This report (as revised November 9, 2004) outlines a framework for a strategic plan that will be dynamic, iterative, and implemented in coordination with the private sector. In addition, this report includes attachments (not included in this case, but available on the web) from the Office of Personnel Management (OPM), the Department of Defense (DoD), and the Department of Veterans Affairs (VA). Collectively, this report and related attachments represent the progress to date on the development and implementation of a comprehensive HIT strategic plan.

### Readiness for Change

There is a great need for information tools to be used in the delivery of health care. Preventable medical errors and treatment variations have recently gained attention. Clinicians may not know the latest treatment options, and practices vary across clinicians and regions. Consumers want to ensure that they have choices in treatment, and when they do, they want to have the information they need to make decisions about their care. Concerns about the privacy and security of personal medical information remain high. Public health monitoring, bioterror surveillance, research, and quality monitoring require data that depends on the widespread adoption of HIT.

### Vision for Consumer-centric and Information-rich Care

Many envision a health care industry that is consumer-centric and information-rich, in which medical information follows the consumer, and information tools guide medical decisions. Clinicians have appropriate access to a patient's complete treatment history, including medical records, medication history, laboratory results, and radiographs, among other information. Clinicians order medications with computerized systems that eliminate handwriting errors and automatically check for doses that are too high or too low, for harmful interactions with other drugs, and for allergies. Prescriptions are also checked against the health plan's formulary, and the out-of-pocket costs of the prescribed drug can be compared with alternative treatments. Clinicians receive electronic reminders in the form of alerts about treatment procedures and medical guidelines. This is a different way of delivering health care than that which currently exists, but one that many have envisioned. This new way will result in fewer medical errors, fewer unnecessary treatments or wasteful care, and fewer variations in care, and will ultimately improve care for all Americans. Care will be centered around the consumer and will be delivered electronically as well as in person. Clinicians can spend more time on patient care, and employers will gain productivity and competitive benefits from health care spending.

## Strategic Framework

In order to realize a new vision for health care made possible through the use of information technology, strategic actions embraced by the public and private health sectors need to be taken over many years. There are four major goals that will be pursued in realizing this vision for improved health care. Each of these goals has a corresponding set of strategies and related specific actions that will advance and focus future efforts. These goals and strategies are summarized below.

### Goal 1: Inform Clinical Practice

Informing clinical practice is fundamental to improving care and making health care delivery more efficient. This goal centers largely around efforts to bring EHRs directly into clinical practice. This will reduce medical errors and duplicative work, and enable clinicians to focus their efforts more directly on improved patient care. Three strategies for realizing this goal are:

- *Strategy 1. Incentivize EHR adoption:* The transition to safe, more consumer-friendly and regionally integrated care delivery will require shared investments in information tools and changes to current clinical practice.
- *Strategy 2. Reduce risk of EHR investment:* Clinicians who purchase EHRs and who attempt to change their clinical practices and office operations face a variety of risks that make this decision unduly challenging. Low-cost support systems that reduce risk, failure, and partial use of EHRs are needed.

- *Strategy 3. Promote EHR diffusion in rural and underserved areas:* Practices and hospitals in rural and other underserved areas lag in EHR adoption. Technology transfer and other support efforts are needed to ensure widespread adoption.

## Goal 2: Interconnect Clinicians

Interconnecting clinicians will allow information to be portable and to move with consumers from one point of care to another. This will require an interoperable infrastructure to help clinicians access critical health care information when their clinical and/or treatment decisions are being made. The three strategies for realizing this goal are:

- *Strategy 1. Foster regional collaborations:* Local oversight of health information exchange that reflects the needs and goals of a population should be developed.
- *Strategy 2. Develop a national health information network:* A set of common intercommunication tools such as mobile authentication, Web services architecture, and security technologies are needed to support data movement that is inexpensive and secure. A national health information network that can provide low-cost and secure data movement is needed, along with a public-private oversight or management function to ensure adherence to public policy objectives.
- *Strategy 3. Coordinate federal health information systems:* There is a need for federal health information systems to be interoperable and to exchange data so that federal care delivery, reimbursement, and oversight are more efficient and cost-effective. Federal health information systems will be interoperable and consistent with the national health information network.

## Goal 3: Personalize Care

Consumer-centric information helps individuals manage their own wellness and assists with their personal health care decisions. The ability to personalize care is a critical component of using health care information in a meaningful manner. The three strategies for realizing this goal are:

- *Strategy 1. Encourage use of Personal Health Records.* Consumers are increasingly seeking information about their care as a means of getting better control over their health care experience, and PHRs that provide customized facts and guidance to them are needed.

- *Strategy 2. Enhance informed consumer choice:* Consumers should have the ability to select clinicians and institutions based on what they value and the information to guide their choice, including but not limited to, the quality of care providers deliver.
- *Strategy 3. Promote use of telehealth systems:* The use of telehealth-remote communication technologies can provide access to health services for consumers and clinicians in rural and underserved areas. Telehealth systems that can support the delivery of health care services when the participants are in different locations are needed.

*Goal 4: Improve Population Health*

Population health improvement requires the collection of timely, accurate, and detailed clinical information to allow for the evaluation of health care delivery and the reporting of critical findings to public health officials, clinical trials and other research, and feedback to clinicians. Three strategies for realizing this goal are:

- *Strategy 1. Unify public health surveillance architectures:* An interoperable public health surveillance system is needed that will allow exchange of information, consistent with current law, between provider organizations, organizations they contract with, and state and federal agencies.
- *Strategy 2. Streamline quality and health status monitoring:* Many different state and local organizations collect subsets of data for specific purposes and use it in different ways. A streamlined quality-monitoring infrastructure that will allow for a complete look at quatity and other issues in real-time and at the point of care is needed.
- *Strategy 3. Accelerate research and dissemination of evidence:* Information tools are needed that can accelerate scientific discoveries and their translation into clinically useful products, applications, and knowledge.

## Key Actions

The Framework for Strategic Action will guide the development of a full strategic plan for widespread HIT adoption. At the same time, a vari-

ety of key actions that have begun to implement this strategy are underway.

*Establishing a Health Information Technology Leadership Panel to eval-
uate the urgency of investments and recommend immediate actions*

As many different options and policies are considered for financing
HIT adoption, the Secretary of HHS is taking immediate action by forming a Health Information Technology Leadership Panel consisting of executives and leaders. This panel will assess the costs and benefits of HIT
to industry and society, and evaluate the urgency of investments in these
tools. These leaders will discuss the immediate steps for both the public
and private sector to take with regard to HIT adoption, based on their individual business experience. The Health Information Technology
Leadership Panel will deliver a synthesized report comprised of these options to the Secretary no later than Fall 2004.

*Private sector certification of health information technology products*

EHRs and even specific components such as decision support software
are unique among clinical tools in that they do not need to meet minimal
standards to be used to deliver care. To increase uptake of EHRs and reduce the risk of product implementation failure, the federal government is
exploring ways to work with the private sector to develop minimal product standards for EHR functionality, interoperability, and security. A private sector ambulatory EHR certification task force is determining the feasibility of certification of EHR products based on functionality, security,
and interoperability.

*Funding community health information exchange demonstrations*

A health information exchange program through Health Resources and
Services Administration, Office of the Advancement of Telehealth
(HRSA/OAT), has a cooperative agreement with the Foundation for
eHealth Initiative to administer contracts to support the Connecting
Communities for Better Health (CCBH) Program totaling $2.3 million.
This program is providing seed funds and support to multistakeholder collaboratives within communities (both geographic and nongeographic) to
implement health information exchanges, including the formation of regional health information organizations (RHIOs) to drive improvements

in health care quality, safety, and efficiency. The specific communities that will receive the funding through this program will be announced and recognized during the Secretarial Summit on July 21.

*Planning the formation of a private interoperability consortium*

To begin the process of movement toward a national health information network, HHS is releasing a request for information (RFI) in the summer of 2004 inviting responses describing the requirements for private sector consortia that would form to plan, develop, and operate a health information network. Members of the consortium would agree to participate in the governance structure and activities and finance the consortium in an equitable manner. The role that HHS could play in facilitating the work of the consortium and assisting in identifying the services that the consortium would provide will be explored, including the standards which the health information network would adhere to in order to ensure that public policy goals are executed and that rapid adoption of interoperable EHRs is advanced. The Federal Health Architecture (FHA) will be coordinated and interoperable with the national health information network.

*Requiring standards to facilitate electronic prescribing*

CMS will be proposing a regulation that will require the first set of widely adopted e-prescribing standards in preparation for the implementation of the new Medicare drug benefit in 2006. When this regulation is final, Medicare Prescription Drug Plan (PDP) Sponsors will be required to offer e-prescribing, which will significantly drive adoption across the United States. Health plans and pharmacy benefit managers that are PDP sponsors could work with RHIOs, including physician offices, to implement private industry-certified interoperable e-prescribing tools and to train and support clinicians.

*Establishing a Medicare beneficiary portal*

An immediate step in improving consumer access to personal and customized health information is CMS' Medicare Beneficiary Portal, which provides secure health information via the Internet. This portal will be hosted by a private company under contract with CMS, and will enable authorized Medicare beneficiaries to have access to their information online or by calling 1-800-MEDICARE. Initially the portal will provide access to fee-for-service claims information, which includes claims type, dates of service, and procedures. The pilot test for the portal will be conducted for the residents of Indiana. In the near term, CMS plans to expand the portal to include prevention information in the form of reminders to beneficiaries to schedule their Medicare-covered preventive health care services. CMS also plans to work toward providing additional electronic health information tools to beneficiaries for their use in improving their health.

*Sharing clinical research data through a secure infrastructure*

FDA and NIH, together with the Clinical Data Interchange Standards Consortium (CDISC), a consortium of over 40 pharmaceutical companies and clinical research organizations, have developed a standard for representing observations made in clinical trials called the Study Data Tabulation Model (SDTM). This model will facilitate the automation of the largely paper-based clinical research process, which will lead to greater efficiencies in industry- and government-sponsored clinical research. The first release of the model and associated implementation guide will be finalized prior to the July 21 Secretarial Summit and represents an important step by government, academia, and industry in working together to accelerate research through the use of standards and HIT.

*Commitment to standards*

A key component of progress in interoperable health information is the development of technically sound and robustly specified interoperability standards and policies. There have been considerable efforts by HHS, DoD, and VA to adopt health information standards for use by all federal health agencies. As part of the Consolidated Health Informatics (CHI) initiative, the agencies have agreed to endorse 20 sets of standards to make it easier for information to be shared across agencies and to serve as a model for the private sector. Additionally, the Public

Health Information Network (PHIN) and the National Electronic Disease Surveillance System (NEDSS), under the leadership of the Centers for Disease Control and Prevention (CDC), have made notable progress in development of shared data models, data standards, and controlled vocabularies for electronic laboratory reporting and health information exchange. With HHS support, Health Level 7 (HL7) has also created a functional model and standards for the EHR.

## PUBLIC–PRIVATE PARTNERSHIP

Leaders across the public and private sector recognize that the adoption and effective use of HIT requires a joint effort between federal, state, and local governments and the private sector. The value of HIT will be best realized under the conditions of a competitive technology industry, privately-operated support services, choice among clinicians and provider organizations, and payers who reward clinicians based on quality. The Federal government has already played an active role in the evolution and use of HIT. In Fiscal Year 2004, total federal spending on HIT was more than $900 million. Initiatives range from supporting research in advanced HIT to the development and use of EHR systems. Much of this work demonstrates that HIT can be used effectively in supporting health care delivery and improving quality and patient safety.

## ROLE OF THE NATIONAL COORDINATOR FOR HEALTH INFORMATION TECHNOLOGY

Executive Order 13335 directed the appointment of the National Coordinator for Health Information Technology to coordinate programs and policies regarding HIT across the federal government. The National Coordinator was charged with directing HIT programs within HHS and coordinating them with those of other relevant Executive Branch agencies. In fulfillment of this, the National Coordinator has taken responsibility for the National Health Information Infrastructure Initiative (NHII), the FHA, and the Consolidated Health Informatics Initiative (CHI), and is currently assessing other health information technology programs and efforts. In addition, the National Coordinator was charged with coordinating outreach and consultation between the federal government and the private sector. As part of this, the National Coordinator was directed to coordinate with the National Committee on Vital Health Statistics (NCVHS) and other advisory committees.

The National Coordinator will collaborate with DoD, VA, and OPM to encourage the widespread adoption of HIT throughout the health care system. To do this, the National Coordinator will gather and disseminate the lessons learned from both DoD and VA in successfully incorporating HIT into the delivery of health care, and facilitate the development and transfer of knowledge and technology to the private sector. OPM, as the purchaser of health care for the federal government, has a unique role and the ability to encourage the use of EHRs through the Federal Employees Health Benefits Program, and the National Coordinator will assist in gaining the complementary alignment of OPM policies with those of the private sector.

## REPORTS FROM OPM, DOD, AND VA

The Executive Order also directs the OPM, the DoD, and the VA to submit reports on HIT to the President through the Secretary of Health and Human Services. These reports are included in this report as Attachments 1 through 3 (which are not included in this case, but are available on the Web at www.hhs.gov/healthit).

OPM administers the Federal Employees Health Benefits Program for the federal government and the more than eight million people it covers. As the nation's largest purchaser of health benefits, OPM is keenly interested in high-quality care and reasonable cost. The adoption of an interoperable HIT infrastructure is a key to achieving both. OPM is currently exploring a variety of options to leverage its purchasing power and alliances to move the adoption of HIT forward. OPM will be strongly encouraging health plans to promote the early adoption of HIT. Details on these options can be found in OPM's report (Attachment 1 of the report), "Federal Employees Health Benefits Program Initiatives to Promote the Use of Health Information Technology."

The VA, collaboratively with DoD, provides joint recommendations to address the special needs of these populations. As mirrored in the DoD Report, these recommendations focus on the capture of lessons learned, the knowledge and technology transfers to be gained from successful VA/DoD data exchange initiatives, the adoption of common standards and terminologies to promote more effective and rapid development of health technologies, and the development of telehealth technologies to improve care in rural and remote areas.

The DoD has significant experience in delivering care in isolated conditions such as those encountered in wartime or overseas peacekeeping missions, which can be compared to the conditions in some rural health care environments. Examples of the technologies used in these conditions include telehealth for radiology, mental health, dermatology, pathology, and dental consultations; online personalized health records for beneficiary use; bed regulation for disaster planning; basic patient encounter documentation; pharmacy, radiology, and laboratory order entry and results retrieval for use in remote areas and small clinics; pharmacy, radiology, and laboratory order entry and results retrieval; admissions and discharges; appointments for use in small hospitals; and online education offerings for health care providers. Technology products, outcomes, benefits, and cumulative knowledge will be shared for use within the private sector and local/state organizations to help guide their planning efforts.

The VA's report (Attachment 2 of the report), "Approaches to Make Health Information Systems Available and Affordable to Rural and Medically Underserved Communities", also highlights its successful strategy to develop high-quality EHR technologies that remain in the public domain. These technologies may be suitable for transfer to rural and medically underserved settings. VA's primary health information systems and EHR (VistA and the Computerized Patient Record System [the current system] and HealtheVet-VistA, the next generation in development) provide leading government/public-owned health information technologies that support the provision, measurement, and improvement "of quality, affordable care" across 1300 VA inpatient and ambulatory settings. The VA continues to make a version of VistA available in the public domain as a means of fostering widespread development of high-performance EHR systems. The VA is also incorporating the CHI approved standards into its next-generation HealtheVet-VistA. Furthermore, the VA is developing PHR technologies such as My HealtheVet, which are consistent with the larger strategic goal of making veterans (persons) the center of health care. Finally, the VA's health information technologies, such as bar code medication administration, VistA Imaging, and telehealth applications, provide the VA with exceptional tools that improve patient safety and enable the increasingly geographically dispersed provision of care to patients in all settings. These and other technologies are proposed as federal technology transfer options in furtherance of the President's goals.

## CONCLUSION

Health information technology has the potential to transform health care delivery, bringing information where it is needed and refocusing health care around the consumer. This can be done without substantial regulation or industry upheaval. It can give us both better care—care that is higher in quality, safer, and more consumer responsive—and more efficient care—care that is less wasteful, more appropriate, and more available. The changes that will accompany the full use of information technology in the health care industry will pose challenges to longstanding assumptions and practices. However, these changes are needed, beneficial, and inevitable. Action should be taken now to achieve the benefits of HIT. A well-planned and coordinated effort, sustained over a number of years, can deliver results that will better support America's health care professionals and better serve the public.

## CASE ANALYSIS

The federal government is by far the largest purchaser of health care in the country, but it has been very slow to demand that providers conform to CQI principles. As Chapters 1 and 10 point out, many political leaders from both parties have called for modernization of the national health care system to bring its information technology up to the level of other information-intensive service industries. This case is the administration's response prior to the 2004 elections. It is written entirely based on public sources.

## ASSIGNMENT QUESTIONS

### Introduction

1. Why does the federal government seem so focused on information technology as the primary lever in its efforts to enhance health care quality improvement?

**Basics**

2. How can the concepts and techniques of quality measurement outlined in the text be adapted to the design, implementation and evaluation of the White House and CHIT strategies as they move ahead?

**Implementation**

3. Chapter 10 on information technology outlines a life cycle approach to analyzing system development, adoption, and implementation. How consistent with that model are the federal government initiatives outlined in the strategic plan?
4. If you were Dr. Brailer or his successor responsible for CHIT, what would you propose for the next iteration of the planning cycle?

**Application**

5. On December 3, 2004 the *New York Times* reported that the $50 million request for funding of Center for Health Information Technology in the budget had been lined out in the FY 2004–05 appropriation bill (Lohr 2004b). What would you do next, if you were responsible for implementing the plan?

**CLASS EXERCISE**

Using the Internet, follow the legislative and executive branch responses to the strategic plan outlined in this case. Does the plan seem to "have legs" or is a new plan needed? Present to the class a revised strategic plan based on recent technological and political developments that you believe will have the greatest potential impact on the quality of the U.S. health care system.

# Malcolm Baldrige Award 2004 Health Care Criteria for Performance Excellence

Health care organizations became eligible to apply for the Malcolm Baldrige National Quality Award for the first time in 1999. In 1995, 46 health care organizations and 19 educational institutions participated in a pilot program in which each organization received feedback on its application from the Baldrige National Quality Program. The Health Care Criteria are intended to have the same framework as the Business and Education Criteria but with health-care-specific issues and language. The first award to a health care organization came in 2002, followed by two more in 2003. Each year's program is outlined on the Baldrige National Quality Program website (www.baldrige.nist.gov), which reviews the program's administration, criteria, core values, and concepts; defines key terms; and offers application instructions and scoring guidelines.

The 2004 Health Care Criteria were designed to help implement the following concepts and values:

- Visionary leadership
- Patient-centered excellence
- Organizational and personal learning
- Valuing staff and partners
- Agility
- Focus on the future
- Managing for innovation
- Social responsibility and community health
- Focus on results and creating value
- Systems perspective

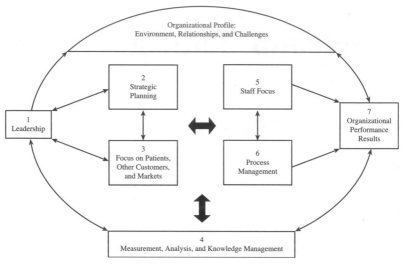

**Figure A–1**  Health Care Criteria

---

These concepts and values are embedded in the seven Health Care Criteria shown in the systems diagram in Figure A-1.

The agency notes that the criteria are not prescriptive; methods of operation, organizational structure, or management approaches are not specified. To a great extent, it is up to the applicant to specify its challenges and requirements in terms of its own strategy and situation.

One key to the application is a five-page organizational profile, which provides a snapshot of the organization, its services, the key influences on its operations, and the key challenges it faces. Within this context, the examiners are expected to apply the appropriate criteria.

### ITEMS FOR 2004 HEALTH CARE CRITERIA

The items used in the 2004 draft of the criteria are as follows:

| **Categories and Terms** | **Point Values** |
|---|---|

Leadership (120)—how senior leadership addresses values, directions, and performance expectations and its social and community responsibilities

| | | |
|---|---|---|
| 1.1 | Organizational Leadership | 70 |
| 1.2 | Social Responsibility | 50 |

Strategic Planning (95)—how strategic objectives and action plans are developed, deployed, and evaluated

| | | |
|---|---|---|
| 2.1 | Strategy Development | 40 |
| 2.2 | Strategy Deployment | 45 |

Focus on Patients, Other Customers, Markets (85)—how requirements, expectations, and preferences of the public are determined and answered

| | | |
|---|---|---|
| 3.1 | Patient, Other Customer and Health Care Market Knowledge | 40 |
| 3.2 | Patient and Other Customer Satisfaction | 45 |

Measurement, Analysis, and Knowledge Management (90)—how the organization selects, gathers, and manages data and knowledge

| | | |
|---|---|---|
| 4.1 | Measurement and Analysis of Organizational Performance | 45 |
| 4.2 | Information and Knowledge Management | 45 |

Staff Focus (85)—how staff work, learn, and are motivated and how these processes align with achieving performance excellence

| | | |
|---|---|---|
| 5.1 | Work Systems | 35 |
| 5.2 | Staff Learning and Motivation | 25 |
| 5.3 | Staff Well-Being and Satisfaction | 25 |

Process Management (85)—how the organization manages processes to create value and quality

| | | |
|---|---|---|
| 6.1 | Health Care Processes | 50 |
| 6.2 | Support Processes | 35 |

Organizational Performance Results (450)—how the organization has actually improved against its requirements and in comparison with similar health care organizations

| | | |
|---|---|---|
| 7.1 | Health Care Results | 75 |
| 7.2 | Patient- and Other Customer-Focused Results | 75 |
| 7.3 | Financial and Market Results | 75 |
| 7.4 | Staff and Work System Results | 75 |
| 7.5 | Organizational Effectiveness Results | 75 |
| 7.6 | Governance and Social Responsibility Results | 75 |

| | |
|---|---|
| TOTAL | 1000 |

## ITEM SCORING

Each item is scored either on (1) Process or (2) Results. Tables A-1 and A-2 show the scoring for each of these items. The tables show the process criteria for each range using four factors—Approach (A), Deployment (D), Learning (L), and Integration (I). The selection within the range is based on the best fit of the overall item response. Scoring within those limits is at the examiner's discretion based on closeness to the next higher or next lower range.

**Table A–1**  Scoring Guidelines—Healthcare Criteria

| Score (%) | Process Categories (1-6) |
|---|---|
| 0% or 5% | • No systematic approach evident, anecdotal information (A)<br>• Little or no deployment of an approach is evident (D)<br>• No evidence of an improvement orientations, responses reactive (L)<br>• No organizational alignment, individual areas operate independently (I) |
| 10%, 15%, 20% or 25% | • Beginnings of a systematic approach to the basic requirements of the item (A)<br>• In early stages of deployment in many units, inhibiting progress in achieving basic requirements of the item (D)<br>• Evidence of early stages of a transition from reacting to problems to a general improvement orientation (L)<br>• Alignment achieve primarily through joint problem-solving (I) |
| 30%, 35%, 40% or 45% | • An effective, systematic approach, responsive to the basic requirements of the item (A)<br>• Approach is deployed, although some areas or work units are in early stages of deployment (D)<br>• Beginning of a systematic approach to evaluation and improvement of key processes (L)<br>• Approach aligned with basic organizational needs cite in other Criteria Categories (I) |
| 50%, 55%, 60% or 65% | • An effective, systematic approach evident, responsive to the overall requirements of the item (A)<br>• Approach is well-deployed, although deployment may vary in some areas or work units (D)<br>• A fact-based, systematic evaluation and improvement process and some organizational learning in place for improving efficiency and effectiveness of key processes (L)<br>• Approach is aligned with basic organizational needs identified in the other Criteria Categories (I) |

**Table A–1** continued

| Score (%) | Process Categories (1-6) |
|---|---|
| 70%, 75%, 80% or 85% | • An effective, systematic approach, responsive to the multiple requirements of the item (A)<br>• Approach is well-deployed with no significant gaps (D)<br>• Fact-based, systematic evaluation and improvement and organizational learning are key management tools; clear evidence of refinement and innovation as the result of organizational-level analysis and sharing (L)<br>• Approach is integrated with organizational needs identified in the other Criteria Categories (I) |
| 90%, 95% or 100% | • An effective, systematic approach, fully responsive to the multiple requirements of the item (A)<br>• Approach is fully deployed without significant weaknesses or gaps in any areas or work units (D)<br>• Fact-based, systematic evaluation and improvement process and extensive organizational learning are key organization-wide tools; refinement and innovation, backed by analysis and sharing, are evident throughout (L)<br>• Approach is well-integrated with organizational needs identified in the other Criteria Categories (I) |

**Table A–2** Ranges and Criteria for Baldrige Award Health Care Results Scores

| Score | Results Category (7) |
|---|---|
| 0% or 5% | • No results or poor results in areas reported<br>• Trend results not reported or show adverse results<br>• Comparative information not reported<br>• Results not reported for any areas of importance to key organizational requirements |
| 10%, 15%, 20% or 25% | • A few organizational performance results reported; some improvements and/or early good performance levels in a few areas<br>• Little or no trend data reported<br>• Little or not comparative data reported<br>• Results reported for a few areas of importance to key organizational requirements. |

*continues*

**Table A–2**　continued

| Score | Results Category (7) |
|---|---|
| 30%, 35%. 40% or 45% | • Improvements *and/or* good performance levels in many areas of importance to key organizational requirements<br>• Early stages of developing trends are evident<br>• Early stages of obtaining comparative information are evident<br>• Results are reported for many to most areas of importance to key organizational requirements. |
| 50%, 55%, 60% or 65% | • Improvement trends *and/or* good performance levels in most areas addressed in item requirements<br>• No pattern of adverse trends and no poor performance levels in areas of importance to key organizational requirements<br>• Some trends *and/or* current performance levels—evaluated against relevant comparisons *and/or* benchmarks—show areas of strength *and/or* good to very good performance levels<br>• Organizational performance results address most key patient and other customer, market and process requirements |
| 70%, 75%, 80% or 85% | • Current performance is good to excellent in areas of importance to Item requirements<br>• Most improvement trends *and/or* current performance levels are sustained<br>• Many to most trends *and/or* current performance levels—evaluated against relevant comparisons *and/or* benchmarks- show areas of leadership and very good relative performance<br>• Organizational performance results address most key patient and other customer, market, process, and action plan requirements |
| 90%, 95% or 100% | • Current performance is excellent in most areas of importance to Item requirements<br>• Excellent improvement trends *and/or* sustained excellent performance levels in most areas<br>• Evidence of health care sector and benchmark leadership demonstrated in many areas<br>• Organizational performance results fully address key patient and other customer, market, process, and action plan requirements. |

## WHAT ONE WINNER OFFERED

2003 award winner Baptist Hospital, Inc. of Pensacola, FL reported the following:

- Multiple, standardized patient satisfaction measures at or near the 99th percentile since 1998
- Employee turnover rates halved since 1997
- Outranked its two major competitors on positive employee morale, perceived consumer value, consumer loyalty, and percent of revenue to indigent patients (6.7 vs. 5.2 and 4%)
- Introduced an extensive system of departmental and hospital-wide indicators (and reported improvements) such as:
  - Medication adverse events (2.5/10,000 in FY2000 to 1.5 in FY2002 vs. benchmark of 18)
  - Patients developing pressure ulcers (7.2% in FY1998 to 3.5 in FY2002 vs. benchmark of 7)
- Instituted a variety of process improvement programs that generated 6,800 suggested changes of which 5,000 were implemented in 2003 up from 1,400 and 350 respectively in 1998
- Improved external and self-reported board effectiveness ratings significantly
- Recognized in 2003 as 15th in *Fortune's* "100 Best Companies to Work For in America" list and in *Training Magazine's* "Top 50". learning organizations with 60 hours per year of training per employee
- Supported these efforts with improvements in hospital information systems, cross-functional process teams, senior management accountability, and integration of planning processes (Source: www.nist.gov/public_affairs/releases/bhitraunma accessed February 25, 2004)

Obviously, these achievements required a great deal of effort and managerial will as well as a substantial investment of money and resources; all of would have been confirmed by on-site examination.

# BIBLIOGRAPHY

Abernathy, W. and J. Utterback. 1978. Patterns of industrial innovations. *Technology Review* 80 (7):40–47.

Accreditation Council for Graduate Medical Education. 1999. Accreditation Council for Graduate Medical Education Outcomes Project: General Competencies. http://www.acgme.org/outcomes/ comptv13.htm.

Ackoff, R. L. 1981. *Creating the Corporate Future.* New York, John Wiley & Sons.

Adams, D. F. *et al.* 1973. The complications of coronary arteriography. *Circulation* 48 (3):609–618.

Adler, P. *et al.* 2003. Performance improvement capability: keys to accelerating performance improvement in hospitals. *California Management Review* 45 (2):12–33.

The Advisory Board Company. 1997. *The Great Product Enterprise: Future State for the American Health System.* Washington, DC.

Agency for Healthcare Research and Quality. 2001. *Patient–Centered Care: Customizing Care to Meet Patient Needs,"* PA-01-124, July 31, 2001. Rockville, MD: Agency for Healthcare Research and Quality.

American Academy of Family Physicians. 2004. Premier Medical Organizations Announce Formation of Physicians Electronic Health Record Coalition, press release, July 22. http://www.aafp.org.

American College of Physicians. 1993. *Enhancing the Physician's Role in Patient-Centered Care.* Philadelphia, PA: American College of Physicians. http://www.acponline.org (accessed March 3, 1999).

American Hospital Assocation. 1996. *Eye on Patients: A Report from the American Hospital Association and the Picker Institute,* Available online at http://www.amphi.com/eyeonpatients/default.html.

American Psychological Association. 2002. New Mexico Governor Signs Landmark Law on Prescription Privileges for Psychologists. *APAOnLine, APA Practice, March 6, 2002.* http://www.apa.org/practice/nm_rxp (accessed September 16, 2002).

American Public Health Association. 1993. *The Guide to Implementing Model Standards. Eleven Steps Toward a Healthy Community.* Washington, DC: American Public Health Association.

Argyris, C. 1990. *Overcoming Organizational Defense: Facilitating Organizational Learning.* Needham Heights, MA: Allyn & Bacon.

Argyris, C. 1991. Teaching Smart People How To Learn. *Harvard Business Review* 69 (3):99–109.

Argyris, C. and D. A. Schon. 1996. *Organizational Learning II: Theory, Method and Practice.* Reading, MA: Addison-Wesley.

Arndt, M. and B. Bigelow. 1995. The implementation of total quality management in hospitals. *Health Care Management Review* 20 (4): 3–14.

Arrow, H. *et al.* 2000. *Small Groups as Complex Systems.* Thousand Oaks, CA: Sage Publications.

Auerbach, S. 1998. Report cards found to improve health care. *Washington Post,* January 6: Z08.

Baker, E. L. *et al.* 1994. Health reform and the health of the public: forging community health partnerships. *JAMA* 272:1276–1282.

Baker, G. R. *et al.* 2004. The Canadian adverse events study: the incidence of adverse events among hospital patients in Canada. *CMAJ* 170:1678–1686.

Baker L. *et al.* 2003.Use of the internet and e-mail for health care information: Results from a national survey. *JAMA* 289:2400–2406.

Baker. L. C. 2005. Benefits of interoperability: A closer look at the estimates. *Health Affairs Web Exclusive* 19 January, W5-22 – W5-25.

Barber, N. 2002. Should we consider noncompliance a medical error? *Quality and Safety in Health Care* 11:81–84.

Barnsley, J. *et al.* 1998. Integrating learning into integrated delivery systems. *Health Care Management Review* 23(1), 18–28.

Batalden, P. B. 1996. *Vision for Change.* Presented at the Interdisciplinary Professional Education Collaborative-Second Milestone Conference, Institute for Healthcare Improvement, Philadelphia, Penn., November 1–2.

Batalden, P. B. 1998. Why focus on health professional development? *Quality Management in Health Care* 6 (2):52–61.

Batalden, P. B. and J. J. Mohr. 1997. Building knowledge of health care as a system. *Quality Management in Health Care* 5 (3):1–12.

Batalden, P. B. and E. C. Nelson. 1990. Hospital quality: Patient, physician and employee judgments. *International Journal of Health Care Quality Assurance* 3 (4): 7–17.

Batalden, P. and P. Stoltz. 1993. Performance improvement in health care organizations. A framework for the continual improvement of health care: Building and applying professional and improvement knowledge to test changes in daily work. *Jt Comm J Qual Improvement* 19: 424–452.

Batalden, P. B. *et al.* 1997. Continually improving the health and value of health care for a population of patients: The panel management process. *Quality Management in Health Care* 5 (3):41–51.

Batalden, P. B. *et al*. 2002. General competencies and accreditation in graduate medical education. *Health Affairs* 21 (5): 103–111.

Batalden, P. B. *et al*. 2003a. Microsystems in health care: Part 9. Developing small clinical units to attain peak performance. *Jt Comm J Qual Safety* 29 (11):575–585.

Batalden, P. B. *et al*. 2003b. Microsystems in health care: Part 5. How leaders are leading. *Jt Comm J Qual Safety* 29 (6):297–308.

Bates, D. W. *et al*. 1995. Evaluation of screening criteria for adverse events in medical patients. *Medical Care* 33 (5):452–62.

Bayley, K. B. *et al*. 2004. Barriers associated with health care hand-offs, *Advances in Patient Safety: From Research to Implementation,* forthcoming AHRQ Publication.

Beaulieu, J. and D. F. Scutchfield. 2003. Content and criterion validity evaluation of national public health performance standards measurement instruments. *Public Health Reports* 8 (6):508–17.

Becher, E. C. and M. R. Chassin. 2001. Improving quality, minimizing error: Making it happen. *Health Affairs* 20(3):69–81.

Benson, M. *et al*. 2000. Comparison of manual and automated documentation of adverse events with an anesthesia information management system (AIMS). *Stud Health Technol Inform.* 77:925–9.

Berger, R. G. and J. P. Kichak. 2004. Computerized physician order entry: Helpful or harmful? *J Am Med Inform Assoc* 11 (2):100–103.

Bertalanffy, L. V. 1968. *General System Theory: Foundations, Development, Applications.* New York: George Braziller, Inc.

Berwick, D. M. 1989. Continuous improvement as an ideal in health care. *N Engl J Med* 320:53–56.

Berwick, D. M. 1991. Controlling variation in health care: A consultation from Walter Shewhart. *Medical Care* 29: 1212–1225.

Berwick, D. M. 1994. Eleven worthy aims for clinical leadership of health system reform. *JAMA* 272 (10): 797–802.

Berwick, D. M. 1996. A primer on leading the improvement of systems. *BMJ* 312: 619–622.

Berwick, D. M. 1998. Developing and testing changes in delivery of care. *Ann Intern Med* 128:651–656.

Berwick, D. M. 2001. Not again! *British Medical J* 322:247–248.

Berwick, D. M. 2004. Lessons from developing nations on improving health care. *British Medical J* 328: 1124–1129.

Berwick, D. M. and T. W. Nolan. 1998. Physicians as leaders in improving health care. *Ann. Int. Med.* 128 (4):289–292.

Berwick, D. M. *et al.* 1990. *Curing Health Care: New Strategies for Quality Improvement.* San Francisco: Jossey-Bass.

Bettcher, D. W. *et al.* 1998. Essential public health functions: results of the international delphi study. *World Health Statistics Quarterly* 51 (1):44–54.

Bigelow, B. and M. Arndt. 1995. Total quality management: field of dreams? *Health Care Manage Rev* 20 (4):15–25.

Blumberg, M. 1986. Risk-adjusting health care outcomes: A methodological review. *Medical Care Review* 43:351–393.

Blumenthal, D. and C. Kilo. 1998. A report card on continuous quality improvement. *Milbank Quarterly* 76:725–648.

Bluth, E. I. *et al.* 1982. Improvement in "stat" laboratory turnaround time: A model continuous improvement project. *Archives of Internal Medicine* 152:837–840.

Bodenheimer, T. 1999. Disease management—promises and pitfalls. *N Engl J Med* 340:1202–1205.

Bohmer, R. and A. Winslow. 1999. *The Dana-Farber Cancer Institute,* Boston, MA: Harvard Business School Publishing. For the many issues under litigation see Crane, M. 2001. Who caused this tragic medication mistake? *Medical Economics* 19:49, Oct. 8.

Borbas, C. *et al.* 1990. The Minnesota clinical comparison and assessment project. *Quality Review Bulletin* 16 (2):87–92.

Bosk, C. L. 1979. *Forgive and Remember: Managing Medical Failure.* Chicago: The University of Chicago Press.

Boynton, A. C. *et al.* 1993. New competitive strategies: Challenges to organizations and information technology. *IBM Systems J.* 32(1): 40–64.

Brailer, D. J. 2005. Interoperability: The key to the future health care system. *Health Affairs Web Exclusive,* 19 January, W5-19 – W5-21.

Braithwaite, R. S. *et al.* 2004. Use of medical emergency team (MET) responses to detect medical errors. *Qual. Safety in Health Care* 13:255–259.

Brassard, M. 1996. *The Memory Jogger Plus Featuring the Seven Management and Planning Tools.* Methuen, MA: Goal/QPC.

Brennan, T. A. and D. M. Berwick. 1996. *New Rules: Regulation, Markets, and the Quality of American Health Care.* San Francisco: Jossey-Bass Inc.

Brennan, T. A. *et al.* 2004. Incidence of adverse events and negligence in hospitalized patients: results of the Harvard medical practice study I. *Qual Safety in Health Care,* 13 (2):145–151.

Breyfogle, F. W. 2003. *Implementing Six Sigma: Smarter Solutions Using Statistical Methods, 2nd edition.* Hoboken, NJ: Wiley.

Britten, N. 2001. Prescribing and the defence of clinical autonomy. *Sociology of Health & Illness*, 23: 478–496.

Brockman, J. 1977. *About Bateson: Essays on Gregory Bateson.* New York: E. P. Dutton.

Brook R. *et al.* 1975. *A Review of the Literature on Cholecystectomy: Findings, Complications, Utilization Rates, Costs, Efficacy, and Indications.* Santa Monica, CA: RAND Corp.

Burrus, W. M. 1993a. How long will CQI take to produce savings? *Quality Matters* 2 (3):3–5.

Burrus, W. M. 1993b. Northwest Hospital counting all the way to the bank. *Quality Matters* 2 (3): 5–7.

Byrne, J. *et al.* 1993. The virtual corporation. *Business Week,* no. 3304: 98–102.

Campbell, S. M. *et al.* 2002. Implementing clinical governance in English primary care groups/trusts: Reconciling quality improvement and quality assurance. *Qual Safety in Health Care* 11:9–14.

Caper, P. 1988. Defining quality in medical care. *Health Affairs* 7 (1): 49–61.

Carey, R. G. and R. C. Lloyd. 2001. *Measuring Quality Improvement in Healthcare: A Guide to Statistical Control Applications.* Milwaukee, WI: American Society for Quality Press.

Carroll, J. S. and A. C. Edmondson. 2002. Leading organizational learning in health care, *Qual. Safety in Health Care* 11:51–56.

Carthey, J. *et al.* 2001. Institutional resistance in healthcare systems. *Quality in Health Care* 10:29–32.

Casalino, L. *et al.* 2003. External incentives, information technology, and organized processes to improve health care quality for patients with chronic diseases. *JAMA* 289:434–441.

Center for Studying Health System Change. 1996. Tracking changes in the public health system: what researchers need to know to monitor and evaluate these changes. *Community Tracking Study Issue Brief* No. 2. Washington, DC: Center for Studying Health System Change. http://www.hschange.org/CONTENT/79/79.pdf (accessed 8/12/04).

Center for Disease Control. National Public Health Performance Standards Program, Local Public Health Performance Assessment Instrument, Version 1.0, Atlanta, GA: CDC, 2003.

CenterWatch Weekly. 1997a. Barnett moves monitor training into university setting. *CenterWatch Weekly 1 (15 September), No. 7.*

CenterWatch Weekly. 1997b. Cleveland Clinic and Quintiles sign mutual preferred provide agreement. *CenterWatch Weekly 1(1 December), No. 18.*

Center Watch Newsletter. 2004. International enthusiasm for EDC. *Center Watch Newsletter,* (February), Vol. 11, Issue 2, Article 350.

Chassin, M. R. 1998. Is health care ready for six sigma quality? *Milbank Quarterly,* 76:565–591.

Chassin, M. R., M. R. Galvin and the National Roundtable on Health Care Quality. 1998. The urgent need to improve health care. *JAMA* 280: 1000–1005.

Chassin, M. R. *et al.* 1996. Benefits and hazards of reporting medical outcomes publicly. *NEJM* 334: 394–398.

Checkland, P. 1981. *Systems Thinking, Systems Practice.* New York: John Wiley & Sons.

Chinn, S. S. 2002. E-health engineering economics. *International J. of Healthcare Technology and Management* 4: 451–455.

Christensen, C. M. *et al.* 2000. Will disruptive innovations cure health care? *Harvard Business Review* 78 (5):102–111.

Churchman, C. W. 1971. *The Design of Inquiring Systems: Basic Concepts of Systems and Organization.* New York: Basic Books.

Classen, D. C. *et al.* 1991. Computerized surveillance of adverse drug events in hospital patients. *JAMA* 266:2847–51.

Cleary, P. D. 2003. A hospitalization from hell: A patient's perspective on quality. *Ann Intern Med* 138 (1):33–9.

Clinton, H. R. 2004. Now can we talk about health care? *New York Times Magazine* April 18: 26–31, 56.

Coddington, D. C. *et al.* 1996. *Making Integrated Health Care Work,* Englewood, CO: Center for Research in Ambulatory Health Care Administration.

Cohen, M. R. *et al.* 1994. Failure mode and effects analysis: A novel approach to avoiding dangerous medication errors and accidents. *Hospital Pharmacy* 29:319–30.

Committee on Understanding and Eliminating Racial and Ethnic Disparities in Health Care, Institute of Medicine, 2003. *Unequal Treatment: Confronting Racial and Ethnic Disparities in Health Care.* Washington, D.C., National Academy Press.

Cook, R. I. and D. D. Woods. 1994. Operating at the sharp end: Complexity of human error in *Human Error in Medicine.* ed. M. S. Bogner. Hillsdale, NJ: Lawrence Erlbaum Associates.

Corso, L. C. *et al*. 2000. Using the essential services as a foundation for performance measurement and assessment of local public health systems. *Journal of Public Health Management and Practice* 6 (5):1–18.

Cotton, P. 1991. Medical schools receive a message: Reform yourselves, then take on health care system. *JAMA* 266:2802–2804.

Counte, M. A. *et al*. 1992. Total quality management in health care organizations: An analysis of employee impacts. *Hospital and Health Services Administration* 37:503–518.

Crane, M. 2001. Who caused this tragic medication mistake? *Medical Economics* 19:49, Oct. 8.

Crosby, P. B. 1979. *Quality is Free: The Art of Making Quality Certain*. New York: Mentor.

Davies, A. R. and J. E.Ware. 1988. Involving consumers in quality of care assessment. *Health Affairs* 7 (1):33–48.

Davies, H. and S. Harrison. 2003. Trends in doctor-manager relationships. *BMJ* 326:646–649.

Davis, D. A. *et al*. 1995. Changing physician performance: a systematic review of the effect of continuing medical education strategies. *JAMA* 274:700–705.

Davis P. *et al*. 2002. Adverse events in New Zealand public hospitals I: Occurance and impact. *New Zealand J. of Medicine* 115(1167): U268.

Davis S. 1987. *Future Perfect*, Cambridge, MA: Perseus Books.

Dekker, S. 2002. *The Field Guide to Human Error Investigations*. Aldershot, UK: Ashgate Publishing Limited.

Deming, W. E. 1986. *Out of the Crisis*. Cambridge: Massachusetts Institute of Technology Center for Advanced Engineering Study.

Deming, W. E. 1993. *The New Economics for Industry, Government, Education*. Cambridge: Massachusetts Institute of Technology Center for Advanced Engineering Study.

Department of Health and Human Services. 2003. *Demonstrating the Value of Health Information Technology*. http://grants2.nih.gov/grants/guide/rft-files/RFA-HS-04-012.

Department of Health, State of Connecticut. 2004. *A Report on Quality of Care in Connecticut Hospitals, April, 2004*. http://www.dph.ct.state.us/OPPE/quality (accessed June 11, 2004).

Derose, S. F. *et al*. 2002a. Public health quality measurement: Concepts and challenges. *Annual Review of Public Health* 23:1–21.

Derose, S. F. *et al*. 2002b. Public health quality measurement: Concepts and challenges. *Journal of Public Health Management and Practice* 3 (3):1–9.

Derose, S. F. *et al.* 2003. Developing quality indicators for local health departments: experience in Los Angeles County. *American Journal of Preventive Medicine* 25 (4):347–357.

DesHarnais, S. *et al.* 1988. The risk-adjusted mortality index: A new measure of hospital performance. *Medical Care* 26:1129–1148.

DesHarnais, S. *et al.* 1990. Measuring hospital performance: The development and validation of risk-adjusted indexes of mortality, readmissions, and complications. *Medical Care* 28:1127–1141.

DesHarnais, S. *et al.* 1991. Measuring outcomes of hospital care using multiple risk adjusted indexes, *Health Services Research* 26:425–445.

DesHarnais, S. *et al.* 1997. Risk-adjusted quality outcome measures: Indexes for benchmarking rates of mortality, complications and readmissions. *Quality Management in Health Care* 5 (2):80–87.

Devers, K. J. and G. Liu. 2004. Leapfrog patient-safety standards are a stretch for most hospitals, *Issue Brief, Center for Studying Health System Change.* February; (77):1–6.

Devers, K. J. *et al.* 2004. What is driving hospitals' Patient-safety efforts? *Health Affairs* 23 (2):103–15.

DiBella, A. J. *et al.* 1996. Understanding organizational learning capability. *Journal of Management Studies* 33 (3):361–379.

DiMasi, J. A. *et al.* 1991. Cost of innovation in the pharmaceutical industry. *Journal of Health Economics* 10 (2):107–142.

Dobyns, L. and C. Crawford-Mason. 1991. *Quality or Else: The Revolution in World Business.* Boston: Houghton Mifflin.

Donabedian, A. 1966. Evaluating the quality of medical care. *Milbank Quarterly* 44 (1):166–203.

Donabedian, A. 1980. The definition of quality and approaches to its assessment. In *Explorations in quality assessment and monitoring.* Vol. 1:95–99. Ann Arbor, MI: Health Administration Press.

Donabedian, A. 1982. *The criteria and standards of quality.* Ann Arbor, MI: Health Administration Press.

Donabedian, A. 1986. Criteria and standards for quality assessment and monitoring. *Quality Review Bulletin,* 14(3):99–108.

Donabedian, A. 1993. Models of quality assurance. *Leonard S. Rosenfeld Memorial Lecture,* School of Public Health, University of North Carolina at Chapel Hill, February 26.

Donabedian, A. 2001. An expert on health care evaluates his own care. *New York Times,* June 12, F7, F12.

Donaldson, M. S. and J. J. Mohr. 2000. *Improvement and Innovation in Health Care Microsystems. A Technical Report for the Institute of Medicine Committee on the Quality of Health Care in America.* Princeton: Robert Wood Johnson Foundation.

Dorner, D. 1996. *The Logic of Failure, Recognizing and Avoiding Error in Complex Situations.* Reading, MA: Perseus Books.

Dotson, M. M. and L. Wallman. 1994. *Applying a value-added Model to a Project Management System.* Presented at the 30th Annual Meeting of the Drug Information Association, Washington, DC, June.

Dreyfus, H. and S. Dreyfus. 1986. *Mind over Machine.* New York: Free Press.

Dumas, R. A. *et al.* 1987. Making quality control theories workable. *Training and Development Journal* 41 (2):30–33.

Dyall, W. W. 1995. Ten organizational practices of public health: A historical perspective. *American Journal of Preventive Medicine* 11:6–8.

Eagle, C. J. *et al.* 1992. Accident analysis of large-scale technical disasters applied to anaesthetic complication. *Canadian J. Anaesth.* 39: 119–122.

Eagle, K. A. *et al.* 2003. Closing the gap between science and practice: The need for professional leadership. *Health Affairs* 22 (2):196–201.

Early, J. F. and A. B. Godfrey. 1995. But it takes too long. *Qual Prog* 28 (7):51–55.

Edmonson A. 1999. Psychological safety and learning behavior in work teams. *Administrative Science Quarterly* 44(4): 350–383.

Edmondson, A. 2003. Framing for learning: lessons in successful technology implementation. *California Management Review* 45 (2):35–54.

Edwards, N. *et al.* 2003. Doctors and managers: A problem without a solution? *BMJ* 326:609–610.

Eilbert, K. W. *et al.* 1997. Public health expenditures: Developing estimates for improved policy-making. *Journal of Public Health Management and Practice* 3 (3):1–9.

Eliastam, M. and T. Mizrahi. 1996. Quality improvement, housestaff, and the role of chief residents. *Academic Medicine* 71(6): 670–674.

Ellwood, P. 1988. Shattuck Lecture: Outcomes management: A technology of patient experience. *NEJM* 318: 1549–1556.

Ellwood, P. 2003. A conversation with Paul Ellwood, MD. *Managed Care Magazine* 12 (3): 38–40,42.

Ellwood, P. M. *et al.* 1971. Health maintenance strategy. *Medical Care* 9:271–298.

Endsley, S. *et al*. 2004. Getting rewards for your results: Pay-for-performance programs. *Fam Pract Manage* 11 (3):45–50.

Epidemiology, Planning, and Evaluation Unit, Seattle-King County Department of Public Health. 1995. *Vista/PH Software for Public Health Assessment: User's Guide*. Seattle, WA.

Epstein, A. M. 2000. Public release of performance data: A progress report from the front. *JAMA* 283:1884–1886.

Epstein, A. M. *et al*. 2004. Paying physicians for high-quality care. *N Engl J Med* 350:406–410.

Evans, R. S. *et al*. 1986. Computer surveillance of hospital-acquired infections and antibiotic use. *JAMA* 256:1007–11.

Farley, D.O. *et al*. 2003. *Regional Health Quality Improvement Coalition's Lessons across the Life Cycle*. Santa Monica, CA: RAND Health: 70.

Feldman S. E. and D. W. Roblin. 1997. Medical accidents in hospital care: Applications of failure analysis to hospital quality appraisal. *Joint Commission J. on Quality Improvement* 23: 567–580.

Felland, L. E. and C. S. Lesser. 2000. Local innovations provide managed care for the uninsured. *Community Tracking Study Issue Brief* No. 25. Washington, DC: Center for Studying Health System Change. http://www.hschange.org/CONTENT/57/57.pdf

Fendt, K. 2004. The case for data quality. *Data Basics* 10(2):1, 3–6.

Fernandopulle, R. *et al*. 2003. A research agenda for bridging the 'quality chasm'. *Health Affairs* 22 (2):178–190.

Ferrini, R. 1997 Screening asymptomatic women for overian cancer: American College of Preventive Medicine practice policy. *American Journal of Preventive Medicine* 13:444–46.

Fielding, J. E. and N. Halfon. 1997. Characteristics of community report cards—United States, 1996. *MMWR* 46 (28):647–55.

Fisher, E. S. *et al*. 1992. The accuracy of Medicare's hospital claims data: Progress has been made but problems remain. *Am J Public Health* 82: 243–248.

Fleeger, M. E. 1993. Assessing organizational culture: A planning strategy. *Nursing Management* 24 (2): 40.

Fletcher, C. E. 1997. Failure mode and effects analysis: An interdisciplinary way to analyze and reduce medication errors. *Journal of Nursing Administration* 27 (12):19–26.

Fletcher, R. H. *et al*. 1983. Patients' priorities for medical care. *Medical Care XXI*:234–242.

Flood, A. *et al*. 1982. Effectiveness in professional organizations: The impact of surgeons and surgical staff organizations on the quality of care in hospitals. *Health Services Research* 17:341–366.

Flood A. B. *et al*. 1998. How do HMOs achieve savings? The effectiveness of one organization's strategies. *Health Services Research* 33 (1):79–99

Food and Drug Administration. 1997. *Title 21 Code of Federal Regulation, Part 11: Electronic Records; Electronic Signatures*. Washington, DC: U.S. Government Printing Office.

Food and Drug Administration. 1999. *Guidance for Computers in Clinical Trials*. Rockville, MD: U.S. Department of Health and Human Services, Food and Drug Administration.

Ford, R. C. *et al*. 1997. Methods of measuring patient satisfaction, *Health Care Management Review* 22 (2):74–89.

Forrester, J. W. 1990. *Principles of Systems*. Portland, OR: Productivity Press.

Frasier, M. 1998. NACCHO survey examines state/local health department relationships. *NACCHO Research Brief* No. 2. Washington, DC: National Association of County and City Health Officials. http://archive.naccho.org/documents/Research_Brief_2.pdf.

French, W. L. 1998. *Human Resources Management*. 4th edition. Boston, MA: Houghton Mifflin Company.

Freidson, E. 1970a. *The Profession of Medicine: a Study of the Sociology of Applied Knowledge,* New York: Dodd, Mead & Company.

Freidson, E. 1970b. *Professional Dominance: The Social Structure of Medical Care*. Chicago: Aldine.

Galbraith, J. 1973. *Designing complex organizations*. Reading, MA: Addison-Wesley.

Galvin, R. S. and E. A. McGlynn. 2003. Using performance measurement to drive improvement: A roadmap for change. *Medical Care* 41 (1): Suppl. I48–I60.

Gardner, E. S., Jr. and C. P. McLaughlin. 1980. Forecasting—A cost control tool for health care managers. *Health Care Management Review* 5 (3):31–38.

Garvin, D. A. 1990. Afterword: Reflections on the future. In *Curing Health Care: New Strategies for Quality Improvement,* by D. M. Berwick, A. B. Godfrey, and J. Roessner, 159–165. San Francisco: Jossey-Bass.

Garvin, D. A. 1993. Building a learning organization. *Harvard Business Review,* 71:(4): 78–91.

Gaucher, E. 1994. *World Class Health Care.* Presentation at the National Conference on Benchmarking Health Care Forum. San Diego, CA, July 17.

Gaucher, E. J., and R. J. Coffey. 1993. *Total Quality in Healthcare: From Theory to Practice.* San Francisco: Jossey-Bass.

Gawande, A. 1999. When doctors make mistakes, *The New Yorker* February 1, 44–55.

Gawande, A. 2004. The Bell Curve. What happens when patients find out how good their doctors really are? *The New Yorker* Dec. 6, 82–91.

Gerteis, M. *et al.* (eds). 1993. *Through the Patient's Eyes: Understanding and Promoting Patient-Centered Care.* San Francisco: Jossey-Bass.

Gerzoff, R. B. 1997. Comparisons: the basis for measuring public health performance. *Journal of Public Health Management and Practice* 3 (5):11–21.

Gibson, R. and J. Prasad. 2003. *Wall of Silence: The Untold Story of Medical Mistakes That Kill and Injure Millions.* Washington, DC: Lifeline Press.

Gillings, D. B. 1997. *Accelerating the Registration Process,* presented at the Institute for International Research.

Gingrich, N. 2003. *Saving Lives and Saving Money.* Washington, DC: Alexis de Tocqueville Institution.

Gingrich, N. and P. Kennedy. 2004. Operating in a vacuum. *New York Times,* May 3, A23.

Gitlow, H. *et al.* 1989. *Tools and Methods for the Improvement of Quality.* Homewood, IL: Irwin.

Glanz, K. *et al.* 1996. *Health Behavior and Health Education: Theory, Research, and Practice,* 2nd Edition. San Francisco: Jossey-Bass.

Glaser, J. P. and M. T. Phillips. 2003. Converting nonbelievers. *Healthcare Informatics* September 2003. http://www.healthcareinformatics.com/issues/2003/09_03/glaser.htm.(accessed 09/28/2003).

Godfrey, M. M. *et al.* 2003. Microsystems in health care: Part 3. Planning patient-centered services. *Jt Comm J Qual Safety* 29 (4):159–170.

Godin S. 1999. *Permission Marketing: Turning Strangers into Friends, and Friends into Customers.* New York: Simon & Schuster, 1999.

Gold, M. 2004. Geographic variation in Medicare per capita spending: Should policymakers be concerned? *Reseach Synthesis Report No. 6.* Princeton, NJ: The Robert Wood Johnson Foundation.

Gold, W. R. and P. R. Kongstvedt. 2003. How broadening DM's focus helped shrink one plan's costs. *Managed Care Magazine* (November).

Goldberg, H. I. 1998. Building healthcare quality: if the future were easy, it would be here by now. *Front Health Serv Manage* 15 (1):40–43.

Goldberg, H. I. *et al.* 1998. A randomized controlled trial of CQI teams and academic detailing: Can they alter compliance with guidelines? *Jt Comm J Qual Improv* 24 (3):130–142.

Goldsmith, J. *et al.* 1995. Managed care comes of age. *Health Forum* 38 (5):14–24.

Goldsmith, J. *et al.* 2003. Federal health information policy: A case of arrested development. *Health Affairs* 22, No. 4: 44–53.

Gordon, R. L. *et al.* 1996. Prevention and the reforming U.S. health system: Changing roles and responsibilities for public health. *Annual Review of Public Health* 17:489–509.

Graham, N. 1990. *Quality Assurance in Hospitals.* Gaithersburg, MD: Aspen Publishers.

Greene, L. W. 1992. PATCH: CDC's planned approach to community health, an application of PRECEED and an inspiration for PROCEED. *Journal of Health Education* 23 (3):140–7.

Greenwood, E. 1957. The Elements of professionalization. *Social Work* 2(3):44–55.

Griffin, S. R. and P. Welch. 1995. Performance-based public health in Texas. *Journal of Public Health Management and Practice* 1 (3):44–49.

Grove, A. S. 1983. *High Output Management.* New York: Vintage Books.

Grumbach, K. and T. Bodenheimer. 2004. Can health care teams improve primary care practice? *JAMA* 291:1246–1251.

Hackman, J. R. 2002. *Leading Teams: Setting the Stage for Great Performances.* Boston: Harvard Business School Press.

Hackman, J. R. & G. R. Oldham. 1990. *Work Redesign.* Reading, MA: Addison-Wesley.

Haddon, W. J. 1972. A logical framework for categorizing highway safety phenomena and activity. *J. Trauma* 12(197).

Hall, L. M. *et al.* 2003. A balanced scorecard approach for nursing report card development. *Outcomes Management* 7 (1):17–22.

Halverson, P. K. and G. P. Mays. 1998. Disease management: A public health perspective. In *A Health Care Professional's Guide to Disease Management.* Couch, J.B. (ed). Gaithersburg, MD: Aspen Publishers.

Halverson, P. K. *et al.* 1996. Performing public health functions: The perceived contribution of public health and other community agencies. *Journal of Health and Human Services Administration* 18 (3):288–303.

Halverson P. K. *et al.* 1997a. Managed care and the public health challenge of TB. *Public Health Reports* 112 (1):22–28.

Halverson, P. K. *et al.* 1997b. Privatizing health services: Alternative models and emerging issues for public health and quality management. *Quality Management in Health Care* 5 (2):1–18.

Halverson, P. K. *et al.* 1998a. Current practices and evolving roles in public health. In *Public Health and Managed Care,* P. K. Halverson, *et al.* 1998. Waithersburg, MD: Aspen Publishers, pp. 11–41.

Halverson, P. K. *et al.* 1998b. *Public Health and Managed Care.* Gaithersburg, MD: Aspen Publishers.

Hammer and Company. 2001. *Post-Sales Support Processes: The Next Competitive Battlefield.* Cambridge, MA: Hammer and Company, March.

Hargraves, J. L. *et al.* 2001. Adjusting for patient characteristics when analyzing reports from patients about hospital care. *Medical Care.* 39:635–41.

Harkey, J., and R. A. Vraciu. 1992. Quality of health care and financial performance: Is there a link? *Health Care Management Review* 17 (4):55–64.

Hart, C. 1993. Handout, Northern Telecom—University Quality Forum, Research Triangle Park, NC, June.

Hatzell, T. A. *et al.* 1996. Improvement strategy for local health departments. *Quality Management in Health Care* 4 (3):79–86.

Headrick, L. *et al.* 1991. Introducing quality improvement thinking to medical students: The Cleveland Asthma Project. *Quality Review Bulletin* 17 (8): 254–260.

Health Grades, Inc. 2004. http://www.HealthGrades.com.

Heard, S. R. *et al.* 2001. Continuous quality improvement: Educating towards a culture of clinical governance. *Quality in Health Care* 10(Suppl.II):ii70–ii78.

Hersey, P. and K. H. Blanchard. 1984. *The Management of Organizational Behavior,* 4th ed. Englewood Cliffs, NJ: Prentice Hall.

Hertz, H. S. *et al.* 1994. The Malcolm Baldrige National Quality Award concept: Could it help stimulate or accelerate health care quality improvement? *Quality Management in Health Care* 2 (4):63–72.

Herzlinger, R. E. 2002. Let's put consumers in charge of health care. *Harvard Business Review* 80 (4):44–55.

Holzer, J. 1990. The advent of clinical standards for professional liability. *Quality Review Bulletin* 16 (2):72–79.

Honigman, B. *et al.* 2001.Using computerized data to identify adverse drug events in outpatients. *J Am Med Inform Assoc.* 8:254–66.

Huber, T. P. *et al.* 2003. Microsystems in health care: Part 8. Developing people and improving work life: What front-line staff told us. *Jt Comm J Qual Safety* 29:512–522.

Hunt, H. K. 1977. CS/D: Overview and future research directions, in *Conceptualization and Measurement of Consumer Satisfaction and Dissatisfaction,* H. K. Hunt, Editor, Cambridge, MS: Marketing Science Institute.

Hurley, R. 1997. Approaching the slippery slope: Managed care as the industrial rationalization of medical practice." In *Rationing Sanity: The Ethics of Mental Health,* edited by P. Boyle. Washington, DC: Georgetown University Press.

Hussey, P. S. *et al.* 2004. How does the quality of care compare in five countries? *Health Affairs* 23 (3):89–99.

Iezzoni, L. I. *et al.* 1994. Identifying complications of care using administrative data. *Medical Care* 32:700–15.

Imai, M. 1986. Kaizen: *The Key to Japan's Competitive Success.* New York: Random House.

Institute of Medicine. 1988. *The Future of Public Health.* Washington, DC: The National Academies Press.

Institute of Medicine. 1997. *Healthy Communities: The Future of Public Health.* Washington, DC: The National Academies Press.

Institute of Medicine, Committee on Using Performance Monitoring to Improve Community Health. 1997. *Improving Health in the Community: A Role for Performance Monitoring.* Washington, DC: The National Academies Press.

Institute of Medicine. 1999. *Roundtable Report, Assuring Data Quality and Validity in Clinical Trials for Regulatory Decisionmaking.* Washington, DC: Workshop Report, The National Academies Press.

Institute of Medicine. 2000. *To Err is Human: Building a Safer Health System.* Washington, DC: The National Academies Press.

Institute of Medicine. 2001. *Crossing the Quality Chasm: A New Health System for the 21st Century.* Washington, DC: The National Academies Press.

Institute of Medicine. 2002a. *The Future of the Public's Health in the 21st Century.* Washington, DC: The National Academies Press.

Institute of Medicine. 2002b. *Fostering Rapid Advances in Health Care: Learning from System Development Demonstrations,* Washington, DC: The National Academies Press.

Institute of Medicine. 2003. *Health Professions Education: A Bridge to Quality.* Washington, DC, The National Academies Press.

Institute of Medicine. 2004. *Patient Safety, Achieving a New Standard for Care,* P. Aspden, J. M. Corrigan, J. Wolcott, S. M. Erickson (Editors), Washington, DC: The National Academies Press.

International Conference on Harmonization (ICH). 1996. ICH Expert Working Group. *Guideline for Good Clinical Practice.* E6, Section 5.1.3.

Ishikawa, K. 1987. *Guide to Quality Control,* trans. Asian Productivity Organization. White Plains, NY: Kraus International Publications.

James, B. 1989. *Quality Management for Healthcare Delivery.* Chicago: The Health Research and Educational Trust of the American Hospital Association.

James, B. 2005. E-Health: Steps on the road to interoperability. *Health Affairs Web Exclusive,* 19 January, W5-26–W5-30.

Jencks, S. *et al.* 2000. Quality of medical care delivered to Medicare beneficiaries: A profile at state and national levels. *JAMA* 284: 1670–1676.

Jencks, S. *et al.* 2003. Change in the quality of care delivered to Medicare beneficiaries, 1998–1999 to 2000–2001. *JAMA,* 289: 305–312.

Jervis, R. 1997. *System Effects.* Princeton, NJ: Princeton University Press.

Jha, A. K. *et al.* 1998. Identifying adverse drug events: Development of a computer-based monitor and comparison with chart review and stimulated voluntary report. *J Am Med Inform Assoc.* 5:305–14.

Joint Commission on Accreditation of Healthcare Organizations. 1992. *Striving Toward Improvement: Six Hospitals in Search of Quality.* Oakbrook Terrace, IL: Joint Commission.

Joint Commission on Accreditation of Healthcare Organizations. 2002. *A Framework for a Root Cause Analysis and Action in Response to a Sentinel Event.* http://www.jcaho.org/accredited+organizations/sentinel+event/se_pp.htm. (Accessed May 20, 2002).

Joint Commission on Accreditation of Healthcare Organizations. 2004. *Facts About the 2005 National Patient Safety Goals* http://www.jcaho.org/accredited+organizations/patient+safety/npsg.htm. (accessed August 3, 2004).

Jollis, J.G. *et al.* 1993. Discordance of databases designed for claims payment vs. clinical information systems: Implications for outcomes research. *Ann Intern Med.* 119:844–850.

Juran, J. 1988. *Juran on Planning for Quality.* New York: Free Press.

Juran, J. M. and A. G. Blanton (Editors). 1999. *Juran's Quality Handbook,* 5th edition, New York: McGraw-Hill.

Kable, A. K. *et al.* 2002. Adverse events in surgical patients in Australia. *Int. J. Qual. Health Care* 14, 269–276.

Kaluzny, A. 1985. Design and management of disciplinary and interdisciplinary groups in health services: Review and critique. *Medical Care Review* 42(1): 77–112.

Kaluzny, A. D. *et al.* 1992. Applying total quality management concepts to public health organizations. *Public Health Reports* 107:257–264.

Kaplan, R. S. and D. P. Norton. 1996. *The Balanced Scorecard, Translating Strategy into Action.* Boston, MA: Harvard Business School Press.

Kaya, S. *et al.* 2003. Comparing patients' and physicians' opinions on quality outpatient care. *Mil Med* 168:1029–33.

Keener, S. R. *et al.* 1997. Providing public health services through an integrated delivery system. *Quality Management in Health Care* 5 (2): 27–34.

Kelly, D. L. 2003. *Applying Quality Management in Healthcare: A Process for Improvement.* Chicago: Health Administration Press.

Ketring, S. P. and J. P. White. 2002. Developing a systemwide approach to patient safety: The first year. *Joint Commission J. on Quality Improvement* 28:287–295.

Kiassi, A. *et al.* 2004. How does the culture of medical group practices influence the types of programs used to assure quality of care? *Health Care Management Review* 29(2):129–138.

Kibbe, D. C. and C. P. McLaughlin. 2004. Getting from A to C: Lifecycle lessons for e-health deployment. *International J. of Electronic Health Care* 1: 127–138.

Kibbe, D. C. and R. M Peters, Jr. 2003. *Removing Gauge Breaks: The Role of Health Information Technology Standards in the Office-Based Medical Practice,* draft, AAFP, available from the authors.

Kibbe, D. C. *et al.* 1993. Continuous quality improvement for continuity of care. *J. of Family Practice* 36:304–308.

Kilbridge, P. and D. Classen. 2002. *Surveillance for Adverse Drug Events: History, Methods and Current Issues.* VHA Research Series Publication, First Consulting Group,

Kilo, C. 1997. Charles Kilo, MD, Director, IHI Breakthrough Series. Personal Communication. September).

Kilo, C. M. 1998. A framework for collaborative improvement: Lessons from the Institute for Healthcare Improvement's Breakthrough Series. *Qual Manage Health Care* 6 (4):1–13.

Knaus, W. *et al.* 1986. An evaluation of outcome from intensive care in major medical centers. *Annals of Internal Medicine* 104:410–418.

Kolata, G. 2004a. Health plan that cuts costs raises doctors' ire. *New York Times* August 11: A1, A17.

Kolata, G. 2004b. Medicare covered new treatments with a catch. *New York Times* November 5: A1, A26.

Kolata, G. 2005. Rapid rise and fall for clinics that market scans to patients. *New York Times* January 23: A1, A18.

Kongstvedt, P. R. 1997. *Essentials of Managed Health Care, 2nd Ed.,* Gaithersburg, MD: Aspen Publishers.

Kosnik, L. and J. A. Espinosa. 2003. Microsystems in health care: Part 7. The microsystem as a platform for merging strategic planning and operations. *Jt Comm J Qual Safety* 29:452–459.

Kotler, P. and G. Armstrong. 1993. Consumer markets and consumer buying behavior, Chapter 5 in M*arketing, An Introduction, Third Edition,* Englewood Cliffs, NJ: Prentice Hall.

Kottke, T. E. *et al.* 1993. Making "time" for preventive services. *Mayo Clinic Proc* 68:785–791.

Kottke, T. E. *et al.* 1997. Preventive services rates in 44 Midwestern primary care clinics: room for improvement. *Proc Mayo Clinic* 72:515–523.

Kuhn, T. S. 1962. *The Structure of Scientific Revolutions.* Chicago: The University of Chicago Press.

Kuperman, G. J. and R. F. Gibson. 2003. Computer physician order entry: Benefits, costs and issues. *Ann Intern Med* 139:31–39.

Kush, R. D. 1999. Electronic data capture: A survey. *The Monitor.* Fall 1999:37–40.

LaBarbara, P. A. and D. Mazursky. 1983. A longitudinal assessment of consumer satisfaction/dissatisfaction: The dynamic aspect of the cognitive process, *Journal of Marketing Research,* 20:393–404.

Labovitz, G. H. and Lowenhaupt, M. 1993. The internal customer. *Quality Management in Health Care* 2 (1):39–45.

Laffel, G. and D. Blumenthal. 1989. The case for using industrial quality management science in health care organizations. *JAMA* 262:2869–2873.

Landon, B. E. *et al.* 2004. Comparison of performance of traditional Medicare versus Medicare Managed Care. *JAMA* 291:1744–52.

Langley, G. J. *et al.* 1994. The foundation of improvement. *Qual Prog* 27: 81–86.

Langley, G. J. *et al.* 1996. *Improvement Guide: A Practical Approach to Enhancing Organizational Performance.* San Francisco: Jossey-Bass.

Lasker, R. 1997. *Medicine and Public Health: The Power of Collaboration.* New York: New York Academy of Medicine.

Lasker, R. D. *et al.* 2001. Partnership synergy: A practical framework for studying and strengthening the collaborative advantage. *The Milbank Quarterly* 79 (2):179–205.

Lawrence, P. R., and J. W. Lorsch. 1967. *Organization and Environment.* Boston: Harvard University Press.

Leape, L. 1987. Unnecessary surgery. *Health Services Research* 24:351–407.

Leape, L. L. 1994. Error in medicine. *JAMA* 272:1851–1857.

Leape, L. L. *et al.* 1998. *Reducing Adverse Drug Events.* Boston, MA: Institute for Healthcare Improvement.

LeapFrogGroup. 2004. http://www.leapfroggroup.org/ (retrieved 6/29/04).

Leatherman, S. and D. McCarthy. 2002. *Quality of Care in the United States: A Chartbook.* New York: The Commonwealth Fund.

Leatherman, S. *et al.* 2003. The business case for quality: Case studies and an analysis. *Health Affairs* 22 (2):17–30.

The Leukemia & Lymphoma Society. 2002. *Annual Report 2002: To Cure.* White Plains, NY.

Levy, M. *et al.* 1999. Computerized surveillance of adverse drug reactions in hospital: implementation. *Eur J Clin Pharmacol* 54:887–92.

Liang, M. H. *et al.* 2002. Measuring clinically important changes with patient-oriented questionnaires. *Medical Care* 40(4 Suppl):II45–51.

Lighter, D. E. and D. C. Fair. 2004. *Principles and Methods of Quality Management in Health Care.* Sudbury, MA: Jones and Bartlett Publishers.

Linder, J. 1991. Outcomes measurement: Compliance tool or strategic initiative. *Health Care Management Review* 16 (4):21–33.

Lohr, K. N. 1997. How Do We Measure Quality? *Health Affairs* 16 (3):22–25.

Lohr, S. 2004a. New economy: Building a medical data network. *New York Times* Nov. 22: C3.

Lohr, S. 2004b. Health care technology is a promise unfinanced. *New York Times* December 3: C5.

Longo, D. R. *et al.* 1997. Consumer reports in health care: Do they make a difference in patient care? *JAMA* 278:1579–1584.

Luft, H. and S. Hunt. 1986. Evaluating individual hospital quality through outcome statistics. JAMA 255:2780–2786.

Macdonald, M. 1998. Using the balanced scorecard to align strategy and performance in long term care. *Healthcare Management Forum* 11 (3):33–38.

Magnan, S. *et al.* 1997. Primary care, process improvement, and turmoil. *J Ambulatory Care Manage* 20 (4):32–38.

Magnan, S. *et al.* 1998. IMPROVE: Bridge over troubled waters. *Jt Comm J Qual Improv* 24:566–578.

Marchibroda, J. A. 2004. *Beyond HIPAA: Building Blocks for a National Health Infrastructure.* Presentation at HIPAA Summit, 03/09. www.ehcaa.com/presentations/HIPAA8/marchibroda (accessed 06/22/05).

Margolis, P. *et al.* 2004. Practice based education to improve delivery systems for prevention in primary care: Randomised trial. *British Medical Journal* 328:388–92.

Marshall, M. and P. Smith. 2003. Rewarding results: Using financial incentives to improve quality. *Quality and Safety in Health Care* 12 (6):397–8.

Marshall, M. N. *et al.* 2000. The public release of performance data: What do we expect to gain? A review of the evidence. *JAMA* 283:1866–1874.

Marshall, M. N. *et al.* 2003. Can health care quality indicators be transferred between countries? *Qual Safety Health Care* 12:8–12.

Masys, D. R. 2002. Effects of current and future information technologies on the health care workforce. *Health Affairs* 21 (5): 33–41.

Mayer, S. M. and D. A. Collier. 1998. Contrasting the original Malcolm Baldrige National Quality Award and the Health Care Pilot Award. *Quality Management in Health Care* 6 (3):12–21.

Mays, G. P. *et al.* 1998a. Collaboration to improve community health: Trends and alternative models. *Joint Commission Journal on Quality Improvement in Health Care* 24:518–540.

Mays G. P. *et al.* 1998b. Assessing the performance of local public health systems: a survey of state health agency efforts. *Journal of Public Health Management and Practice* 4 (4):63–78.

Mays, G. P. *et al.* 2000. *Local Public Health Practice: Trends and Models.* Washington, DC: American Public Health Association.

Mays, G. P. *et al.* 2004a. Identifying dimensions of performance in local public health systems: Results from the nNational public health performance standards program *Journal of Public Health Management and Practice* 10 (3):193–203.

Mays, G. P. *et al.* 2004b. Getting what you pay for: Public health spending and the performance of essential public health services. *Journal of Public Health Management and Practice* 10 (5):441–9.

Mays, G. P. *et al.* 2004c. Availability and perceived effectiveness of public health activities in the nation's most populous areas. *American Journal of Public Health* 94 (6):1019–1026.

McAninch, M. 1988. Accrediting agencies and the search for quality in health care. In *Handbook of Quality Assurance in Mental Health,* ed. G. Stricker and A. Rodriguez, New York: Plenum.

McDermott, R. E. *et al.* 1996. *The Basics of FMEA.* New York: Quality Resources.

McEachern, J. E. and D. B. Neuhauser. 1989. The continuous improvement of quality at the Hospital Corporation of America. *Health Matrix* 7: 5–11.

McEachern, J. E. *et al.* 1995. Medical leadership in an era of managed care and continual improvement. *Health Care Management* 2:19–32.

McGlynn, E. A. 1997. Six challenges for measuring the quality of health care. *Health Affairs* 16 (3):7–21.

McGlynn, E. A. *et al.* 2003. The quality of health care delivered to adults in the United States. *N Engl J Med* 348:2635–2645.

McLaughlin, C. P. 1968. Personal recollections from site visit interviews.

McLaughlin, C. P. 1995. Balanced collaboration and competition: The Kingsport, Tennessee experience, *Joint Commission J. on Quality Improvement* 21: 646–655.

McLaughlin, C. P. 1996. Why variation reduction is not everything: A new paradigm for service operations." *International Journal of Service Industry Management* 7 (3): 17–30.

McLaughlin, C. P. 1998. Rebuilding community and regional collaboration: The Kingsport, Tennessee experience, *Joint Commission J. on Quality Improvement* 24: 601–608.

McLaughlin, C. P and C. Q. Fitzgerald. 2001. Converging genetics and information technologies and the emerging health care system. *International J. of Healthcare Technology and Management,* 3: 498–518.

McLaughlin, C. P. and S. P. Johnson. 1995. Inherent variability in service operations: Identification, measurement and implications. In *Services Management: New Directions and Perspectives.* C. G. Armistead and G. Teare, Eds. London: Cassell plc, pp. 226–229.

McLaughlin, C. P. *et al.* 1995. Professional service organizations and focus. *Management Science* 41: 1185–1193.

McLaughlin, C. P. and A. D. Kaluzny, Eds. 1999. *Continuous quality improvement in medicine,* 2nd Ed. Gaithersburg, MD: Aspen Publishers, Inc.

McLaughlin, C. P. and A. D. Kaluzny. 2002. Missing the middleman: Disintermediation challenges to the doctor-patient relationship, *MGMA Connexion* 2 (4):48–52.

McLaughlin, C. P. and A. D. Kaluzny. 1997. Total quality management issues in managed care, *Journal of Healthcare Financial Management* 24(1):10–16.

McLaughlin, C. P. and K. N. Simpson. 1994. Holston Valley Hospital and Medical Center. In *Continuous Quality Improvement in Health Care,* 2nd Ed., McLaughlin, C. P. and A. D. Kaluzny. (eds.), Gaithersburg, MD: Aspen Publishers, pp. 335–360.

McLaughlin, C. P. *et al.* 2005. Addressing relationship challenges like 'Direct to Consumer' marketing: Future roles in primary care practice, *Healthcare Quarterly* 8 (2):70–78.

McNeese-Smith, D. 1996. Increasing employee productivity, job satisfaction, and organizational commitment. *Hosp. Health Serv. Adm.* 41 (2):160–175.

Mehrotra, A. *et al.* 2003. Employers' efforts to measure and improve hospital quality determinants of success, *Health Affairs* 22 (2):60–71.

Mehta, R. H. *et al.* 2000. Quality improvement initiative and its impact on the management of patients with acute myocardial infarction. *Archives of Internal Medicine* 160: 3057–3062.

Mello, M. M *et al.* 2003. The Leapfrog Standards: Ready to jump from marketplace to courtroom, *Health Affair,* 22 (2):46–59.

Melum, M. M. and M. K. Sinioris. 1992. *Total Quality Management—The Health Care Pioneers.* Chicago: American Hospital Publishing.

Mendelson, D. N. and E. M. Salinsky. 1997. Health information systems and the role of state government. *Health Affairs* 16 (3):106–119.

Meurier, C. E. 2000. Understanding the nature of errors in nursing: Using a model to analyze critical incident reports of errors which had resulted in an adverse or potentially adverse event. *J. of Advanced Nursing* 32:202–207.

Meyerson, D. E. 2001. *Tempered Radicals: How People Use Difference to Inspire Change at Work.* Cambridge: Harvard Business School Press.

Michaels, A. 2001. Schering hit by FDA ruling on Claratin sales. *Financial Times,* May 12/13, 2001. Also see *Transcript of Joint Meeting, Nonprescription Drugs Advisory Committee and Pulmonary-Allergy Drugs Advisory Committee, Food and Drug Administration Center for Drug Evaluation and Research, DHHS, May 11, 2001,* prepared by Miller Reporting Company, Inc., Washington, D.C.

Millenson, M. L. 2002. Pushing the profession: How the news media turned patient safety into a priority. *Quality & Safety in Health Care* 11:57–63.

Millenson, M. L. 2003. The silence on clinical quality failure, *Health Affairs* 22 (2):103–112.

Miller, C. A. *et al.* 1994a. A proposed method for assessing public health functions and practices. *American Journal of Public Health* 84:1743–1749.

Miller, C. A. *et al.* 1994b. A screening survey to assess local public health performance. *Public Health Reports* 109:659–664.

Miller, L. and L. G. Millstein. 1996. The FDA and the regulatory oversight of the clinical research process in drug development. In *Clinical Research in Pharmaceutical Development.* B. Bleidt and M. Montagne, eds., 79–95. New York: Marcel Dekkar.

Miller, R. H. and H. S. Luft. 2002. HMO plan performance update: An analysis of the literature, 1997–2001. *Health Affairs* 21 (4):63–85.

Mitchell, S. M. and S. M. Shortell. 2000. The governance and management of effective community health partnerships. *The Milbank Quarterly* 78 (2):241–289.

Mitroff, I. I. and L. A. Linstone. 1993. *The Unbounded Mind: Breaking the Chains of Traditional Thinking.* New York: Oxford University Press.

Mittman, B. S. 2004. Creating the evidence base for quality improvement collaboratives. *Ann Intern Med* 140:887–896.

Mizuno, S. 1988. *Company-Wide Total Quality Control.* Tokyo, Japan: Nordica International Limited.

Mohr, J. 2000. *Forming, Operating, and Improving Microsystems of Care.* Hanover, NH: Center for the Evaluative Clinical Sciences, Dartmouth College.

Mohr, J. J. and P. Batalden. 2002. Improving safety at the front lines: The role of clinical microsystems. *Quality and Safety in Health Care* 11 (1):45–50.

Mohr, J. J. *et al.* 2003a. Microsystems in health care: Part 6. Designing patient safety into the microsystem. *Jt Comm J Qual Safety* 29:401–408.

Mohr, J. J. *et al.* 2003b. Integrating improvement competencies into residency education: A pilot project from a pediatric continuity clinic. *Ambulatory Pediatrics* 3(3):131–136.

Moingeon, B. and A. Edmonson. 1996. *Organizational Learning and Competitive Advantage.* Thousand Oaks, CA: Sage.

Morris, A. H. 1992. Protocols, ECOO2R, and the evaluation of new ARDS therapy. *Japanese Journal of Intensive Care Medicine* 16:61–63.

Moses, L. and F. Mosteller. 1968. Institutional differences in postoperative death rates: Commentary on some of the findings of the National Halothane Study. *JAMA* 203:492–494.

Mosquera, M. 2004. On-line extra: HHS Grants go to health IT. *Government Computer News* 23(15) June 21. www.appserv.gcn.com/ 23_15/news/26295 06/21/05.

Mosser, G. M. and J. L. Reinertsen. 1996. Healthcare guidelines as engines for improvement. *Preventive Med.* 100:15–18.

Moynihan, J. J. and M. L. McLure. 2000. HIPAA brings new requirements, new opportunities. *Healthcare Financial Management* 54 (3):52–56.

Murray, E. *et al.* 2003. The impact of health information on the internet on the physician-patient relationship. *Arch Intern Med* 163:1727–34.

National Association of County and City Health Officials. 1991. *Assessment Protocol for Excellence in Public Health* (APEXPH). Washington, DC: National Association of County and City Health Officials.

National Association of County and City Health Officials. 2004. *The MAPP Demonstration Site Process: Description of Sites and Early Stages of Implementation.* Washington, DC: NACCHO. http://mapp. naccho.org/Demo_Sites_Overview.pdf (accessed 8/12/04).

National Center for Health Statistics. 1991. Consensus set of health status indicators for the general assessment of community health status— United States. *MMWR* 40(27):449–451.

National Committee for Quality Assessment. 2003. *The State of Health Care Quality: Industry Trends and Analysis.* Washington, DC: NCQA.

National Committee on Quality Assurance. 1995. *Report Card Pilot Project.* Washington, DC: National Committee on Quality Assurance.

National Quality Forum (NQF). 2003. *Safe Practices for Better Healthcare: A Consensus Report,* Washington, DC: NQF.

Nelson, D. E. *et al*. 1995. Outcome-based management and public health: The Oregon Benchmarks experience. *Journal of Public Health Management and Practice,* 1(2):8–17.

Nelson, E. C. and P. B. Batalden. 1993. Patient-based quality measurement systems. *Quality Management in Health Care* 2(1):18–30.

Nelson, E. C. *et al*. 1992. The relationship between patient perceptions of quality and hospital financial performance. *Journal of Healthcare Marketing* 12 (4):6–14.

Nelson, E. C. *et al*. 1998. Building a Quality Future. *Frontiers of Health Services Management* 15 (1):3–32.

Nelson, E. C. *et al*. 2002. Microsystems in Health Care: Part 1. Learning from High-Performing Front-Line Clinical Units. *Joint Commission Journal on Quality Improvement* 28(9):472–93.

Nelson, E. C. *et al*. 2003. Microsystems in health care: Part 2. Creating a rich information environment. *Jt Comm J Qual Safety* 29 (1):5–15.

New York Times. 1995. Health care report cards. *New York Times,* July 10:A12.

Nolan, T. 1997. Accelerating the pace of improvement: An interview with Thomas Nolan. *Jt Comm J Qual Improv* 23 (4):217–222.

Norman, D. A. 1988. *The Psychology of Everyday Things.* New York: Basic Books.

Ogrinc, G. *et al*. 2004. Teaching and assessing resident competence in practice-based learning and improvement. *Journal of General Internal Medicine,* 19: 496–500.

O'Kane, M. E. 2004. Trust but verify. *Health Affairs* 23 (3):280–281.

Oliveira, J. 2001. The balanced scorecard: An integrative approach to performance evaluation. *Healthcare Financial Management* 55:42–6.

Oshel, R. E. *et al*. 1997. Use of national practitioner data bank disclosure information for decision making, *Quality Management in Health Care* 5 (4):34–42.

Ovretreit, J. and D. Gustafson. 2002. Evaluation of quality improvement programmes. *Quality Safety in Health Care* 11:270–275.

Ovretveit, J. *et al*. 2002. Quality collaboratives: Lessons from research. *Qual Saf Health Care* 11:345–351.

Pacific Business Group on Health. 2004. http://pbgh.org.

Pan, E. *et al*. 2004. *The Value of Healthcare Information Exchange and Operability.* Boston, MA: Center for Information Technology Leadership.

Pappaioanou, M. and C. Evans. 1998. Development of the guide to community preventive services: A U.S. Public Health Service initiative. *Journal of Public Health Management and Practice* 4 (2):48–54.

Pascale, R. T. *et al.* 1997. Changing the way we change. *Harvard Business Review* 75 (6):126–139.

Pascoe, G. C. 1983. Patient satisfaction in primary health care: A literature review and analysis. *Evaluation and Program Planning* 6:185–210.

Patel, R. and L. Kinginger. 1997. Childhood immunizations: American College of Preventive Medicine practice policy. *American Journal of Preventive Medicine* 13 (2):74–77.

Paul Shaheen, P. 1987. Small area analysis: A review of the North American literature. *American Journal of Health Politics, Policy and Law* 12:741–809.

Pennsylvania Health Care Cost Containment Council. 1991. *A Consumer Guide to Coronary Artery Bypass Graft Surgery: Pennsylvania's Declaration of Health Care Information.* Harrisburg: Pennsylvania Health Care Cost Containment Council.

Perneger, T. V. *et al.* 2003. A randomized trial of four patient satisfaction questionnaires. *Med Care* 41:1343–52.

Perrin, E. B. and J. J. Koshel (eds). 1997. *Assessment of Performance Measures for Public Health, Substance Abuse, and Mental Health.* Washington, DC: National Academy Press.

Peters, T. 1987. *Thriving on Chaos: Handbook for a Management Revolution.* New York: Harper & Row.

Pharmaceutical Research and Manufacturers of America. 1998. *Industry Profile, 1998.* Washington, DC: Pharmaceutical Research and Manufacturer's Association of America.

Picker Institute Europe. 2003. Picker NHS Inpatient Questionnaire. http://www.pickereurope.org http://www.nhssurveys.org.

Pineno, C. J. 2002. The balanced scorecard: An incremental approach model to health care management. *J Health Care Finance* 28 (4): 69–80.

Pink, G. H. *et al.* 2001. Creating a balanced scorecard for a hospital system. *J Health Care Finance* 24 (1):55–8.

Plsek, P. E. and T. Greenhalgh. 2001. Complexity science: The challenge of complexity in health care. *British Medical J.* 323(7313):625–8.

Plsek, P. E. and T. Wilson. 2001. Complexity, leadership, and management in healthcare organisations. *British Medical J.* 323(7315):746–9.

Pocock, S. J. 1983. *Clinical Trial: A Practical Approach.* New York: John Wiley and Sons.

Pollack, M. *et al.* 1987. Accurate prediction of the outcome of pediatric intensive care: A new quantitative method. *NEJM* 316:134–139.

Porter, M. and E. O. Teisberg. 2004. Redefining competition in health care. *Harvard Business Review* 82 (6):64–76,136.

Press, Ganey Associates, Inc. 2001. Inpatient Survey, 2001. http://www.pressganey.com.

Public Health Foundation. 2002A. *From Silos to Systems: Using Performance Management to Improve Public Health.* Seattle, WA: Turning Point National Program Office at the University of Washington.

Public Health Foundation. 2002B. *Survey on Performance Management Practices in States.* Seattle, WA: Turning Point National Program Office at the University of Washington. http://www.turningpointprogram.org/Pages/pmc_state_survey.pdf (accessed 8/12/04).

Public Health Functions Steering Committee. 1994. *Public Health in America.* Atlanta, GA: Centers for Disease Control and Prevention.

Quinn, J. B. 1992. *The Intelligent Enterprise.* New York: Free Press.

Quintiles Transnational Corp. 1997. *Annual Report.*

Raschke, R. A. *et al.* 1998. A computer alert system to prevent injury from adverse drug events: Development and evaluation in a community teaching hospital. *JAMA* 280:1317–20.

Rastegar, D. A. 2004. Health care becomes an industry. *Ann Family Med* 22:79–83.

Reason, J. 1990. *Human Error.* Cambridge, UK: Cambridge University Press.

Reason, J. 1995. Understanding adverse events: Human factors. In *Clinical Risk Management.* C. Vincent, Editor. London: British Medical J. Publications, pp. 31–54.

Reason, J. 2000. Human error: Models and management. *British Medical J.* 320:768–770.

Reason, J. 2002. Combating omission errors through task analysis and good reminders. *Quality & Safety in Health Care* 11:40–44.

Reason, J. T. *et al.* 2001. Diagnosing "vulnerable system syndrome": An essential prerequisite to effective risk management. *Quality in Health Care* 10 (Suppl II):ii21–ii25.

Redman, T. C. 1992. *Data Quality Management and Technology.* New York: Bantam Books.

Reed, R. and D. Evans. 1987. The deprofessionalization of medicine: Causes, effects, and responses. *JAMA* 258:3279–3282.

Rehm, S. and S. Kraft. 2001. Electronic medical records: The FPM vendor survey. *Family Practice Management* 8 (1):45–54.

Reinertsen, J. L. 1995. Collaborating outside the box: When employers and providers take on environmental barriers to guideline implementation. *Jt Comm J Qual Improv* 21:612–618.

Robinson, J. C. and L. P. Casalino. 2001. Reevaluation of capitation contracting in New York and California. *Health Affairs* Suppl.Web Exclusive:W11–9.

Rocha, B. H. *et al.* 1994. Computerized detection of nosocomial infections in newborns. *Proceedings of the Annual Symposium on Computer Applications in Medical Care,* 684–688.

Roemer, M. I. *et al.* 1968. A proposed hospital quality index: Hospital death rates adjusted for case severity. *Health Services Research* 3 (2):96–118.

Roos, L. *et al.* 1985. Using computers to identify complications after surgery. *American Journal of Public Health* 75:1288–1295.

Roos, L. L. *et al.* 1991. Comparing clinical information with claims data: Some similarities and differences. *J Clin Epidemiol* 44:881–888.

Roper, W. L. and G. P. Mays. 1999. GIS and public health policy: A new frontier for improving community health. *Journal of Public Health Management and Practice* 5,(2):vi–vii.

Rosenthal, M. B. *et al.* 2004. Paying for quality: Providers' incentives for quality improvement. *Health Affairs* 23 (2):127–141.

Rudy, L. J. 1996. The CRO of the future. *Scrip Magazine,* July/August: 42–44.

Russo, F. 1999. The clinical trials bottleneck. *The Atlantic Monthly.* May, 30–36.

Sarudi, D. 2001. The Leapfrog Effect. *Hospitals and Health Networks* May/June: 32–36.

Savitz, L. A. 1994. *The Influence of Maternal Employment on Obstetrical Health Care Seeking Behavior.* Ann Arbor, MI: UMI Press.

Scalise, D. 2003. The patient experience. *Hosp Health Network* 77 (12):41–8.

Schechter, M. and Margolis, P. 2004. *Improving Healthcare in Subspecialty Healthcare: The Example of Cystic Fibrosis.* Unpublished manuscript.

Schein, E. H. and W. Bennis. 1965. *Personal and Organizational Change via Group Methods.* New York: Wiley.

Scherger, J. E. 2004. Communicating with your patients online. *Family Practice Management* March, 47.

Schlesinger, M. 2002. A loss of faith: The source of reduced political legitimacy for the american medical profession. *The Milbank Quarterly* 80 (2):185–235.

Schmittdiel, J. *et al.* 1997. Choice of a personal physician and patient satisfaction in a health maintenance organization. *The Journal of the American Medical Association* 278: 1596–1599.

Schuring, R. W. and T. A. M. Spil. 2002. Explaining plateaued diffusion by combining the user-IT-success factors (USIT) and adopter categories: The case of electronic prescription systems for general practitioners. *International J. of Healthcare Technology and Management* 4: 303–318.

Schwarz, R. M. 1989. Understanding and changing the culture of an organization. *Popular Government* 45 (2): 23–26.

Schweikhart, S. B. *et al.* 1993. Service Recovery in health service organizations, *Hospital and Health Services Administration* 38 (1):3–23.

Schweitzer, S. O. 1997. *Pharmaceutical Economics and Policy.* New York: Oxford University Press.

Scutchfield, F. D. *et al.* 1997. The presence of total quality management and continuous quality improvement processes in California public health clinics. *Journal of Public Health Management and Practice* 3 (3):57–60.

Selby, J. V. *et al.* 2003. Determininng the value of disease management programs. *Jt Comm J Qual Safety* 29:491–499.

Senge, P. 1990. *The Fifth Discipline.* New York, Doubleday.

Senge, P. M. *et al.* 1994. *The Fifth Discipline Fieldbook: Strategies and Tools for Building a Learning Organization.* New York: Doubleday/Currency.

Sharma, R. K. 2003. Putting the community back in community health assessment: A process and outcome approach with a review of some major issues for public health professionals. *Journal of Health and Social Policy* 16 (3):19–33.

Shojania, K. G. *et al.*, eds. 2001. *Making Health Care Safer: A Critical Analysis of Patient Safety Practices, Evidence Report/ Technology Assessment No. 43,* prepared by the University of California at San Francisco-Stanford Evidence-based Practice Center under Contract No. 290-97-0013, AHRQ Publication No. 01-E058, Rockville, MD: Agency for Healthcare Research and Quality.

Shortell, S. M. and A. D. Kaluzny 2006. *Health Care Management: Organization Design and Behavior,* 5th Ed. Albany, NY: Thomson Delmar Learning, 2006.

Shortell, S. M. *et al.* 1995. Assessing the evidence on CQI: Is the glass half empty or half full? *Hosp Health Serv Adm* 40 (1):4–24.

Shortell, S. M. *et al.* 1998. Assessing the impact of continuous quality improvement on clinical practice: What will it take to accelerate programs. *Milbank Quarterly* 76:593–624.

Simone, P. M. 1995. Essential components of a tuberculosis prevention and control program: Recommendations of the Advisory Council for the Elimination of Tuberculosis. *MMWR* 44(RR-11):1–16.

Sitzia, J. 1999. How valid and reliable are patient satisfaction data? An analysis of 195 studies. *International Soc for Qual in Health Care* 11 (4):319–328.

Slovensky, D. J. and B. Morin. 1997. Learning through simulation: The next step in quality improvement. *Quality Improvement in Health Care* 5(3):72–79.

Society for Clinical Data Management (SCDM). 2003. *Good Clinical Data Management Practices,* Version 3, September. Available from www.scdm.org.

Solberg, L. 1993. Improving disease prevention in primary care. Washington, DC: AHCPR Working Paper.

Solberg, L. I. 2000. Guideline implementation: What the literature doesn't tell us. *Jt Comm J Qual Improv* 26:525–537.

Solberg, L. I. *et al.* 1997a. How important are clinician and nurse attitudes to the delivery of clinical preventive services? *J Fam Pract* 44:451–461.

Solberg, L. I. *et al.* 1997b. Delivering clinical preventive services is a systems problem. *Ann Behav Med* 19 (3):271–278.

Solberg, L. I. *et al.* 1997c. The three faces of performance measurement: Improvement, accountability, and research. *Jt Comm J Qual Improv* 23:135–147.

Solberg, L. I. *et al.* 1998. The case of the missing clinical preventive services systems. *Eff Clin Pract* 1 (1):33–38.

Solberg, L. I. *et al.* 2000a. Lessons from experienced guideline implementers: Attend to many factors and use multiple strategies. *Jt Comm J Qual Improv* 26 (4):171–188.

Solberg, L. I. *et al.* 2000b. Failure of a trial of continuous quality improvement and systems intervention to increase the delivery of clinical preventive services. *Eff Clin Pract* 3:105–115.

Sollecito, W. A. and M. M. Dotson. 1994. *Getting the Most from a Contract Research Organization.* Proceedings of the Annual Project Management Institute Symposium.

Sollecito, W. A. and M. M. Dotson. 1995. *Communications Guidelines and Networks for Drug Development Teams.* Proceeding of the Annual Project Management Institute Symposium.

Sollecito, W. A. and A. D. Kalusny. 1999. "Continuous quality improvement in contrast research organizations—The customer focus," *Quality Management in Health Care,* Vol 7, No. 7, pp. 7–11.

Spath, P. L. ed. 2000. *Error Reduction in Health Care: A Systems Approach to Improving Patient Safety,* San Francisco: Jossey-Bass Publishers.

Speake, D. L. *et al.* 1995. Integrating indicators into a public health quality improvement system. *American Journal of Public Health* 85:1448–9.

Stamatis, D.H. 1995. *Failure Model and Effect Analysis, FMEA from Theory to Execution,* Milwaukee, WI:. American Society for Quality.

Starr, P. 1982. *The Social Transformation of American Medicine.* New York: Basic Books.

Starr, P. 1997. Smart technology, stunted policy: developing health information networks. *Health Affairs* 16 (3):91–105.

Steiber, S. R. 1988. How consumers perceive health care quality, *Hospitals* 62, (7):84.

Steinhauer, J. 2001. So, the tumor is on the left, right? Seeking ways to reduce operating room errors. *New York Times* Sunday, April 1, Section 1, Page 27.

Stewart, D. M. and J. R. Grout. 2001. The human side of mistake-proofing. *Production and Operations Management* 10:440–459.

Streibel, B. J. *et al.* 2003. *The Team Handbook,* 3rd edition. Madison, WI: Joiner/Oriel, Inc.

Striener, D. L. and G. R. Norman. 1989. *Health Measurement Scales. A Practical Guide to their Development and Use.* Oxford: Oxford University Press.

Studnicki, J. *et al.* 1997. A community health report card: Comprehensive assessment for tracking community health (CATCH). *Best Practices and Benchmarking in Healthcare.* 2 (5):196–207.

Studnicki, J. *et al.* 2001. A minimum data set and empirical model for population health status assessment. *American Journal of Preventive Medicine* 20 (1):40–9.

Tan, J. K. 1995. *Health Management Information Systems: Theories, Methods, and Applications.* Gaithersburg, MD: Aspen Publishers.

Tarlov, A. E. *et al.* 1989. The Medical Outcomes Study: An application of methods for monitoring the results of medical care. *JAMA* 262: 925–930.

Tassignon, J. 1992. *The Contract Clinical Research Market.* Brussels: Tassignon and Partners, S.A.

Taylor, R. J. and S. B. Taylor. 1994. *The AUPHA Manual of Health Services Management.* Gaithersburg, MD: Aspen Publishers.

Tichy, N. 1997. *The Leadership Engine.* New York: Harper Business.

Tucker, A. and A. Edmondson. 2003. Why hospitals don't learn from failures: Organizational and psychological dynamics that inhibit system change. *California Management Review* 45 (2):55–72.

Turnock, B. J., A. S. Handlet, C. A. Miller. CA. 1998. Care function related local public health practice effectiveness. *Journal of Public Health Managment and Practice* 4(5):26–32.

Turnock, B. J. and A. S. Handler. 1997. From measuring to improving public health practice. *Annual Review of Public Health* 18:261–82.

Turnock, B.J. *et al.* 1994. Local Health Department effectiveness in addressing the core functions of public health. *Public Health Reports* 109:653–658.

Tversky, A. and D. Kahneman. 1974. Judgment under uncertainty: Heuristics and biases. *Science* 185:1124–1131.

U.S. Agency for Toxic Substances and Disease Registry. 1992. *ATSDR Public Health Assessment Guidance Manual.* Boca Raton, FL: Lewis Publishers.

U.S. Congress, Office of Technology Assessment. 1993. *Pharmaceutical R and D: Costs, Risks and Rewards.* Washington, DC: U.S. Government Printing Office.

U.S. Congress, Senate. Permanent Subcommittee on Investigations on Government Affairs. *Patient Safety: Instilling Hospitals with a Culture of Continuous Improvement.* Testimony by S. Delbanco, June 11, 2003. http://www.senate.gov/~gov_affairs/061103delbanco.pdf.

U.S. Department of Health and Human Services. 1990. *Healthy People 2000: National Health Promotion and Disease Prevention Objectives.* Washington, DC: DHHS.

U.S. Department of Health and Human Services. 2001. *Healthy People 2010: National Health Objectives for the Year 2010.* Washington, DC: DHHS.

U.S. Environmental Protection Agency. 1998. *The Changing Nature of Environmental and Public Health Protection: An Annual Report on Reinvention.* Washington, DC: Government Printing Office.

U.S. General Accounting Office. 1994. *Report Cards Are Useful But Significant Issues Need to Be Addressed.* Washington, DC: U.S. General Accounting Office.

U.S. General Accounting Office (GAO). 1997. *Performance Budgeting: Past Initiatives Offer Insights for GPRA.* Washington, DC: GAO, March.

U.S. Office of Technology Assessment (OTA). 1988. *The quality of medical care: Information for consumers.* OTA-H-386. Washington, DC: U.S. Government Printing Office, June.

U.S. Preventive Services Task Force. 1989. *Guide to Clinical Preventive Services: An Assessment of the Effectiveness of 169 Interventions.* Baltimore, MD: Williams & Wilkens.

Vaughan, D. 1996. *The Challenger Launch Decision, Risky Technology, Culture, and Deviance at NASA.* Chicago, IL: The University of Chicago Press.

Vaughn, E. H. *et al.* 1994. An information manager for the Assessment Protocol for Excellence in Public Health. *Public Health Nursing* 11 (6): 399–405.

Victor, B. and A. C. Boynton. 1998. *Invented Here: Maximizing Your Organization's Internal Growth and Profitability,* Boston, MA: Harvard Business School Press.

Vincent, C. 2003. Understanding and responding to adverse events. [see comment]. *New England Journal of Medicine* 348:1051–6.

Vincent, C. *et al.* 1998. Framework for analysing risk and safety in clinical medicine. *British Medical J.,* 316(7138):1154–7.

Wagner, D. *et al.* 1986. The case for adjusting hospital death rates for severity of illness. *Health Affairs* 5 (2):148–153.

Wagner, E. H. *et al.* 2001, Improving chronic illness care: Translating evidence into action, *Health Affairs* 20(6):64–78.

Wagner, M. 2004. Under the Knife. *Business 2.0* 5(1):84–89.

Walker, J. *et al.* 2005. The value of health care information exchange and interoperability. *Health Affairs Web Exclusive,* 19 January, W5-10 W5-18.

Walley, P. and C. Davies. 2002. Implementing IT in NHS hospitals: Internal barriers to technological advancement. *International J. of Healthcare Technology and Management* 4:258–272.

Walshe, K. and S. M. Shortell. 2004. When Things Go Wrong: How Health Care Organizations Deal With Major Failures. *Health Affairs* 23 (3):103–109.

Walton, M. 1990. *Deming Management at Work.* New York: G.P. Putnam's Sons.

Washington State Department of Health. 1996. *Public Health Improvement Plan: A Blueprint for Action.* Olympia, WA: Washington State Department of Health.

Wasson, J. H. *et al.* 2003. Microsystems in health care: Part 4. planning patient-centered care. *Jt Comm J Qual Safety* 29 (5):227–237.

Weick, K. E. 1976. Educational systems as loosely coupled organizations. *Administrative Science Quarterly* 21:1–19.

Weick, K. E. 1993. The Collapse of Sensemaking in organizations: The Mann Gulch Disaster. *Administrative Science Quarterly* 38:628–652.

Weick, K. E. 1995. *Sensemaking in Organizations*. 1995. Thousand Oaks, CA: Sage Publications.

Weick, K. E. 1996. Prepare your organization to fight fires. *Harvard Business Review* 74 (3):143–148.

Weick, K. E. and K. M. Sutcliffe. 2001. *Managing the Unexpected: Assuring High Performance in an Age of Complexity.* San Francisco, CA: Jossey-Bass.

Weick, K. and K. Sutcliffe. 2003. Hospitals as cultures of entrapment: A re-analysis of the Bristol Infirmary. *California Management Review* 45:75–84.

Weingart, S. 1996. House officer education and organizational obstacles to quality improvement. *The Joint Commission Journal on Quality Improvement,* 22 (9): 640–646.

Weingart, S. 1998. A house officer-sponsored quality improvement initiative: Leadership lessons and liabilities. *Joint Commission Journal on Quality Improvement* 24:371–378.

Weingart, S. N. *et al.* 2000. Use of administrative data to find substandard care: Validation of the complications screening program. *Medical Care* 38:796–806.

Wennberg, J. E. *et al.* 1996. *The Dartmouth Atlas of Health Care.* Chicago: American Hospital Association.

Wennberg, J. and A. Gittelsohn. 1973. Small area variations in health care delivery. *Science* 182:1102–1108.

Wensing, M. and G. Elwyn. 2002. Research on patients' views in the evaluation and improvement of quality of care. *Qual Saf Health Care* 11:153–157.

Wensing, M. and G. Elwyn. 2003. Improving the quality of health care: Methods for incorporating patients' views in health care. *BMJ* 326:877–9.

West, E. 2000. Organizational sources of safety and danger: Sociological contributions to the study of adverse events. *Quality in Health Care* 9:120–126.

Westert, G. P. and R. J. Lagoe, 1995. Evaluation of hospital stays for total hip replacement. *Quality Management in Health Care* 3 (3):62–71.

Wheatley, M. 1992. *Leadership and the New Science: Learning About Organization from an Orderly Universe.* San Francisco, CA: Berrett-Koehler.

Wheeler, D. J. 2000. *Understanding Variation: The Key to Managing Chaos.* Knoxville, TN: SPC Press.

Whittle, J. *et al.* 1991. Accuracy of Medicare claims for estimation of cancer incidence and resection rates among elderly Americans. *Medical Care.* 29:1226–1236.

Wilf-Miron, R. *et al.* 2003. From aviation to medicine: Applying concepts of aviation safety to risk management in ambulatory care. *Quality and Safety in Health Care,* 12:35–39.

Williams, E. and R. Talley. 1994. The use of failure mode effect and criticality analysis in a medication error subcommittee. *Hospital Pharmacy,* 29:331–7.

Woodbury, D. *et al.* 1997. Does considering severity of illness improve interpretation of patient satisfaction data? *Journal for Healthcare Quality* 20 (4):33–40.

Zifko-Baliga, G. M. and R. F. Krampf. 1997. Managing perceptions of hospital quality. *Marketing Health Services* 17 (11):28–35.

Zimmerman, B. and B. Hayday. 1999. A board's journey into complexity science. *Group Decision Making and Negotiations* 8:281–303.

# INDEX